Unicompartmental Knee Arthroplasty

Arnaud Clavé · Frédéric Dubrana

Editors

Unicompartmental Knee Arthroplasty

A New Paradigm?

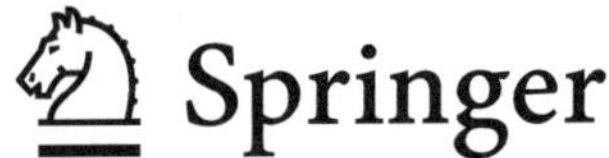

Springer

Editors
Arnaud Clavé
Service de Chirurgie Orthopédique
Clinique Saint George
Nice, France

Frédéric Dubrana
Service de Chirurgie Orthopédique
CHU Cavale Blanche
Brest, France

ISBN 978-3-031-48334-9   ISBN 978-3-031-48332-5   (eBook)
https://doi.org/10.1007/978-3-031-48332-5

Original French edition published by Sauramps Medical, Montpellier, France, 2020

Translation from the French language edition: "La prothèse unicompartimentale de genou - Vers un nouveau paradigme " by Arnaud Clavé and Frédéric Dubrana, © Sauramps Médical, Montpellier, France, 2020. Published by Sauramps Médical. All Rights Reserved.

This Springer imprint is published by the registered company Springer Nature Switzerland AG
The registered company address is: Gewerbestrasse 11, 6330 Cham, Switzerland

Paper in this product is recyclable

Foreword

Unicompartmental knee arthroplasties (UKA) have a long history in the treatment of degenerative knee disease. Initially described in the early 1970s as an alternative to total knee arthroplasty, the concept of a resurfacing option limited to one of the three knee compartments continues to play an essential role in managing knee osteoarthritis (OA). The current renewed interest in UKA is completely justified first for their delivery of a less invasive procedure with faster recovery and, secondly, their improved results and patient satisfaction compared to total knee arthroplasty. They represent a significant proportion of the so-called forgotten knees that every surgeon and patient dreams of obtaining after a surgical procedure, and modern prosthetic knee surgery cannot be considered without precise knowledge of mono- or bicompartmental arthroplasty. Of course, we must not forget technological advances, such as computer-assisted and robotic surgery, which have made this procedure even more reliable and reassured its most reluctant opponents.

As we enter the fifth decade of its use, Arnaud Clavé and Frédéric Dubrana have sought in this work entitled *Unicompartmental Knee Arthroplasty* towards a new paradigm to present a modern vision of UKA, supported by long-term results that equal, and in many cases are better than total knee arthroplasty. In this book, they have brought together a group of French and international experts in the field, asking them to present the state of the art in monocompartmental knee surgery without, of course, overlooking the historical aspects, which make it possible to better comprehend the current strategies.

The book naturally starts with the history and biomechanical concepts of OA and monocompartmental arthroplasty. The conventional indications and modern approach to them will then be detailed before the principles for performing fixed and mobile plateau arthroplasty, as well as the different alignment philosophies, are comprehensively reviewed. Ambulatory management and complications will be described, as will UKA revision. Innovative technologies will receive special attention before specific situations such as bilateral arthroplasty, external UKA, or resumption of athletic activities are examined. Lastly, the registers will provide exclusive insights into current objective data.

From indications for the surgical technique to the results, the reader will have access to the latest reviews and opinions on this fascinating topic, and we must thank Arnaud Clavé and Frédéric Dubrana as well as the authors for all their hard work summarising them.

I know that this book will be an invaluable resource for anyone interested in knee surgery and I hope that you will enjoy reading it.

Lyon, France   Sébastien Lustig

Preface

After almost half a century of reflection, hesitation, and research, unicompartmental knee arthroplasty is finally reaching maturity. It was the Oxford school that bravely carried the torch for its resurrection. A renaissance, because orthopedists, distracted from their history, had, for a time, forgotten the very origin of modern TKAs: quite simply, two unicompartmental knee implants! This book is not a new paradigm because the truth it defends may be false tomorrow. However, it is a change of references, an opening of the mind, and a hope for many patients.

Through the photography of their activities, we must thank the forty (or so) authors who participated in its creation and shared their knowledge and expertise.

Nice, France

Brest, France

Arnaud Clavé

Frédéric Dubrana

Contents

History of Unicompartmental Prostheses

Frédéric Dubrana and Hoel Letissier

1.1 Arthroplastic Resection Eighteenth–Nineteenth Century

It was not until the eighteenth century that the first descriptions of arthroplastic resections were described and taught. This intervention was not without risk for the patient, yet there are two historical evocations, one of Hippocrates (460–377) and the other of Paul D'Égine (VIIth century). If Hippocratic corpus is vague and cautious, Paul of Aegina mentions it and recommends it without specifying the indication and the technique:

> *The resection by the saw of the protrusion of the bone is controlled by the following conditions: if it cannot be reduced, if it is only a little needed that it does not fit in, and if it is possible to remove it; it is still a case of resection when it causes inconvenience, injures the wattles in some way, makes the position of the limb bad, and at the same time is stripped naked. In other circumstances, it does not matter whether or not to resect; because it is necessary to know that all the bones, which are completely stripped* [1]
> *Similarly, if the tip of the bone near a joint is sick, it must be resected* [2]

It was in 1768 that the first surgical description of arthroplastic resection was reported. It was Charles White (1728–1813) who took care of a 16-year-old boy with infectious necrosis of his left shoulder [3, 4]. However, primacy is not certain, because a year earlier Professor Barthelemi Vigarous of Montpellier would have made the same intervention on a young man of 17 year old. This is described in a posthumous book published in 1820 by her son Professor Joseph-Marie Vigarous [5, 6]. However, there is an even older description of 1730 (Fig. 1.1). This is a clinical case published by Johanne Daniele Schlichting. This surgeon removed the carious head of the femur in a 14-year-old girl by dilating a fistulous opening on the hip (Fig. 1.2). Schlichting mentioned that his patient recovered in 6 weeks: [7]

> *In 1973. A 14-year-old girl's hip joint is swollen, painful, suppurative and disturbed. The surgeon, due to the nature of the large hole, removes the entire head of the femoral bone, then inserts into the bone cavity a tincture of myrrh, and a juice... Finally, he binds the wound with a tight tie, and secures her for 6 weeks, so that after that the girl can walk freely. Here is the figure roughly sketched by this surgeon:*
> *1. It designates an unnamed dish.*
> *2. of the head, which must be removed from the ulceration.*
> *3. the bone cavity, etc.*

The first arthroplastic resection of the knee was made in 1781 by Dr. Henry Park of Liverpool:
"Suffice it to note that the case caused him a lot of problems and was accompanied by many embarrassing circumstances, resulting mainly from the difficulty of keeping the limb in a fixed

F. Dubrana · H. Letissier (✉)
Department of Orthopaedic & Trauma Surgery,
University Hospital La Cavale Blanche,
Brest cedex, France

A. Clavé, F. Dubrana (eds.), *Unicompartmental Knee Arthroplasty*,
https://doi.org/10.1007/978-3-031-48332-5_1

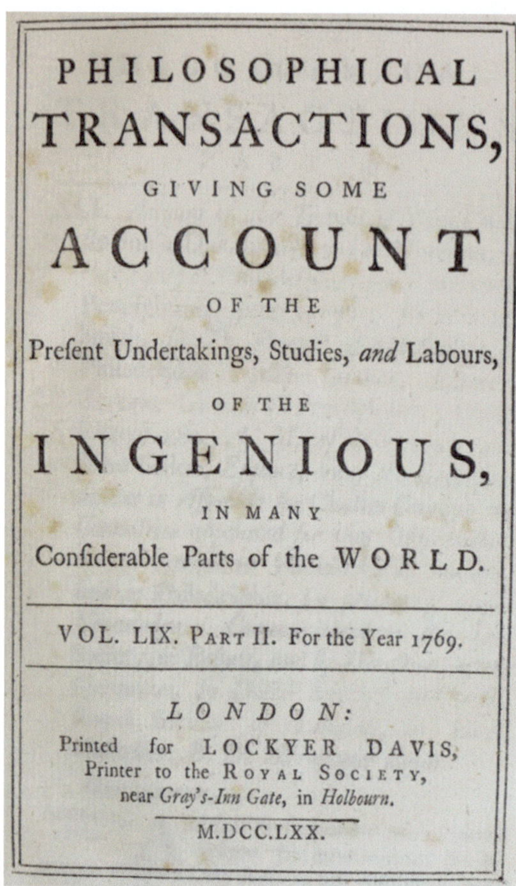

Fig. 1.1 Front page of philosophical transactions. Royal Society London

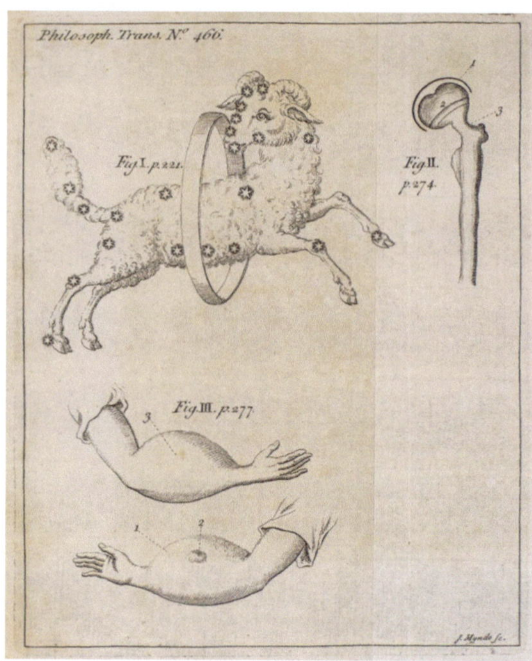

Fig. 1.2 Carious head of the femur in a 14-year-old girl

ends of the femur and tibia. Three months later the limb was very solid, and the operated on was good enough to no longer need care. He was still living in 1782. 'The person still lives,' filkin Jr. said in his letter to Binns (of Liverpool), and sometimes goes to Liverpool, where, if I may, I will ask her to go see you [10].

This intervention was widely distributed, in 1862 Dr. Heyfelder counted more than 176 cases of arthroplastic knee resections in the world (Fig. 1.3). He devotes to it in his book *Treatise on Resections* the tenth chapter: *Joint resections or in contiguity* [11]. For the hip, the arthroplastic resection procedure was less frequent, in 1860 Professor Léon Le Fort made an exhaustive inventory, he found 86 publications of arthroplastic hip resections. It was not until the work of Léopold Ollier [12, 13] at the end of the nineteenth century that a scientific approach to arthroplastic resection developed. Léopold Ollier developed the concept of arthroplastic resection sub-capsulo-periosteal. This concept interested the shoulder, elbow, hip and knee. But, unlike the elbow the goal for the knee was not to obtain a

position [8]...*" This* intervention was published 20 years later by Samuel Cooper; following this publication Dr. Filkin claimed the anteriority of the technique (Northwich, Cheshire), in a letter he wrote to Park he specified its anteriority of 20 years (1762) [9]:

Filkin operated on a subject who had been carrying a white tumor of the knee for several years, and who, in a fall from a horse, fractured his kneecap. The result was a suppuration of the article for which amputation of the thigh was proposed. Despite the subject's dilapidated health, Filkin proposed the resection of the decayed parts. After practicing on the corpse, he performed resection on 23 Aug. 1702. He found the ligaments very affected, the cartilage very compromised, and the articular extremities severely impaired, especially those of the tibia. He removed the patella and the

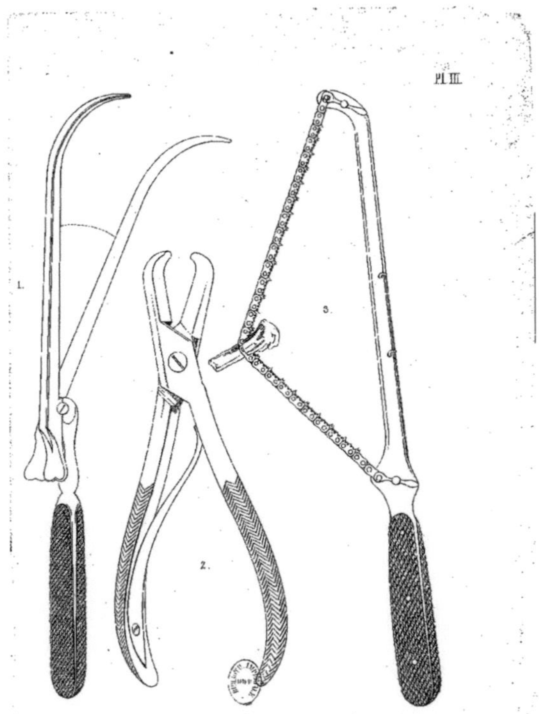

Fig. 1.3 Treatise of resections. O. Heyfelder: 1863. fig. 1. Mr. Billroth's apparatus for resection of the knee (p. 93). fig. 2. Apparatus of M. Esmarch for resections in general. fig. 3. Apparatus of M. Bceckel for the resection of the instep (p. 127)

neo joint, but a bone fusion or even a stable fibrous ankylosis. However, Ollier specified that the surgical risk (death, complications) was important during resection of the knee:

The frequency of surgical shock after knee resection has long been reported (Holmes). Even before the absorption of toxic substances could be blamed, it was considered more dangerous from this point of view than other joint resections [14].

In Ollier's work, two notions are important to remember the scientific basis based on experimental studies and the notion of partial resection of the knee: *"We had well demonstrated that it is possible in young animals to reconstitute, after a subperiosteal resection, distinct femoral condyles, which can be articulated with a tibial plateau of new formation, and play on it in flexion movements and of more or less extensive extensions. But we did not propose to pursue the same*

result in human beings... Instead of cutting the lateral ligaments, we carefully preserved them, and we also spared everything that was healthy from the perio-capsular sheath to accumulate around the healing line of the bones as much ossifiable tissue as possible. In this way, we considerably increased the chances of bone healing, and, in the event that mobility persisted, we would have retained the tendon-muscular belt of this new joint, that is, its means of resistance and its organs of movement." [15]

We will then have the semi-articular resections, either femoral or tibial, and the partial resections... Partial resections of the knee will include, according to the general division that we have given of the resections, operations in which one will remove either a condyle of femur or a condyle of the tibia, or even a part only of the two opposite ends by maintaining the contact of the two bones by a certain extent of their normal articular surfaces. In this classification the total removal of the patella will constitute a partial resection of the knee [16].

1.2 From Osteotomy to Arthroplastic Interposition

The first osteotomies of relaxations are due to J. Rhea Barton who performed two osteotomies, one for the hip in 1827 (Fig. 1.4) and one for the knee in 1837 (Fig. 1.5). These straightening osteotomies were done in a very short time, 7 min for the hip and 5 min for the knee. For the femur, it was a subtrochanteric osteotomy and for the knee a supracondylar osteotomy [4, 17, 18]. Barton hoped that after creating a neo joint, the bone fusion would take place. For the hip, it was not so and the patient resumed his work with his neo joint:

The patient, upon whom this operation was performed, enjoyed the use of his artificial joint for 6 years; during which period he pursued a business (trunk- making) with great industry, earning for himself a comfortable subsistence, and a small annual surplus [18].

On the other hand, for the osteotomy of the knee, he obtained a consolidation by keeping a

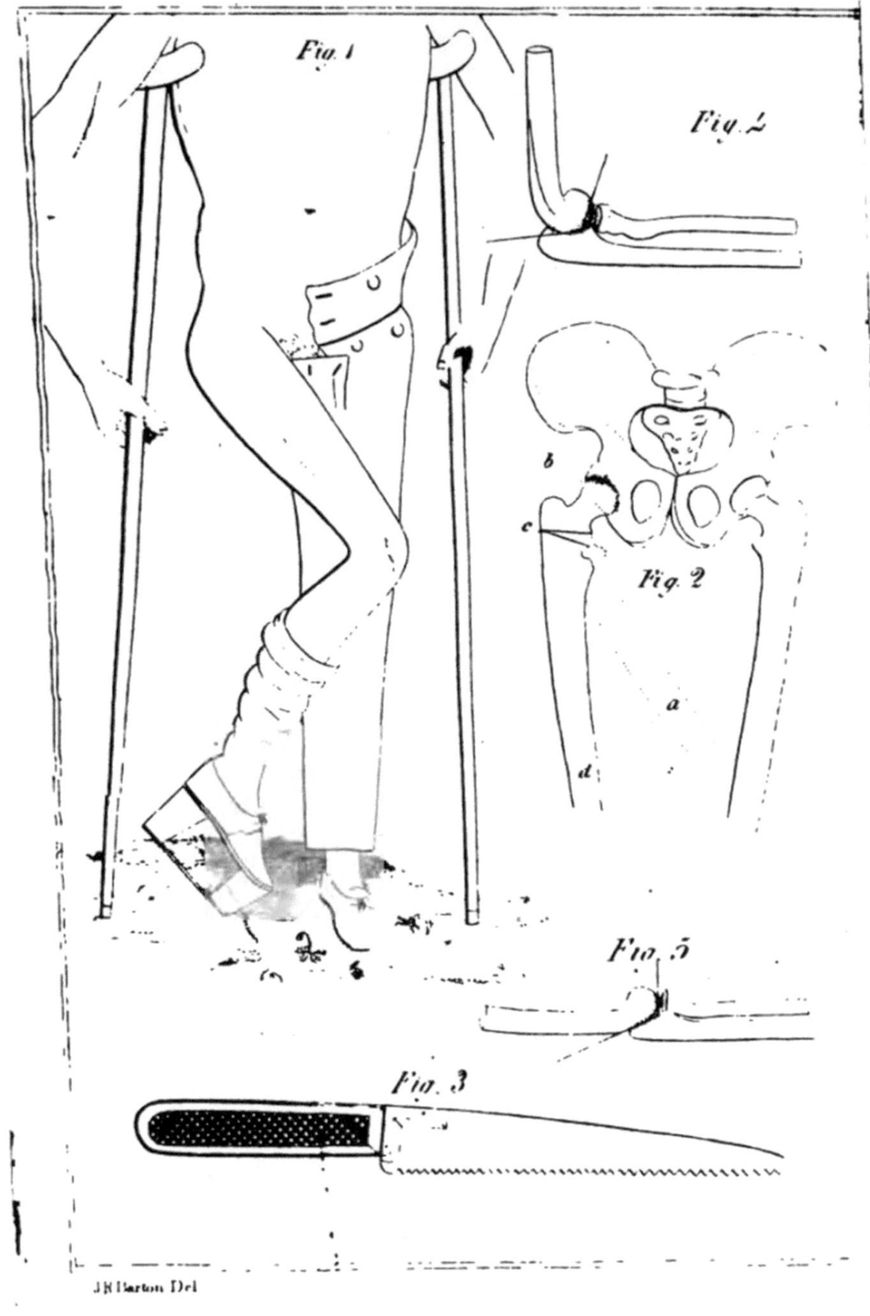

Fig. 1.4 J. Rhea Barton hip osteotomy in 1827

splint for 4 months. Six months before the operation, the patient (Mr. Seaman Deas) sent a long letter to his surgeon:

Charleston, November sixth, 1837. My dear sir, — Your letter of the eighth October, directed to me at Mobile, has just reached me at this place, where I am on a visit to my Parents... Letter of the eighth is the first information I have had of your return. I have the satisfaction and pleasure of saying to you now, that the operation you performed on my leg has been completely successful and has more than realized my most sanguine anticipations. The small abscess, which you dressed the day before we

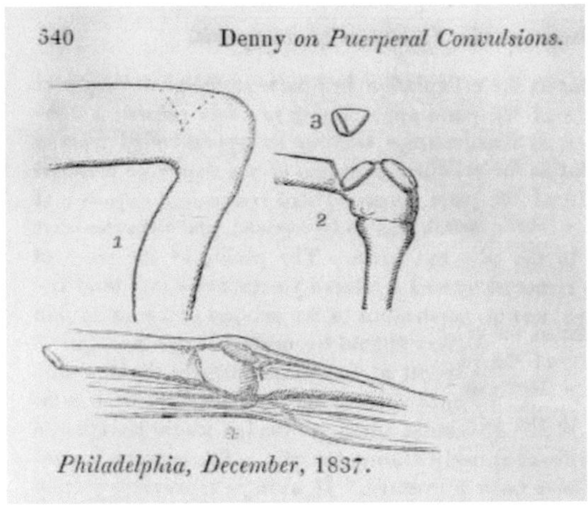

Fig. 1.5 J. Rhea Barton osteotomies of the knee in 1837

parted at Norfolk, continued open, and threw out, from time to time, small pieces of bone, until the August after, when the last piece was discharged; the orifice then closed, and I have suffered no material inconvenience from it since. I am at present well; the wound sound; and I feel no other inconvenience in riding or walking, than what arises from my knee joint being stiff, which was the case before you performed the operation. I walk without a stick or other aid, with the sole of the foot to the ground, and my friends tell me, with but a slight limp; and I have great pleasure in adding that the leg and foot have increased considerably in size, so as now to be nearly equal to the other.... Adieu and I am, my dear sir, very sincerely, your friend. Seaman Deas. To Dr. J. Rhea Barton [19].

Certainly resecting, allowed to give mobility in the neo joint of the hip, but quickly the surgeons wanted to put an interposition tissue to facilitate the movement while limiting the risk of bone ankylosis. Aristide Verneuil (1823–1895) is falsely credited with the first peripheral interposition during the resection of the temporomandibular joint. This ambiguity is linked to the concept of anaplasty and autoplasty that Verneuil is developing and where he can consider one of the founders of modern plastic and reconstructive surgery. For Verneuil, anaplasty is synonymous with reconstructive surgery by natural means and autoplasty with the help of prosthesis. However, one does not find his writings the description of tissue interposition in the temporomandibular joint. In his text of 1860, it is as Verneuil specifies the description of the clinical cases of Professor

Rizzoli between 1853 and 1857. These interventions consisted of a mandibular resection osteotomy without interposition during the initial resection: *"It has been several years since chance provided Mr. Rizzoli with the opportunity to surgically treat the immobility of the jaw. His first observation dates back to 1853."* [20]

The notion of tissue interposition is found at the end of the nineteenth century in Ollier's book (Fig. 1.6) [21]:

We can, after extracting it, reconstitute the shape of the region by suturing the palatine periosteum at the periosteum of the outer side of the bone. By thus joining the horizontal palatine plane to the external vertical plane, the separation of the nasal and oral cavities is restored, which is very important from the point of view of the functioning of the organs of phonation and swallowing.

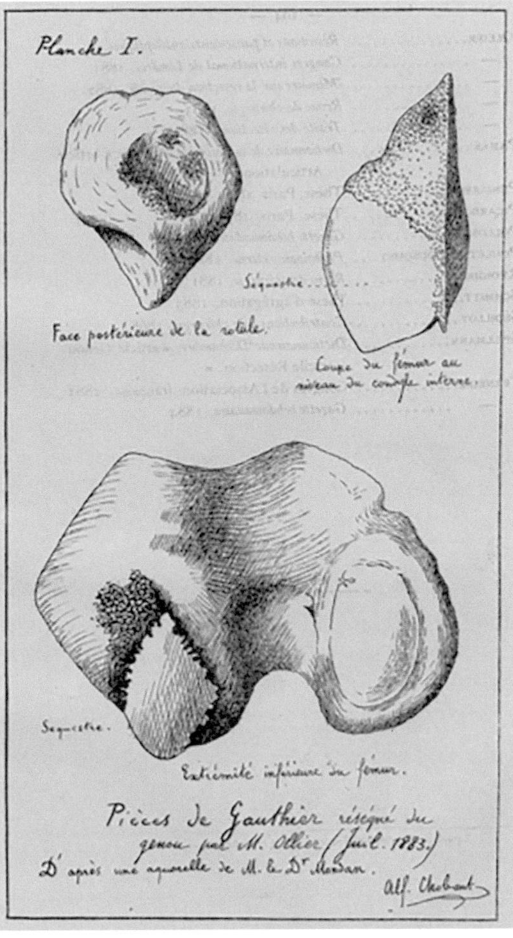

Fig. 1.6 Resection specimen on tuberculosis of the knee: 1883. Pr L. Ollier

1.3 Tissue Interposition

In 1886, Ollier proposed tissue interposition by periosteum for the hip and a few years later Gluck proposed to use skin. In 1918, Erich Lexer of the University of Jena took stock of the interpositions of tissue, especially fatty in the hip and knee joints. Concerning the interpositions of fascia lata, the author specifies that the indications are numerous [22]:

To prevent adhesions: In this connection, from my own experiences, fat transplantation plays a very important role. Fat insertion to prevent rigidity of the joint after operations for ankylosis succeeds with best results in the loose joints of the arm, although favourable results. I have also been obtained in the hip and knee (Murphy, Lexer, Ropke). In operations on the knee, fat pads prevented recurrence of the fixation of the patella. Likewise, fat implantation on the freshened acetabulum has relieved the ankylosis of congenital dislocation of the hip due to haemorrhage (Lexer). What changes take place in the flap of fat introduced into the joint is not known. There was no sign of the oft-mentioned watery-like fluid. Whether or not it will make its appearance later, I cannot say... The indications are numerous ... application of fascial flaps between articular surfaces after postoperative injury to the synovial membrane; in mobilisation of joints; as a base for haemostatic sutures in organs...

John Murphy stated in an article in 1913 that he and his team had performed more than 60 arthroplasties including all joints, including 28 knees [23]: *"The knee is the most difficult joint in which to secure the perfect restoration of function and restoration of nearly normal joint anatomy."*

In another article, John Murphy describes surgical techniques and publishes many photographs [24]. In 1918, Melvin Henderson of the Mayo Clinic grouped cases from several centers and published results for 121 patients. At a longer setback, 80 patients were evaluated as successful. Nevertheless, at the end of his career, Henderson was reserved about this type of surgery about conservative arthroplastic surgery he wrote [25]:

I am free to confess that my own experience leaves me still far from satisfied with my efforts along these so-called reconstructive lines... I have used all the operations mentioned, with the result that

function has been, on the whole disappointing, although the aim was lessened, the results were not such as to awaken my enthusiasm.

Willis Campbell in 1922 also focused on the different techniques of interposition, he advised against interpositions by animal tissue in favor of pediculated shreds (Fig. 1.7) [26]:

Pedunculated fascial flaps have been extensively employed between the articular surfaces, after remodelling or carving out a new joint. The procedure has been discarded by a majority of experienced operators in this field, interposition of animal membranes specially prepared, such as the fragile membrane, Baer's pig's bladder, Allison's fascia, etc. While successes have been reported, the disadvantage is that foreign body irritation invites infection and the material is often excluded. Transplantation of free fascia lata, extensively used by Putti, of Italy, and Russell Mac Ausland, of Boston.

In the same year, Campbell published a series of 24 cases [flap of pediculated and free fascia lata, pig bladder] (Figs. 1.8 and 1.9), of the 13 patients who could be assessed only five patients

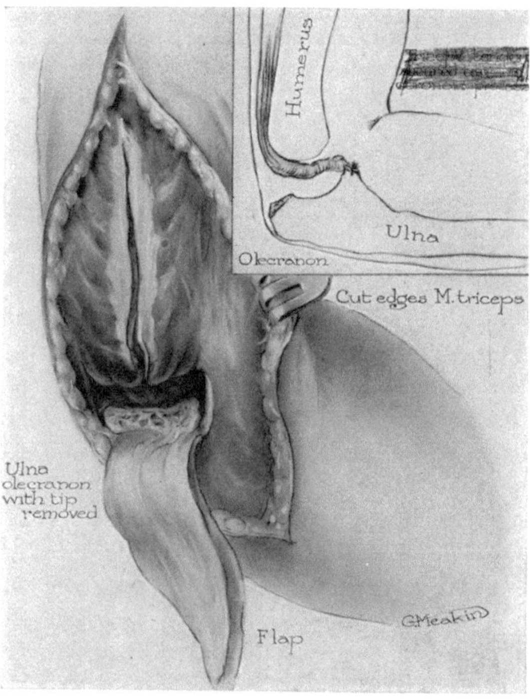

Fig. 1.7 Elbow interposition flap for arthrolysis. Willis C. Campbell. 1922

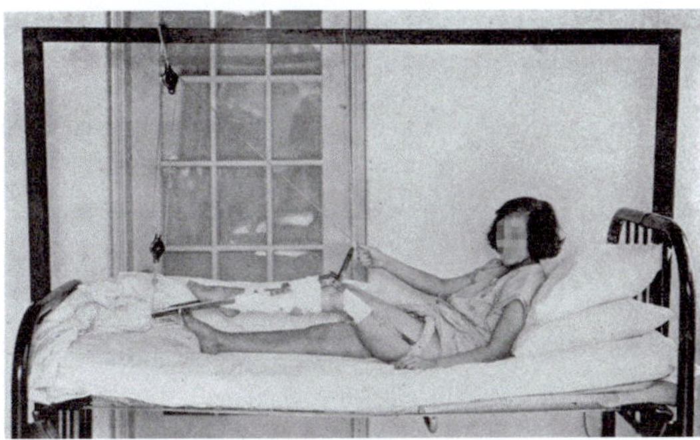

Fig. 1.8 Knee mobilization device after arthrolysis of the knee joint. Willis C. Campbell. 1924

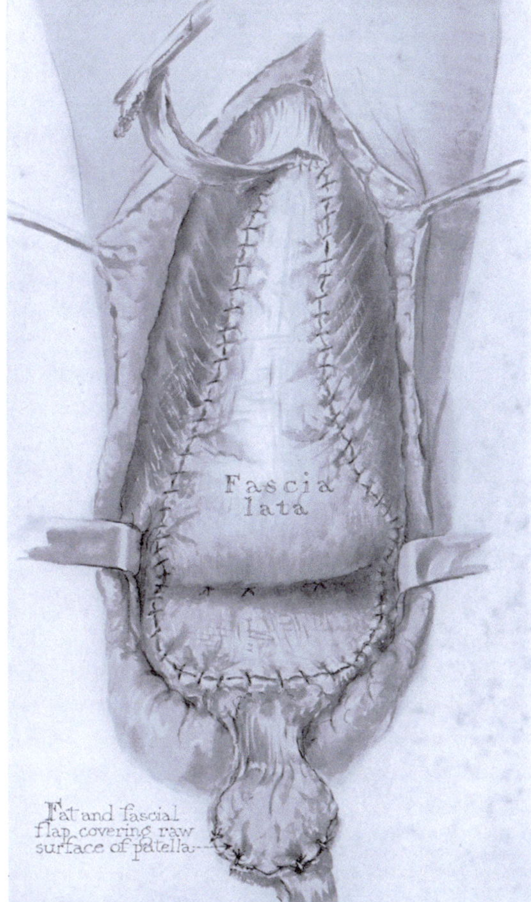

Fig. 1.9 Fascia lata flap. contralateral: William C. Campbell. 1924

had a mobility considered as good. In his last publication of 1924, Campbell described an original technique for contralateral lata fascia trans-

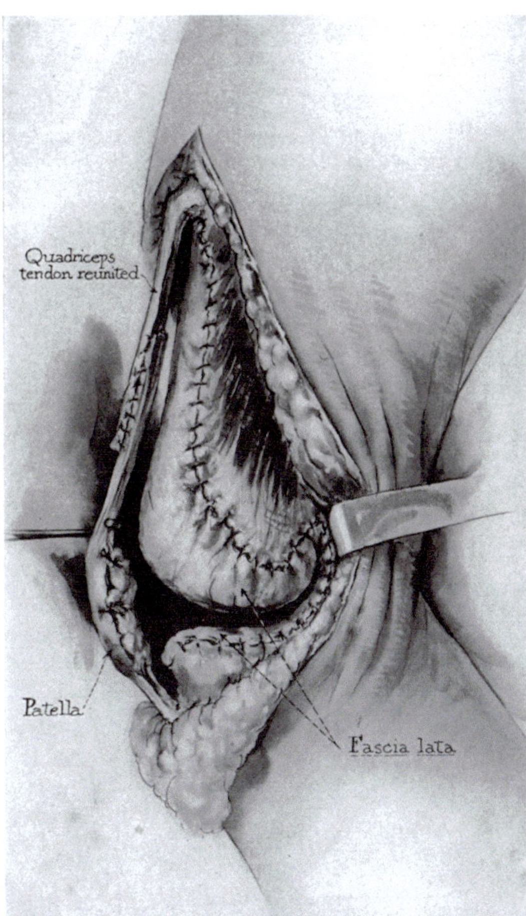

Fig. 1.10 Fascia lata flap. ipsilateral: William C. Campbell. 1924

fer (Figs. 1.9 and 1.10) and [27] stated that he had operated on 16 patients in recent years with homo or contralateral transplants. Only 12 patients could be evaluated, he had ten good results and two failures, his conclusion is as follows [28]: *"My first report was by no means encouraging but from results obtain, especially during the last year, arthroplasty of the knee is justifiable in well-selected cases, with an excellent chance of obtaining satisfactory motion."*

These results led him to develop another concept, the joint interposition of inert materials. Following Smith-Petersen's work on the hip, he opted for vitallium. Smith-Petersen had made many tests before vitallium with the following materials: glass, pyrex glass, viscaloids, Bakeites. In 1940, Campbell published his first two clinical cases of interposition of vitallium plate also called cap. It was a cast of the lower end of the femur whose size was evaluated by [29] X-rays. The fixation was made by two posterior hooks and an anterior screw. He specified in his publication that he is also working on a tibial plate. These interposition trays [30] had always been used in 1970 by Ranawat and Sbarbaro. From the 1950s, many types of arthroplasty will see the light of day and some anecdotal models testify however to the medical reflection engaged, C. Rocher in 1952 proposed an arthroplasty of the knee by two femoral heads in Judet acrylic [31]. However, all these attempts were disappointing.

1.4 Synthetic Interposition

From the 1950s, three surgeons modified Campbell's concept by proposing interposition trays such as Mc Keever in 1953, Mc Intosh in 1954 and Spotarno.

1. Mc Keever.

    In 1949, Mc Keever set up two patellofemoral prostheses (left and right), and in 1955, he published 40 cases. In 1960 in a posthumous article, Robert Elliot published the work of Mc Keever on the placement of unicompartmental tibial prosthesis about 76 interventions (Fig. 1.11). The first surgery was

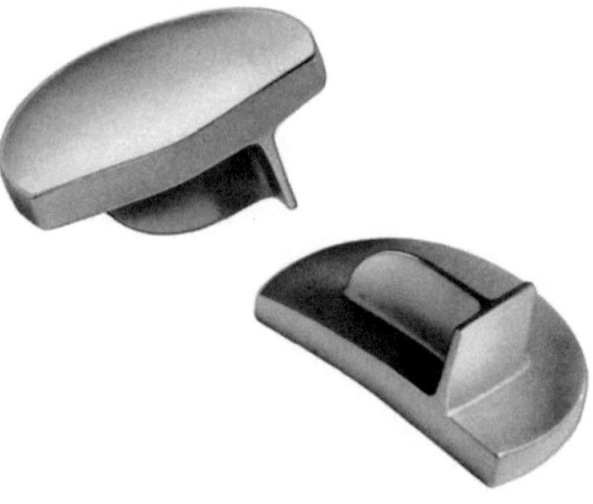

Fig. 1.11 McKeever prosthesis

performed in 1952 for a villonodular synovitis, it was a single tibial piece fixed by a blade [32]:

He had a restoration of both tibial plateaus by a prosthesis, a patellar prosthesis and an extensive joint debridement. Cellophane was interposed to restore the periarticular gliding surfaces and the suprapatellar pouch. The conclusions are as follows: *"With this prosthesis it is possible to restore satisfactory function to most of the badly damaged knee joints that ordinarily would be subjected to an arthrodesis. If this prosthesis will function satisfactorily in these severely damaged knee joints, it will function in any case other than that with an infection.*

2. Mac Intosh published his first cases in 1966 [33], then in a second publication in 1972 about 130 surgeries. Mac Intosh [34] [Toronto] was the first prosthesis which was implanted in 1954. He made an oral presentation in 1965 at the annual meeting of the British Orthopaedists' Association, on 58 cases, 51 of which were bilateral. For Mac Intosh, the ideal indication is rheumatoid arthritis, for osteoarthritis he prefers to do arthrodesis of the knee.

    In a 1972 publication, Mac Intosh described how in 1954 he made his first case: *"A 73-year-old woman was operated on at Toronto General Hospital for knee arthrodesis."* During surgery, she realized that the valgus deformity could be reduced and the tension of the lateral collateral ligament improved stability to the knee. He decided intraoperatively to put a hemiprosthesis, for this he saws in two a knee prosthesis and implanted only the external part. It was an acrylic prosthesis from Dr. Sven Kiaer, Kund Jansen from Copenhagen. The patient lived 12 years with this hemiprosthesis. Six other patients were operated, four patients on six had a result considered as good at 10 years. The acrylic initially used for hip prostheses following the work of the Judet brothers was abandoned after reactions to foreign bodies at the hip. The conclusion of the article is in rheumatoid arthritis, hemi arthroplasty was the procedure of choice, since tibial osteotomy was not a reasonable alternative.

All these implants were based on the concept of joint improvement related to the restoration of joint line and the tension of collateral ligaments. The prostheses of Mc Keever and Sbarbaro were stabilized by a keel or blade inserted into a groove of the tibial plateau. Mac Intosh's device was free placed on a prepared tibia, the shape of the prosthesis allowed a ligament tension stabilizing the joint (Fig. 1.12). The procedure for implanting the devices was demanding and relatively lengthy. However, two major problems persisted: the lack of secondary fixation of the implants and femoral cartilage wear. The last experiments with this type of implant date back to the 2000s with the development of the Unispacer™ (Zimmer, Warsaw, USA). The results were dissapointing: Cartier et al. [35]. performed six surgical revisions on the 17 surgeries, so they did not recommend the use of this implant and commercialization was stopped (Fig. 1.13).

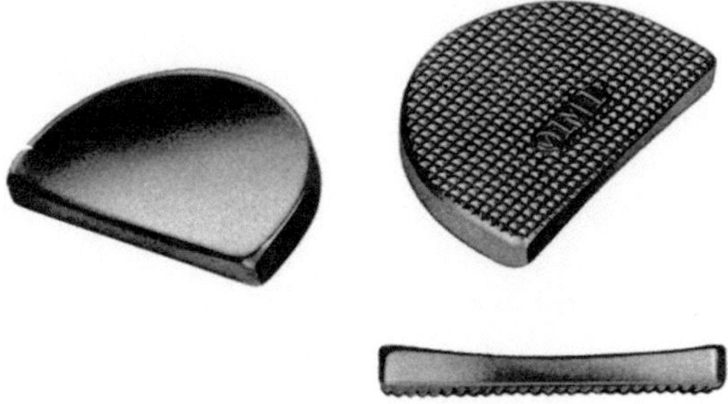

Fig. 1.12 Mac Intosh prosthesis

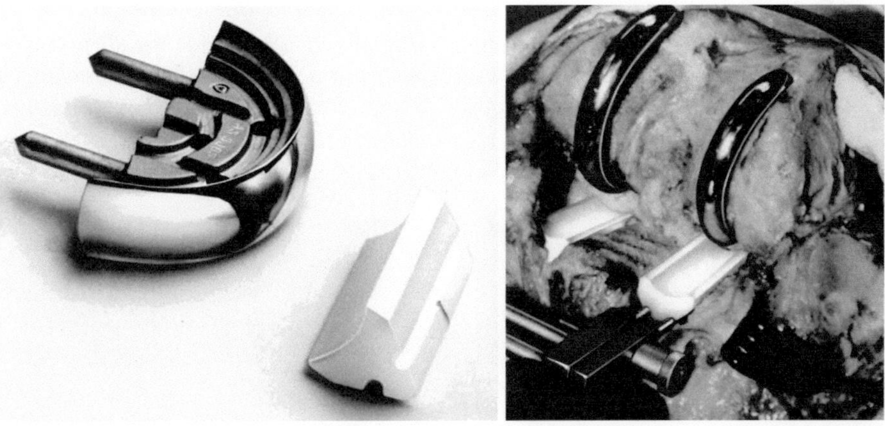

Fig. 1.13 Gunston Polycentric Knee Prosthesis

1.5 The Unicompartmental Prosthesis

1.5.1 Cement

Frank H. Gunston, (Winnipeg, Canada) was awarded a travel grant to study hip replacement in Wrightington with Sir John Charnley in 1966. During this period, he worked on a concept of arthroplasty of the cemented knee and published in 1966 a biomechanical and clinical work on the polycentric prosthesis (prosthetic simulation of normal knee movement). This prosthesis was cemented, it was two cemented unicompartmental prostheses for femur and tibia. Upon his return to Canada, he worked with Peterson of the Mayo Clinic to develop a polycentric knee prosthesis (Howmedica [36], Rutherford, New Jersey, USA) in 1970. This prosthesis was technically difficult to implant, and the clinical results were unsatisfactory in long term (Fig. 1.14). In 1984, Lewallen published the results of the Mayo Clinic with 10 years of follow-up, the survival rate was 66%. Patients had 13% instability due to ligament lax-

ity, 7% incidence of loosening, 3% incidence of infection, and 4% incidence of tibiofemoral joint pain. This double prosthesis was abandoned; however, surgeons at the Mayo Clinic used it for unicompartmental damage. During surgery if only one side was worn, the prosthesis was implanted on the worn side. Bryan et al. published a series of 207 knees, with 3 years of follow-up, 83% of patients were satisfied [37]. However, at the same time, other cemented unicompartmental arthroplasties were developed, such as Geomedic, Savastano, and Marmor.

1.5.2 Insall's Articles

John Insall in the 1970s and 1980s was in a dilemma, his position about unicompartmental prostheses was ambiguous while remaining open [38]: *"Unicompartmental replacement for osteoarthritis of the knee is an attractive concept. It seems reasonable that limited replacement would come closest to normal functional restoration."* The confusion was total, because the same year

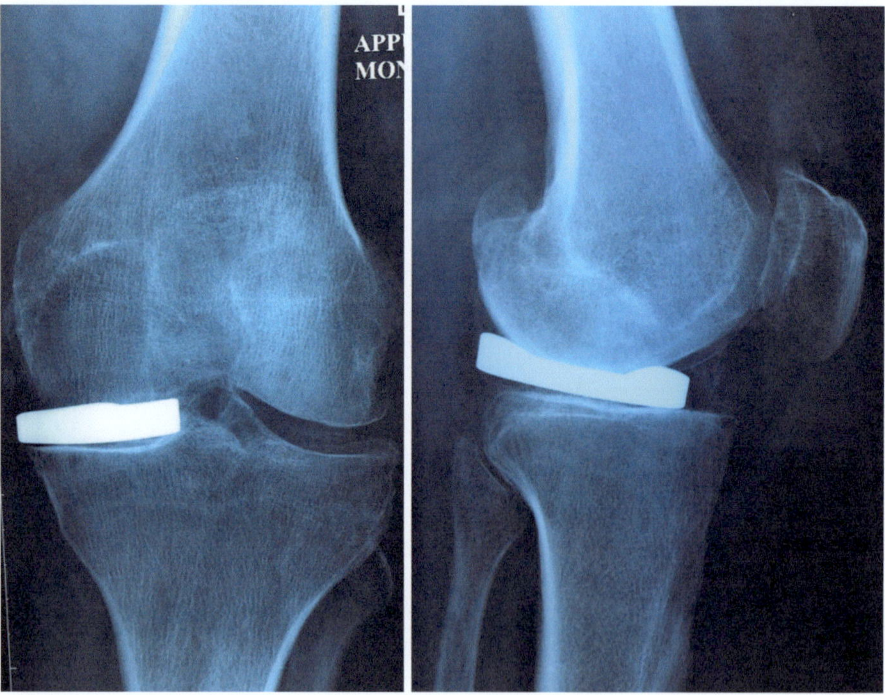

Fig. 1.14 Unispacer™

he published two contradictory articles! In October 1976, an article with P. Walker [38], in this article, his conclusion about the unicondylar prosthesis was as follows:

The best results were seen in the lateral compartment arthroplasties. Such deformities may be the only future indication for the use of this operation as these knees do not do well when treated by tibial osteotomy. However, when only the medial compartment is involved, osteotomy may still remain in the treatment of choice.

In the second article of 1976 [39], where he compared four models of prostheses his conclusion was without appeal: *"We now think that there is no indication for this type of prosthesis and that the tibial osteotomy or the bicondylar prosthesis should be chosen preferentially."*

In 1980, Insall et al. confirmed the impressions of 1976 and in a study of a series of 32 unicompartmental prostheses at 5 years of hindsight, they showed that despite the good results of the initial clinical results deteriorate over time [40]: *"Unicompartmental prostheses are used in the least advanced cases that give the least complications, but the clinical results are not superior to other prostheses."*

Following these publications, even if Insall moderated his remarks in his book *Surgery of the knee. Total knee replacement* [41] we can say that for Insall that a good knee prostheses is a total knee arthroplasty.

1.5.3 Kozinn and Scott's Criteria

In an article that will serve as a reference: Stuart Kozinn, Clare Marx, and Richard Scott proposed an algorithm of indications. In their [42] series, they reported 92% excellent and good results at 5.5 years of follow-up by respecting the following selection criteria:

- Over 60 years.
- Less than 67 kg.
- Moderate activity.
- Little pain at rest.
- Flexum less than 5° and flexion greater than 90°.

- Reducible frontal deformity: in varus less than 10° and in valgus less than 15°.

These extremely restrictive criteria carried by the *Robert Breck Brigham hospital* team will be taken up by John Insall, then relayed in France by the Lyon teams, including Gérard Deschamps and Chol [43]:

Summary: Unicompartmental knee arthroplasty – UKA – is designed for patients presenting arthritic wear limited to a single medial or lateral tibiofemoral compartment. The indication is based on strict criteria. Wear must stem from degenerative osteoarthritis or be secondary to aseptic necrosis of the medial condyle. Inflammatory rheumatism is a contraindication. Age and activity level should be compatible with an indication for arthroplasty. The body mass index should be less than 30 kg/m². The ligament system must be intact, particularly both cruciate ligaments. Any pre-existing axis deformity should be moderate and the residual axis deformity, after correction of wear with a unicompartmental tibial augmentation spacer, should not exceed 7–10° varus or valgus.

For more than four decades, these criteria will become paradigmatic, defining a new global standard of indications.

1.5.4 The 1980s: The Awakening

Léonard Marmor for the Anglo-Saxon countries then Philippe Cartier in France extracted the UKA from ostracism where John Insall and his collaborators had locked it up. But it is the Oxford team that is pulling the UKAs out of the New York rut while reviewing, thanks to a continuous and scientific work spanning more than 30 years, the indications, the surgical technique, and the prosthetic models.

1.5.4.1 Marmor

Léonard Mamor developed a unicompartmental prosthesis that he implanted in 1974. The first publications were encouraging with 88% of patients satisfied at 2 years. However, considering the wear and tear he advised against using polyethylenes with a thickness of less than six millimeters [44]:

A follow-up of 2 years or more on 105 patients with the Modular – Marmor – knee replacement revealed that 88 per cent of the patients had a successful result. The complications and failures are analysed in depth. Late loosening of the components were not observed except with the 6 mm tibial plateau. Pain relief was dramatic as well as improved function, stability and motion.

His second major publication dates from 1988, about 60 prostheses more than 10 years of follow-up. Marmor in introduction clarified the scope of the UKAs [45]:

In the past decade, two concepts have caused considerable controversy in orthopedic surgery of the knee. Some orthopedic centers contend that osteotomy of the tibia is the procedure of choice for unicompartmental gonarthrosis of the knee and resist the concept of unicompartmental arthroplasty."The other concept is that if unicompartmental arthroplasty is necessary, the entire joint should be replaced, since the uninvolved compartment may develop arthritis in the future.

At 11 years of hindsight, he had in his series 70% satisfied patients and 87 painless knees. However, a resounding trial will damage the image of Marmor's UKA. In June 1983, Richard was ordered to pay Dr. Marmor $25,000 on the prosthesis patent and $500,000 in personal damages. The Richard company was condemned following the manufacture between January 1973 and April 1973 of 4000 medium tibial parts not corresponding to the sizes of the concept. This modification may lead to difficulties in surgical placement and affect the clinical results, and a patient complaint will be filed [46].

1.5.4.2 Philippe Cartier

A few years later, Philippe Cartier in France reported a positive experience, with more than 90%, excellent or good results at less than 5 years of decline. This author will successively use the Marmor, the Mod III condylar, the Mansat Uni,

and the Genesis. In 2007, in an oral publication [GECO] on 2170 cases, he detailed the factors of recovery of UKAs. In his experiment, the failures of the models of the 1970s had [47, 48] essentially a technical cause [instrumentation and surgeons], for the models of the 1980s, the failures were essentially mechanical linked in particular to the poor quality of polyethylene (sterilization with gamma rays, polyethylene too fine, metal back too rigid ...).

In his practice from the 90s complications were rare, in total 46 surgical repetitions out of 1170 UKAs, the main causes of failures are the defects of initial indications.

1.5.4.3 The Oxfordian Revolution

In a remarkable study of the biomechanics of the Knee, John Goodfellow laid the foundations of the prosthesis with a movable plate in 1978. He first observes, as Aldabert Kapandji had done before him, that the tension of the cruciate ligaments constrains the flexion/extension movement of the knee. Goodfellow completed Kapandji's model by associating the menisci movement. He attributed to the menisci a double role: stabilization of the condyles and increase of the contact surface between the femur and the tibia. To illustrate his point, he made a model (Fig. 1.15) that served as a two-dimensional model and introduced between the femur and the tibia a *"meniscal washer."* Meniscus substitutes by increasing the contact surfaces decrease the stresses. Starting from this model and following his articles on hip and elbow constraints [49], he developed the concept of the Oxford [50] prosthesis and filed a patent [1977, US, patent 21,905] (Fig. 1.16) jointly with John O'Connor of Oxford and Nigel Shrive of Calgary [51]. For these designers, the Oxford prosthesis met the following specifications: con-

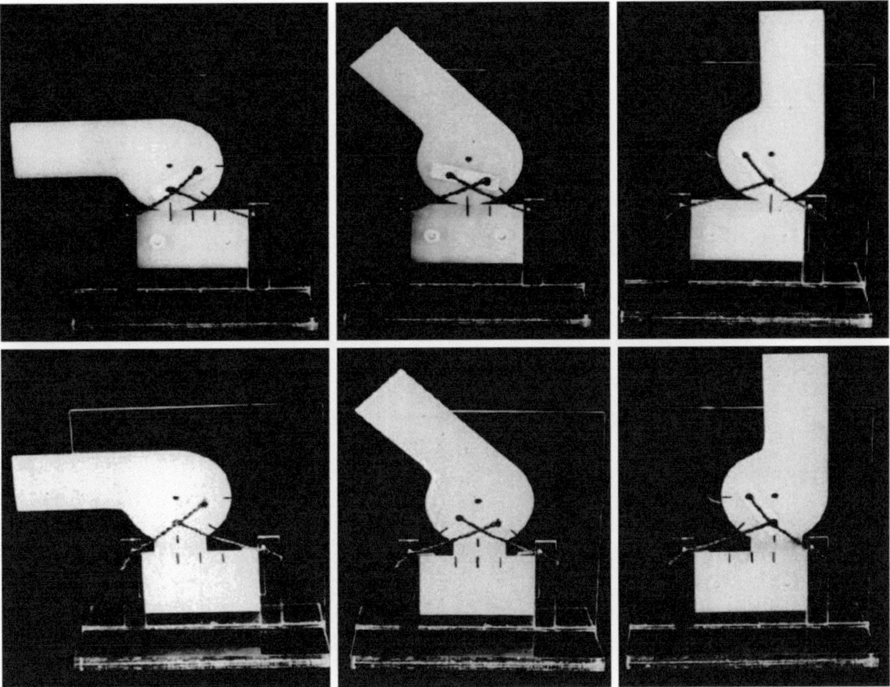

Fig. 1.15 Biomechanical model: importance of the mobile meniscal wedge between the femur and the tibia

gruence during bending movements, little stress at the interfaces, and reduced wear.

Initially, this prosthesis is implanted in bilateral osteoarthritis, but from 1982 it was implanted in isolated unicompartmental osteoarthritis. In 1988, Goodfellow et al. published their first clinical results, 36 months of follow-up [52], and then 10 years of follow-up. The authors confirmed the very good clinical results and show that prosthetic wear was minimal, thus standing out from other prostheses, for example, the Lotus [53]. For these authors, the rate of wear of the Oxford prosthesis remained negligible, well below other arthroplasties:

The mean wear rate of 0.02 mm/year measured in the vivo study compares favorably with the published results of polyethylene penetration for other forms of arthroplasty which use a metal-on-polyethylene bearing. The value is approximately ten times less than the penetration rates of 0.1–0.2 mm/year reported for total hip arthroplasty [54].

At 15 years of decline, the clinical results of the Oxford 3 prosthesis remain excellent [55] confirming the results of Price and Svard [56] and Liddle [57] who found a survival of the prostheses of 92% at 20 years of follow-up for the Oxford models 1 and 2 prosthesis (Figs. 1.17 and 1.18).

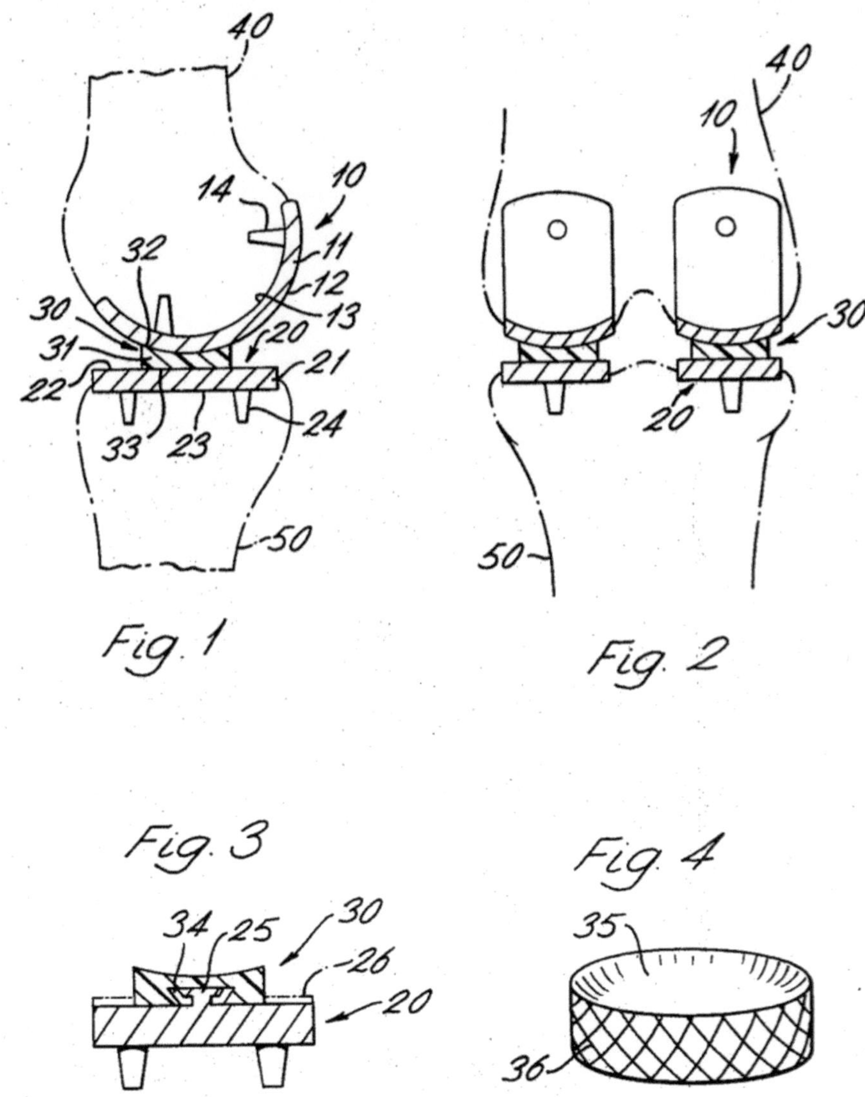

Fig. 1.16 Oxford prosthesis: 1978 patent drawings

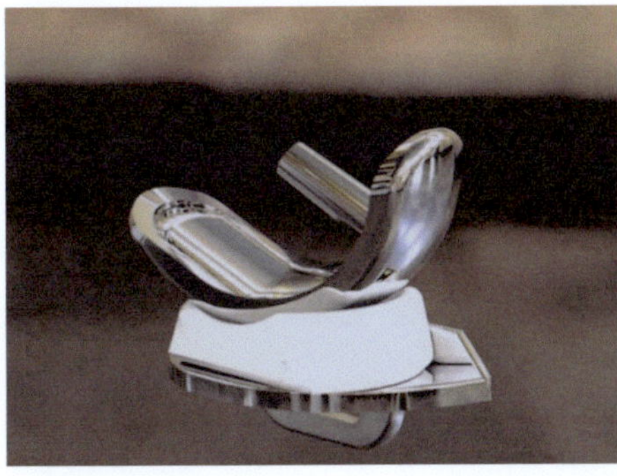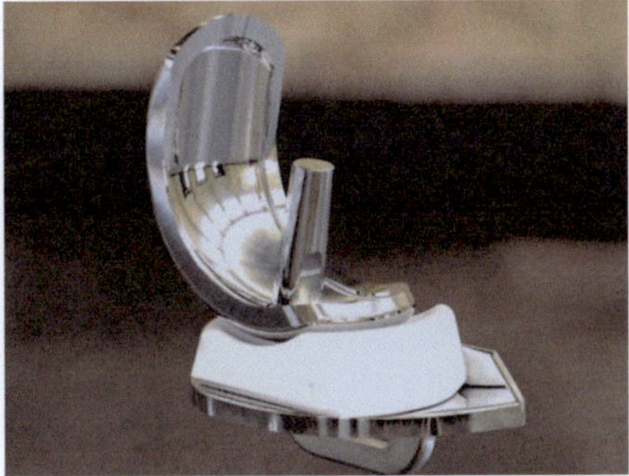

Fig. 1.17 Oxford 3 prosthesis

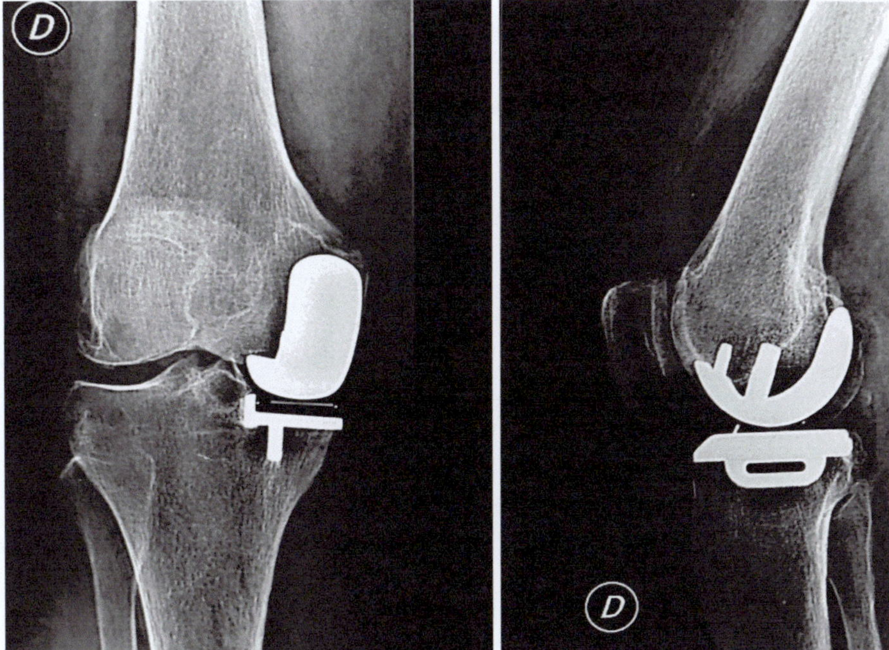

Fig. 1.18 Oxford 3 prosthesis

1.6   Conclusion

The concept of unicompartmental prosthesis was built over the past century, it is the emergence of an inventive, prudent, and respectful surgery, as evidenced by the clinical and philosophical descriptions of our elders.

We must not forget the ancient interventions, all of which aimed at function, with empathy as a corollary; from Anthony White to Léopold Ollier, the surgeons wanted to be correctors, functionals, and humans.

At the dawn of this twenty-first century, the unicompartmental prosthesis has just acquired its letters of nobility, it is safe and reproducible. We can say with Ahmadou Kourouma looking at the path traced and the finality:

When you don't know where you're going, let you know where you're coming from [58].

References

1. Hippocrates. Complete works. Fractures. Literary and artistic union, Paris. 1955, p. 44.
2. Surgery of Paul of Aegina. Trad. by M. René Briau. Paris. Ed. Victor Masson. 1855, pp. 315–7.
3. Philosophical Transactions. 1769, vol. LIX, pp. 39–45.
4. Barton JR. On the treatment of anchylosis by the formation of artificial joints. North Am Med Surg J. 1827;3:279–92.
5. Works surgery—practical, civil and military. Barthelemi Vigarous. Ed. Tournel, Montpellier. 1812, pp. 431–3.
6. The analysis of Vigarous Sr.'s book, however, raises doubts about his son's words, because Barthelemi Vigarous perfectly described all the clinical cases he cites and arranges them by chronology. In his book he quotes and describes White's description before his own case.
7. Observations variœ medico-chirurgicœ a Johanne Daniele Schlichting, Med. & Chir. Doctore. Obserrationis rarie medico chirurgica, Philosophical Transactions, London. 1742, vol. XLII, p. 274.
8. A Dictionary of Practical Surgery – Samuel Cooper. Ed. J. Harper, New York. 1818, pp. 53–5.
9. Barton J. On the treatment of anchylosis by the formation of artificial joints. North Am Med Surg Newspaper. 1827;3:279–92.
10. Treaty of resections and conservatives operations that can be practiced on the system bony. T3, l. Ollier. Ed. G. Masson. Paris. 1891, p. 207.
11. Treatise on resections. O. Heyfelder Ed Baillère, Translated from German, with additions and notes, by Dr. Eug. Boekel. Strasbourg. 1863, pp. 45–58.
12. Hip resection in cases of coxalgia. Leon the Strong. Dissertation read at the Imperial Academy of Medicine. 1860, vol. XXV, pp. 445–583.
13. Hip resection in cases of coxalgia. Leon the Strong. Ed. Baillière, Paris. 1862, pp. 3–5.
14. Treated with resections and conservative operations that can be performed on the bone system. T. Ollier. Ed. G. Masson, Paris. 1891; T3, l. p. 243.
15. Treated with resections and conservative operations that can be performed on the bone system. Leopold Ollier. Ed. G. Masson, Paris. 1891; T3, p. 210.
16. Leopold Ollier. Treatise of resections and conservative operations that can be performed on the bone system. T3, l. Ed. G. Masson, Paris. 1891, pp. 220–1.
17. J. Rhea Barton. A new treatment in a case of anchyloses. The American Journal of the Medical Science. Philadelphia. Ed Carey, Lea, Blanchard. 1837, pp. 332–40.
18. J. Rhea Barton. A new treatment in a case of anchyloses. The American Journal of the Medical Science. Philadelphia. Ed Carey, Lea, Blanchard. 1837, p. 333.
19. J. Rhea Barton. A new treatment in a case of anchyloses. The American Journal of the Medical Science. Philadelphia. Ed Carey, Lea, Blanchard. 1837, pp. 337–8.
20. Aristide Verneuil. The creation of a false joint by section or partial resection of the lower maxillary bone, as a means of remedying a true or false ankylosis of the lower jaw. Ed Labé. Arch Gen Med 15, Paris. 1860; vol. 1, pp. 174–88.
21. Treaty of resections and operations preservatives that can be performed on the bone system. Leopold Ollier. Ed. G. Masson, Paris. 1891; T3, l. p. 777.
22. Lexer E. Free transplantation. Ann Surg. 1914;60(2):77–182.
23. Murphy JB. Original memories. Arthroplasty. Ann Surg. 1913;57:611.
24. Murphy JB. The classic: ankylosis: arthroplasty—clinical and experimental. Clin Orthop Relat Res. 2008;466:2573–8.
25. Henderson MS. Role of fusion operations as applied to the hip-joint. Br Med J. 1933;19(2):3789.
26. Campbell WC. Arthroplasty of the elbow. Ann Surg. 1922;76(5):615–23.
27. Campbell WC. Arthroplasty of the knee. Report of cases. Am J Orth Surg. 1921;3(9):430–4.
28. Campbell WC. Arthroplasty of the knee. Ann Surg. 1924;76(5):615–23.
29. Smith-Petersen MN. Arthroplasty of the hip. A new method. J Bone Joint Surg. 1939;21:269. (We were unable to view the original).
30. Campbell WC. Interposition of vitallium plate sin arthroplasties of the knee. Report. Am J Surg. 1940;47:639–41.
31. Rock. Knee arthroplasty by femoral heads in acrylic. Bordeaux Elit. 1952;1:48. (We were unable to view the original).
32. Dc. MC Keever. Tibial plateau prosthesis. Blinking. Orthop Relat Res. 1960;18:86–95. This is a posthumous article that was written by Dr. Robert B. Elliott (Houston), a year after Mc's death. Keever. Republished in 2005: *The classic. Tibial plateau prothesis. Duncan C. Mc Keever. Blinking Orthop Relat Res. 2005;440:4–9.*
33. Mac Intosh D. Arthroplasty of the knee in rheumatoid arthritis. J Bone Joint Surg. 1966;48B:179.
34. Myc Intosh D. The use of the hemiarthroplasty prothesis for advanced osteoarthritis and rheumatoid arthritis of the knee. J Bone Joint Surg Br. 1972;54:244.
35. Catier C, Turcat M, Jacquel A, Baulot E. The Unispacer ᵀᵐ unicompartmental knee implant: it's outcomes in medial compartment knee osteoarthritis. Orthop Traumatol Surg Res. 2011;97:410–7.
36. Gunston F. Polycentric knee arthroplasty. Prosthetic simulation of normal knee movement. J Bone Joint Surg Br. 1971;53:272–7.
37. Jones W, Bryan R, Peterson LF, Ilstrup D. Unicompartmental knee arthroplasty using polycentric and geometric hemicomponents. J Bone Joint Surg Am. 1981;63(6):946–54.
38. Insall J, Walker P. Unicondylar knee replacement. Clin Orthop Relat Res. 1976;120:83–5.
39. Insall J, Ranawat C, Aglietti P, Shine J. A comparison of four models of the total knee replacement protheses. JBJS. 1976;58-A(6):754–65.

40. Insall J, Aglietti P. A five to seven-year follow-up of unicondylar arthroplasty. J Bone Joint Surg Am. 1980;62(8):1329–37.
41. J. Insall. Surgery of the knee. Total knee replacement. Ed. Churchill Livingstone, New York. 1984, p. 615.
42. Kozinn S, Marx C, Scott R. Unicompartmental knee arthroplasty. A 4.5-6-year follow-up study with a metal-backed tibial component. J Arthroplast. 1989;4(Suppl):S1–S10.
43. Deschamps G, Chol C. Fixed-bearing unicompartmental knee arthroplasty. Patients' selection and operative technique. Orthop Traumatol Surg Res. 2011;97(6):648–61.
44. Marmor L. The modular (Marmor) knee. Clin Orthop Relat Res. 1976;120:86–94.
45. Marmor L. Unicompartmental knee arthroplasty. Ten- to 13-year follow-up study. Clin Orthop Relat Res. 1988;226:14–20.
46. Nellie Vossler, Plaintiff and respondent, v. Richards Manufacturing Company, Inc., Defendant and Appellant. Docket No. 6436. Court of Appeals of California, Fifth District. June 15, 1983.
47. Cartier P, Cheaib S. Unicondylar knee arthroplasty: 2–10 years of follow-up evaluation. J Arthroplasty. 1987;2:157–62.
48. https://docplayer.fr/128712875-Reprise-de-p-u-c-geco-2007-chirurgie-de-reprise-janvier-2007.html.
49. Bullough P, et al. The relationship between degenerative changes and load-bearing in the human hip. J Bone Joint Surg Br. 1973;55B:746.
50. Goodfellow J, O'Connor J. The mechanics of the knee and prosthesis design. J Bone Joint Surg (Br). 1978;6G-8:358–69.
51. https://patentimages.storage.googleapis.com/1a/94/a9/71e1f4ea6a25cc/US4085466.pdf.
52. Goodfellow J, Kershaw C, D'A Benson M, Connor JO. The Oxford knee for unicompartmental osteoarthritis. The first 103 cases. J Bone Joint Surg (Br). 1988;70(5):692–701.
53. Witvoët J, Peyrache M, Nizard R. Single-compartment "Lotus" type knee prosthesis in the treatment of lateralized gonarthrosis: results in 135 cases with a mean follow-up of 4.6 years. Rev Chir Orthop Reparatrice Appar Mot. 1993;79(7):565–76.
54. Price A, et al. Ten years in vivo wear measurement of a fully congruent mobile bearing unicompartmental knee arthroplasty. J Bone Joint Surg (Br). 2005;87-B:1493–7.
55. Pandit H, Hamilton T, Jenkins C, Mellon S, Dodd C, Murray D. The clinical outcome of minimally invasive phase 3 Oxford unicompartmental knee arthroplasty: a 15-year follow-up of 1000 UKAs. Bone Joint J. 2015;97B:1493–500.
56. Price A, Svard U. A second decade lifetable survival analysis of the Oxford uni-compartmental knee arthroplasty. Clin Orthop Relat Res. 2011;469:174–9.
57. Liddle A, Judge A, Pandit H, Murray D. Determinants of revision and functional outcome following unicompartmental knee replacement. Osteoarthr Cartil. 2014;22:1241–50.
58. Ahmadou Kourouma : Ivorian writer (1927/1994) born in Côte d'Ivoire, he comes from the Malinké ethnic group. He was an infantryman in Indochina from 1950 to 1954. "Waiting for the vote of the wild beasts" Seuil, 2000.

The Disappearing Unicompartmental Knee Prostheses

2

Samuel Laurent, Baptiste Montbardon, Arnaud Clavé, and Frédéric Dubrana

2.1 Introduction

The improvement in the functional results of unicompartmental knee surgery over the last three decades is closely linked to the development of prosthetic implants, but also to the reproducibility of this surgery thanks to more efficient ancillary equipment.

These improvements have been made possible by the existing demand for these new prostheses, but also because of financial competition between the different laboratories involved in the market.

The first versions of these prostheses have now given way to new-generation implants that more faithfully reproduce the anatomical and biomechanical characteristics of the knee joint.

This chapter will focus on the discontinued unicompartmental prostheses.

There are many reasons for the discontinuation of these devices: poor clinical results, lack of financial profitability, technological innovation, laboratory consolidation or restructuring, etc.

Unfortunately, the literature on this subject is very poor and unlike Australia or the Scandinavian countries, we do not have quality registers on unicompartmental implants.

We will present some of these unicompartmental prostheses (UKA) that have disappeared, while trying to understand if their disappearance is linked to a design defect or to the tumult of the world economy, punctuated by the takeover bids and counter-takeovers of the world giants producing our orthopaedic equipment.

This chapter does not pretend to be exhaustive or to be a peremptory judgement on the implants mentioned.

2.2 History of Major Chip Companies

The choice of these different companies was made on the basis of data that some laboratories have communicated to us (Table 2.1).

2.2.1 Depuy Synthès

At the beginning of the 90s, several laboratories were producing unicompartmental prostheses of French design. Among them, the LANDANGER laboratories which produced *the **Goeland***, and the Roannais MEDINOV AMP which produced the ***Gonometric.***

S. Laurent · B. Montbardon · F. Dubrana
Department of Orthopaedic Surgery and Traumatology, Brest University Teaching Hospital "La Cavale Blanche", Brest, France

A. Clavé (✉)
Department of Orthopaedic Surgery and Traumatology, Saint George Private Hospital, Nice, France

LaTIM, INSERM-UBO UMR 1101, Brest, France

A. Clavé, F. Dubrana (eds.), *Unicompartmental Knee Arthroplasty*,
https://doi.org/10.1007/978-3-031-48332-5_2

Table 2.1 UKA status in 2020

UKA		
NK-Uni	Then allegretto	Now Alpina Uni
Repicci		
Miller Galante Uni	Now ZUK	Commercialized by LIMA
Oxford UKA	Commercialized by Zimmer Biomet	
Persona UKA		
Alpina UKA		

These two laboratories were bought in 1996, by the American-Swiss group SYNTHES, which then decided to stop the production of Gonometric in 1997 to rationalize its range.

With the acquisition of the Depuy Synthès laboratory by the American pharmaceutical group Johnson and Johnson, the unicompartmental prostheses of French design have been abandoned, the project was to create a new prosthesis with American surgeons, the *Preservation.*

2.2.2   Zimmer Biomet

At the origin of this giant we find 2 companies belonging to the Swiss Group SULZER: ALLOPRO which produced the *Uni NK2* and PROTEK: which produced the *Uni Allegretto.*

These two companies were merged in 1995 to create the Swiss group: SULZER MEDICA.

At the beginning of the year 2000, SULZER MEDICA decided to create the company CENTERPULSE in order to manage only its Orthopaedic branch. This was also a way to make disappear SULZER's name in the United States, which had become embarrassing due to lawsuits over defective hip prostheses and for which the group was condemned by the American justice system and suffered a loss of 793 million euros in 2001.

Two years later, the ZIMMER company, which was already producing the *Miller Gallante*

II and the *ZUK (Zimmer Uni Knee)*, bought the CENTERPULSE company.

In order to rationalize its ranges, the production of the *uni NK2* and *Allegretto* has been stopped, these will be replaced by the *ZUK.*

In 2014, ZIMMER bought out BIOMET, which produced two unicompartmental the Oxford and the Alpina Uni, and the creation of the giant ZIMMER BIOMET.

Following the takeover of BIOMET and due to anti-trust laws, in some countries ZIMMER had to cede the exploitation rights of ZUK, acquired in 2015 by the Italian company LIMA.

From now on, ZIMMER BIOMET markets 3 unicompartmentals:

- Oxford.
- PPK (evolution of the ZUK through the Persona range).
- Alpina Uni.

Thus, with globalization, we are witnessing a progressive takeover of companies producing French and European unicompartmentals, which are gradually coming under the American flag.

American flag. But their conception remains for the most part European *(Oxford of English conception, Alpina uni France, and PPK of French design).*

For example, Zimmer manufactures most of its EMEA products in Winterthur, Switzerland with subcontractors in France.

2.2.3   Smith & Nephew

Among the laboratories that still produce unicompartmental implants in Europe, we find SMITH AND NEPHEW, which produced the Marmor Modular Knee, the MOD 3 and then the Genesis, and recently the Genesis and more recently the Accuris Uni and the Journey Uni for which the technique, the ancillary, and the shape of the implant have been revised in a new version to be more guiding and reproducible.

2.3 Unicompartmental Devices Withdrawn from the Market

The choice of these examples was based on the existence of articles in the scientific literature, allowing us to support our discussion. This list is not exhaustive.

2.3.1 Goeland

The Goeland was a cup prosthesis, produced from 1988 to 1998. The femoral implant could be cemented or unsealed, and consisted of an anchoring pin associated with an anti-rotational fin and a flat polyethylene insert fixed on a tibial metal-back.

2.3.2 Gonometric

The Gonometric (Fig. 2.1) was a cemented prosthesis with a cup made of a Chrome- Cobalt alloy, produced from 1991 to 1997.

The Gonometric line included:

- 5 sizes of internal and 4 sizes of external femoral condyles
- 5 sizes of internal or external tibial bases
- 5 polyethylene thicknesses ranging from 8 to 12 mm

2.3.3 Preservation

Preservation was marketed in the United States from 2001 to 2007 by DePuy (Johnson & Johnson).

This prosthesis was composed of a femur made of a chrome-cobalt alloy associated with tibial implant with a full polyethylene or metal-back with a polyethylene insert that could be either fixed or mobile.

In the series by Marini [1], out of 38 Uni Preservation cases, 15 had to be rehabilitated for loosening of the femoral component. No correlation was found between failure and preoperative or postoperative flexion, the difference obtained,

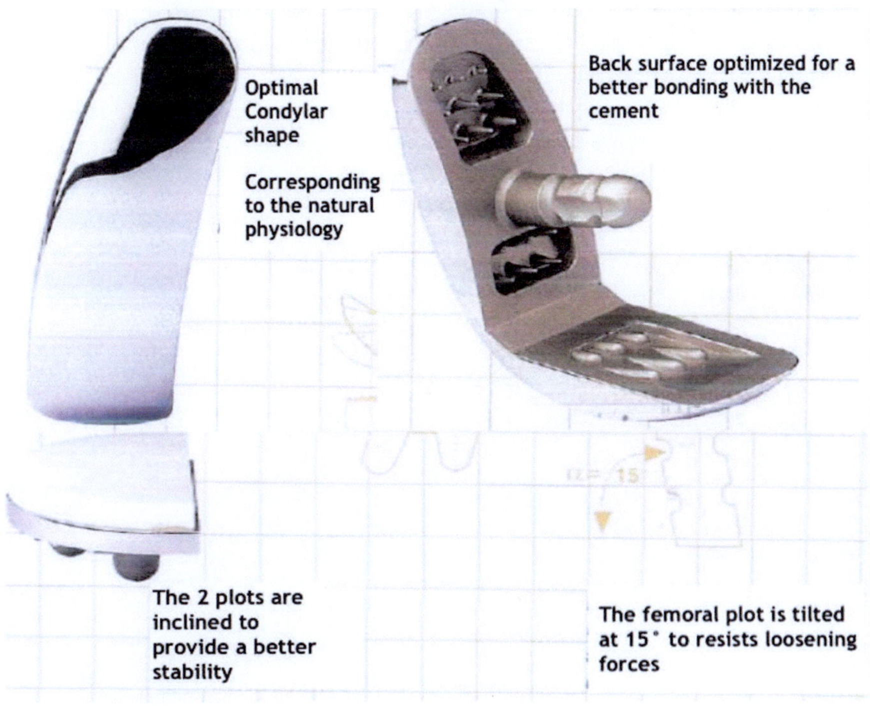

Fig. 2.1 Gonometric UKA

the postoperative tibial slope, the alignment of the femoral component, postoperative range of motion, gender or BMI of the patient.

2.3.4 Miller-Galante II

Marketed by Zimmer (Warsaw, Ind. USA) between 1992 and 2008, this was a cemented, fixed-plate, cup prosthesis (Fig. 2.2).

The Miller-Galante II was designed to be cemented only. For this purpose, it had benefited from two studs on the femoral component and three on the tibial component, to improve stability. The thinnest polyethylene that could be used was 8 mm thick and was sterilized by gamma irradiation.

The series of Koskinen [2], on the medium-term survival of Miller-Galante II showed poor results with 86% survival at 7 years. In fact, 8 out of 46 prostheses had to be revised for premature wear of the polyethylene, with the hypothesis of a poor quality of the polyethylene due to sterilization by gamma irradiation.

However, Berger et al. [3] showed very good results in their prospective series with 98% survival at 10 years average follow-up.

The marketing of the Miller-Gallante II was stopped in 2008 in favour of the Physica ZUK® prosthesis (Zimmer and nowadays LIMA Corporate. UD, Italy).

2.3.5 PCA

Designed by two Swedish surgeons, A. Lindstrand and A. Stenstrom [4], it was commercialized by Stryker Howmedica Osteonics in 1983.

This cut prosthesis could be inserted with or without cement. The bone-prosthesis interface was equipped with a PCA microbead blasting system using 800-micron balls.

The femoral component, thanks to its anatomical shape, ensured good compatibility between the prosthesis and the patella in a range of flexion from 0° to 130°.

There were 4 sizes for the femoral, tibial, and polyethylene implant.

The femoral and tibial parts were designed to be compatible with each other regardless of their size.

The series by Gacon [5] showed a 9.5% revision rate (65/772) at 2 years follow-up. The failures were mainly due to femoral loosening (35 cases) and premature wear of the polyethylene (20 cases).

Skyrme's series [6], showed a revision rate of 42% at 4 years, with also as main failures main failures: loosening of the femoral implant and rapid degradation of the polyethylene (Figs. 2.3 and 2.4). The hypothesis of this wear was the poor quality of the polyethylene which was hot-pressed during its manufacture to obtain a smooth polyethylene. This manufacturing process caused

Fig. 2.2 Miller-Galante II (courtesy of Zimmer Biomet)

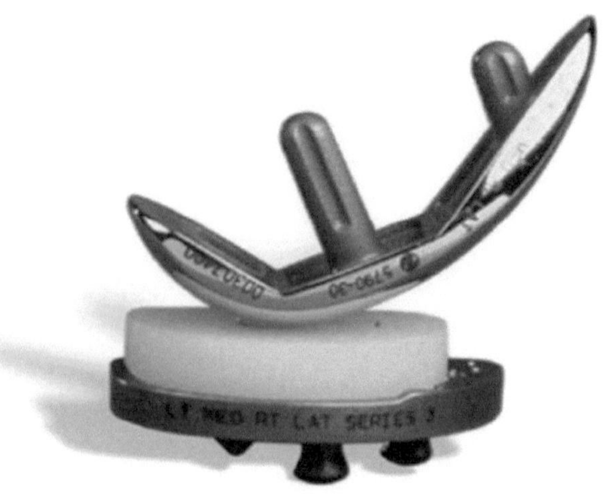

Fig. 2.3 Loosening of the femoral component of a PCA Uni

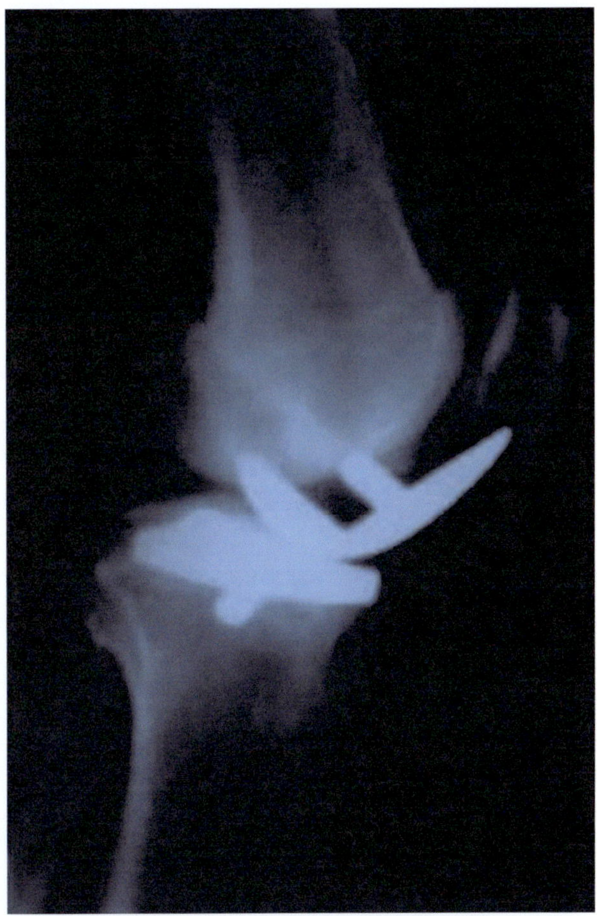

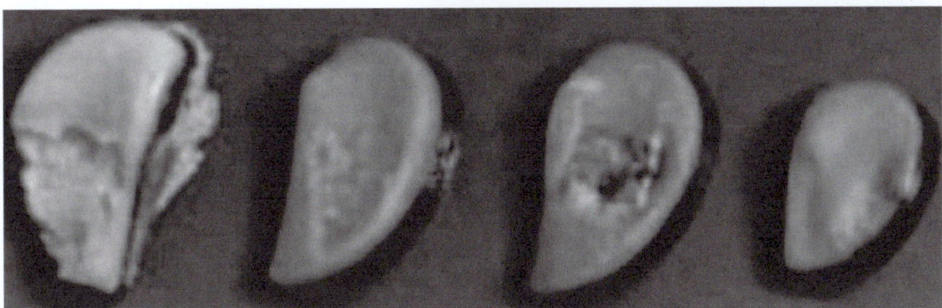

Fig. 2.4 Polyethylene wear of tibial component found during a revision procedure

early delamination of the polyethylene. The thickness of the polyethylene has also been blamed.

Other series, notably those of Christensen [7] and Lindstrand [8], have recommended the discontinuation of the PCA prosthesis due to the wear rate of the polyethylene and the resulting high revision rate.

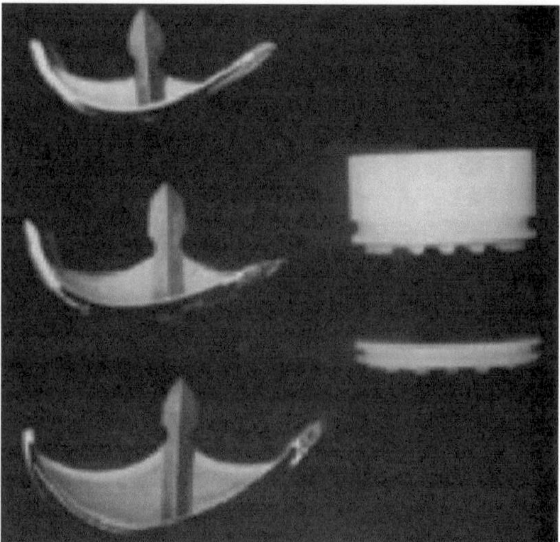

Fig. 2.5 Marmor UKA

2.3.6 Marmor Modular Knee

Between 1970 and 1972, Dr. Leonard Marmor, in association with Richards Manufacturing Corporation, developed a prosthesis known at the time as the Marmor Modular Knee (Fig. 2.5).

This was a pure resurfacing prosthesis, with minimal condylar femoral resection. The implants were cemented, and the femoral implant had a central stud [9].

The tibial tray was made of 6 mm thick PE.

This implant was developed with the philosophy that "a unicompartmental prosthesis is not half of a total prosthesis" [10].

The widespread use of the Marmor Modular Knee was halted in 1973 by an unfortunate engineering error, as the final implants were larger than the trial ones. This led to lawsuits.

In 1976, Marmor published a series with a 2-year follow-up with a stable and pain-free joint in 88% of cases [11], and a few years later a series at 13 years follow-up with 86% good results [12].

Cazanave and Cartier [13], in their series of 69 Marmor PUCs, showed a survival rate of 93% at 12 years' follow-up. The functional scores at the same follow-up were excellent in 57% of cases, good in 20%, fair in 7%, and poor in 7%.

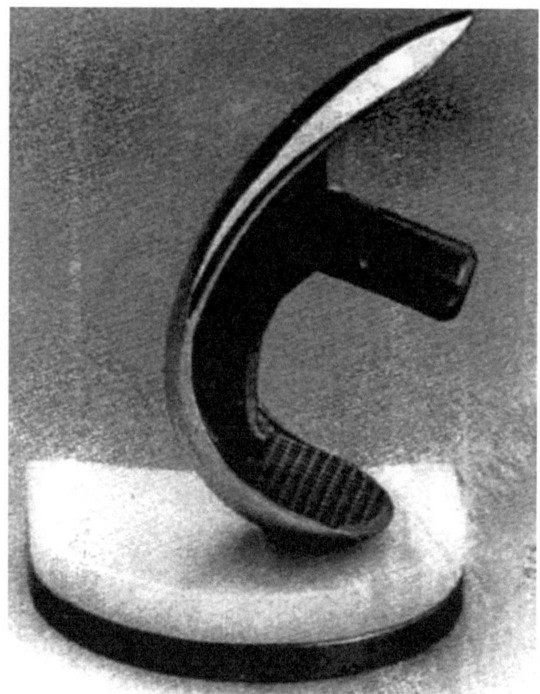

Fig. 2.6 MOD3 UKA

According to Dr. Leonard Marmor, the main causes of failure of the Marmor Modular Knee [14] were as follows:

– At the level of the femoral implant, the evidence of a stress on the posterior edge of the implant at 90°, as well as a posterior gap most often filled by cement.
– In the tibial implant, the cemented full polyethylene component was only 6 mm thick and was also a source of loosening.
– Given Dr. Leonard Marmor's contributions and innovation in the design of the components and surgical technique, he is still considered by many to be the father of the modern CUP [9].
– The Marmor CUP was replaced in 1984 by the MOD3 (Fig. 2.6).

2.3.7 MOD 3

This was the evolution of the Marmor Modular Knee (Fig. 2.7 and Table 2.2), marketed by Smith

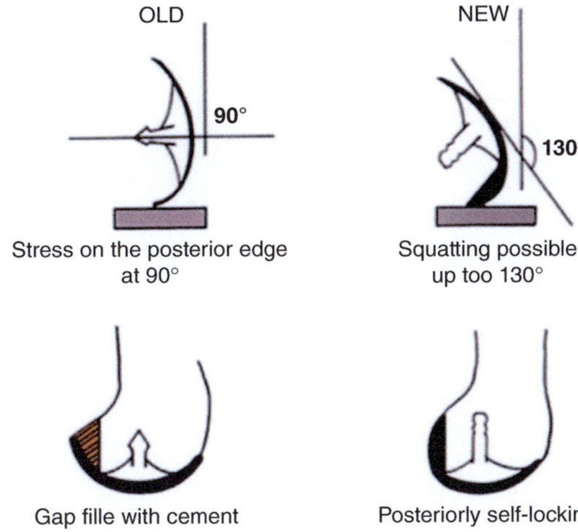

Fig. 2.7 Evolution of the Marmor design towards the MOD3 UKA

Table 2.2 Differences between Marmor and MOD3 UKAs

Evolution of the Marmor UKA to the MOD3		
Implant	MARMOR	MOD3
Femoral	Constraint on the posterior wall of the implant at 90° Posterior gap between implant and bone was filled up by cement	Flexion >130° without any constraint Posterior design with an auto locking system Central keel with a press-fit fixation.
Tibia	9 mm cemented full PE Tibial cut has to be ≥9 mm	Chrome cobalt metal back Tibial tray of 7.5 mm

& Nephew (France) from 1984 to 1994. It was bought by Richards Manufacturing Corporation in 1986.

Modifications to the femoral implant were intended to allow for more than 130° of unconstrained flexion, as well as a self-locking posterior design with a central keel with a central pin for press-fit fixation (Fig. 2.7 and Table 2.2).

In the tibial implant, the main change was an improved fixation with a metal-back support in chrome-cobalt, and a fixed 7.5 mm polyethylene (Fig. 2.7 and Table 2.2).

According to Cartier [15], MOD3 could be used in younger and more active patients.

However, the results obtained were not as expected. Out of 790 implants of this type, an early failure rate of 6% has been demonstrated. The real rate would probably be even closer to probably even closer to double if we took into account the information provided by other centres.

However, Cohen [16] reported a 95% survival rate at 8 years, with only one case of early malposition requiring revision by total prosthesis.

The main causes found for these failures were mechanical with accelerated wear of the polyethylene.

The primary reasons put forward and highlighted at the time were gamma ray sterilization (instead of ethylene oxide) [17], a polyethylene that was too thin (7.5 mm) and a metal-backed CrCo too rigid.

These failures led to new reflections concerning the design of the implants with the replacement of the MOD3 by the Genesis (Fig. 2.8):

2.3.8 Genesis

Marketed between 1991 and 2006 by Smith & Nephew, (Watford, UK). At the femoral level, the main differences with MOD3 were as follows:

– Between each size, a proportional increase between the width and length of the implant.
– A tapered and superiorly contoured component appearance to minimize the risk of patellar impingement.
– A wide range of sizes, offering seven possibilities, each with two implant thicknesses femoral implants: standard 4 mm and 7.5 mm for lateral condylar dysplasia or post-traumatic reconstruction.

At the tibial level, the main evolution was the use of titanium for metal-back where the advantages over chrome-cobalt were greater strength and less rigidity [18].

The aim was to limit the thickness of the metal-back in favour of polyethylene [15].

Cazenave [13] reported a survival rate of 94% at 10 years, followed by a progressive decrease to

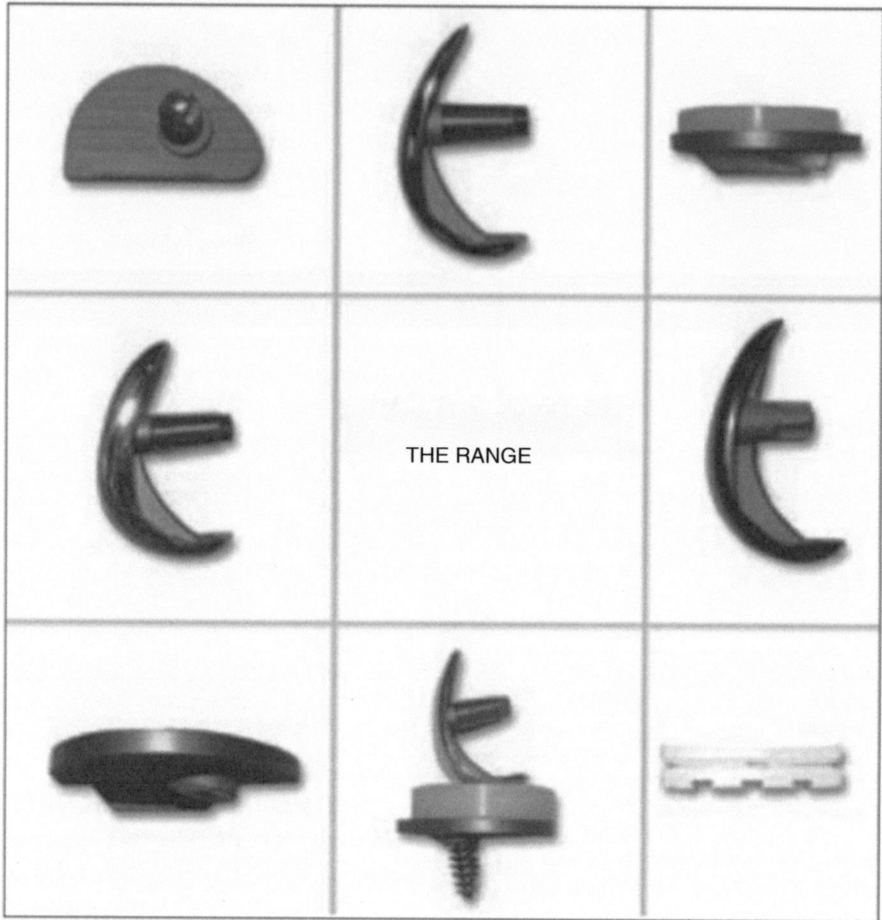

Fig. 2.8 Genesis (courtesy of Smith and Nephew)

88% at 12 years in his series of 1173 knees operated on from 1991 to 2006.

The main complications could be divided into two categories: problems of technical origin and inappropriate surgical indications.

The study of polyethylene wear, on the other hand, was quite reassuring, with wear not exceeding of 1 mm at any time during the revision.

All of these complications had in common the simplicity of their revision, contrary to the opinion expressed by Douglas, Padgett, and Stern [19], due to the use of a resurfacing implant, the very small amounts of cement used, and the early diagnosis of loosening follow-up.

The Genesis was replaced in the early 2000s by the Accuris (Fig. 2.9), developed for a minimally invasive approach by Leo Pinczewski [15].

It represents a considerable advance in the technical reproducibility of unicompartmental prosthesis implantation. This prosthesis is still on the market.

Notable advantages over previous ancillaries:

- Pre-balancing of the knee joint is performed before the bone cuts with the help of intra-articular wedges.
- Posterior femoral and tibial resection is performed at the same time and at the ideal level.
- The parallelism between the tibial cutting surface and the femoral resurfacing level is respected, by using an electric femoral resurfacing drill that can be adapted to the tibial trial base.

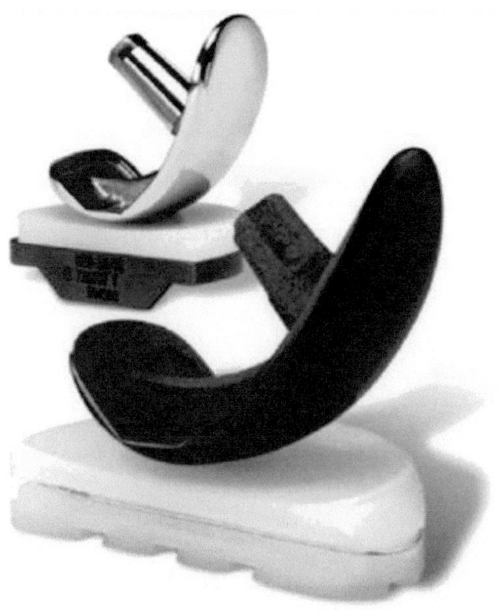

Fig. 2.9 Accuris UKA (courtesy of Smith et Nephew)

Concerning the implants, the femur is made of oxidized zirconium, which seems to cause less wear of the polyethylene than cobalt-chromium [20].

2.4   Conclusion

The various data analysed show us that the discontinuation of the marketing of a unicompartmental prosthesis results from a combination of several factors:

Factors Related to the Implant
Its components

- Type of sterilization
- Thickness of the polyethylene
- Characteristics of certain components (e.g. rigidity of CrCo)

Its evolution in time

- Survival
- Mechanical loosening of femoral and tibial implants
- Premature wear of polyethylene

Human Factors
For the patient and his surgeon

- Functional results
- Importance of the revision rate

For the surgeon

- Simplicity in its use
- Reliability
- Reproducibility
- Revision rate

Economic factors
Probably the most important for companies.

The great paucity of literature in this field leads us to wonder about the lack of serious evaluation by these different companies.

In addition, we note an impoverishment of design companies in the field of orthopaedics in France and in Europe.

The acquisition of French and European SMEs with technological innovations has been a strong trend for several years.

There are many examples of this: the takeover by an American firm of the Montpellier- based company Medtech, specialized in biotechnology, or the Aube-based company LDR Medical, specialized in spine surgery.

In another register, we can mention IMASCAP created in 2009, by Jean CHAOUI, in the field of computer-assisted shoulder surgery at the laboratory of medical information (LaTIM-Telecom Bretagne, Brest).

His initiative was supported by surgeons experts in shoulder surgery and by Telecom Bretagne. This work aroused the interest of several major players in the shoulder arthroplasty market and in 2018 IMASCAP was acquired by a world leader in shoulder prostheses: the American company.

Wright Medical (the latter having itself been acquired more recently by Stryker).

Most of these conglomerates are under American leadership, and more than 2/3 of the world market for orthopaedic implants is held by six companies.

This situation may lead to fears of a future and progressive sidelining of French and European designers, which could lead to an impoverishment of both the industrial and intellectual of the design of prosthetic implants.

There is also a risk linked to a standardization of products and concepts by American companies, sometimes focused on dogmatic ideas and concepts.

Historically, this does not reflect their culture but may have been dictated by judicial influence, resulting in a certain chilliness, a lack of ingenuity and evolution both in terms of surgical techniques but also in terms of solutions.

All orthopaedic surgeons need to think deeply in order to consider strong actions, necesasary to reverse a potentially disastrous trend.

References

1. Mariani EM, Bourne MH, Jackson RT, Jackson ST, Jones P. Early failure of unicompartmental knee arthroplasty. J Arthroplasty. 2007;22(6):81–4.
2. Koskinen E, Paavolainen P, Eskelinen A, Harilainen A, Sandelin J, Ylinen P, et al. Medial unicompartmental knee arthroplasty with Miller-Galante II prosthesis: mid-term clinical and radiographic results. Arch Orthop Trauma Surg. 2009;129(5):617–24.
3. Berger RA, Meneghini RM, Jacobs JJ, Sheinkop MB, Della Valle CJ, Rosenberg AG, et al. Results of unicompartmental knee arthroplasty at a minimum of ten years of follow-up. J Bone Joint Surg Am. 2005;87(5):999–1006.
4. Lindstr A, Stenström A, Lewold S. Multicenter study of unicompartmental knee revision: PCA, Marmor, and St Georg compared in 3,777 cases of arthrosis. Acta Orthop Scand. 1992;63(3):256–9.
5. Gacon G. Résultats des prothèses unicompartimentales PCA du genou. Orthopédie Traumatol. 1992;2(1):61–70.
6. Skyrme AD, Mencia MM, Skinner PW. Early failure of the porous-coated anatomic cemented unicompartmental knee arthroplasty: a 5- to 9-year follow-up study. J Arthroplasty. 2002;17(2):201–5.
7. Christensen OM, Christiansen TG, Johansen T. Polyethylene failure in a PCA unicompartmental knee prosthesis. Acta Orthop Scand. 1990;61(6):578–9.
8. Lindstr A, Stenström A. Polyethylene wear of the PCA unicompartmental knee: rospective 5 (4-8) year study of 120 arthrosis knees. Acta Orthop Scand. 1992;63(3):260–2.
9. Johannes Plate MD, Ali Mofidi MB, Sandeep Mannava MD, Cara Lorentzen MD, Beth Smith P, Thorsten Seyler MD, et al. Unicompartmental knee arthroplasty: past, present, future. Reconstr Rev. [cité 10 mai 2020];2(1). Disponible sur: http://reconstructiveview.org/ojs/index.php/rr/article/view/15
10. Grelsamer RP, Cartier P. A unicompartmental knee replacement is not "half a total knee": five major differences. Orthop Rev. 1992;21(11):1350–6.
11. Marmor L. The Modular (Marmor) knee: case report with a minimum follow-up of 2 years. Clin Orthop Relat Res. 1976;120:86–94.
12. Marmor L. Unicompartmental knee arthroplasty. Ten-to 13-year follow-up study. Clin Orthop Relat Res. 1988;226:14–20.
13. Cazenave A. Cazenave A, Cartier P- prothèse unicompartimentale marmor évolution genesis- In « Arthroplastie du genou de 1°intention : expériences cliniques ». Ed SAURAMPS médical 2008, pp. 155–162. 7.
14. Marmor L. Unicompartmental arthroplasty of the knee with a minimum ten-year follow-up period. Clin Orthop Relat Res. 1988;228:171–7.
15. Cartier P, Khefacha A. Fixed-bearing unicompartmental knee arthroplasty. In: Bellemans J, Ries MD, Victor JMK, éditeurs. Total knee arthroplasty [Internet]. Berlin/Heidelberg: Springer-Verlag; 2005 [cité 10 avr 2019], pp. 317–21. Disponible sur: http://springer.com/10.1007/3-540-276580_50
16. Cohen I, Zeev F, Hendel D, Blankstein A, Chechick A, Rzetelny V. Unikompartimenteller kniegelenkersatz mit zementierter MOD3TM-prothese: a prospective study. Eur J Trauma Emerg Surg. 1999;25:287–93.
17. Chaigneau M. [Advantages and disadvantages of ethylene oxide sterilization of medicosurgical equipment and pharmaceutical products]. Bull Acad Natl Med. 1983;167(6):627–31.
18. Mezache F, Mazouz H, Amrani H. Principes biomécanique de la prothèse du genou. 2013;5.
19. Padgett DE, Stern SH, Insall JN. Revision total knee arthroplasty for failed unicompartmental replacement. J Bone Joint Surg Am. 1991;73(2):186–90.
20. Spector BM, Ries MD, Bourne RB, Sauer WS, Long M, Hunter G. Wear performance of ultra-high molecular weight polyethylene on oxidized zirconium total knee femoral components. J Bone Joint Surg Am. 2001;83-A(Suppl 2 Pt 2):80–6.

Samuel W. King, Bernard H. Van Duren,
and Hemant Pandit

3.1 Introduction

Symptomatic knee osteoarthritis occurs in up to 16.7% of people over 45 years of age [1]. Total knee arthroplasty (TKA) is an extremely successful and popular procedure for the treatment of end-stage knee osteoarthritis, and demand continues to increase significantly [2, 3]. It involves the replacement of both tibiofemoral articular compartments but disease is often only present in one. In approximately 60% of patients knee osteoarthritis is restricted to the medial compartment only [4–7]. A significant proportion of these patients may be treated with a unicompartmental knee arthroplasty (UKA) providing they fulfil certain criteria. Its primary indication is anteromedial osteoarthritis of the knee, and requirements include an intact anterior cruciate ligament (ACL). Proponents of UKA cite its improved clinical outcomes and fewer side effects. Rates of

S. W. King · B. H. Van Duren
Leeds Institute of Rheumatic and Musculoskeletal
Medicine, University of Leeds,
Leeds, West Yorkshire, UK

H. Pandit (✉)
Leeds Institute of Rheumatic and Musculoskeletal
Medicine, University of Leeds,
Leeds, West Yorkshire, UK

Nuffield Department of Orthopaedics, Rheumatology
and Musculoskeletal Sciences (NDORMS),
University of Oxford, Oxford, UK
e-mail: h.pandit@leeds.ac.uk

UKA are increasing but the procedure still only represents 8–12% of all knee arthroplasties [8–10]. This chapter discusses the history of anteromedial osteoarthritis, the development of the UKA, and its results, indications, and contraindications.

3.2 Anteromedial Osteoarthritis

Knee osteoarthritis is often present only in the anterior part of the medial tibiofemoral compartment. Ahlback et al. studied 370 knees with osteoarthritis and found that 85% of these had degeneration limited to only one compartment, and that the medial compartment was 10 times more likely to be affected than the lateral [6]. Further radiographical study of 94 patients with symptomatic knee osteoarthritis by Hernborg and Nilsson also demonstrated a predominance of medial compartment disease. Ninety percent of patients had disease isolated to this region with very little long-term progression laterally [11]. Studies of the knee at this time generally used anteroposterior plain knee radiographs and lateral films were rarely utilised, often suggested to be of little clinical use [12].

Anteromedial osteoarthritis of the knee (also known as anteromedial gonarthrosis) was first proposed as a distinct clinicopathological entity by White et al. in their 1991 study [13]. They studied resected tibial plateaus in 46 patients who had undergone UKA for medial compartment osteoarthritis. The ACL was intact in all specimens, degenerative lesions were centred anteriorly on the medial tibial plateau, and posterior cartilage was spared. These degenerative findings were consistent with changes noted on lateral knee radiographs. The authors hypothesised that the anatomical findings explained their clinical examination. In anteromedial osteoarthritis, genu varum is present on extension but is correctable with knee flexion. Intact cruciate ligaments and lateral articular surfaces allow the medial femoral condyle to roll posteriorly in flexion and articulate with the posterior medial tibial plateau. The articular cartilage, and therefore also tibial plateau height, is preserved here. Preservation of tibial plateau height allows the varus deformity to correct when the knee flexes. The correction tensions the medial collateral ligament (MCL) to full length, preventing its contracture over time. No soft tissue release is therefore required to correct MCL length intra-operatively.

The presence of an intact ACL in all knees undergoing UKA described by White et al. is of key importance [13]. In chronic rupture due to osteoarthritis, the ACL first loses its synovial covering, then splits longitudinally. After this collagen bundles begin to stretch and lose strength, before the ACL finally ruptures [14]. Following this the ligament may eventually be absorbed and disappear. A later study investigated the effects of damage to functionally intact ACL. Knees undergoing UKA with higher grades of ACL damage had more full thickness loss of cartilage in the anteromedial region of the tibial plateau. Cartilage loss migrated laterally and posteriorly with increasing ACL damage [15], Harman et al. studied 143 tibial plateaus resected during TKA for osteoarthritis and demonstrated the effects of functionally impaired ACLs [16]. They tested ACL integrity intra-operatively and used digital imaging to study plateau wear patterns. In varus knees with intact ACL, their findings were consistent with intra-operative reports of knees with intact ACL during UKA; wear was present in the middle to anterior aspect of the medial plateau. In varus knees with ACL deficiency, wear areas were larger and had migrated more posteriorly and progressed to the lateral compartment. As the authors hypothesised, this suggests that ACL rupture allows posterior femoral subluxation, posterior tibiofemoral contact, and posterior progression of medial compartment wear. Radiographical correlation has also been noted. A study of 200 knees demonstrated a 95% correlation between preservation of posterior medial tibial plateau on lateral radiograph and intra-operative findings of an intact ACL. The authors also found that 100% of knees with degenerative changes noted on lateral radiograph had a deficient ACL [17].

The mechanism of chronic ACL rupture in knee osteoarthritis is believed to be both mechanical and nutritional [14]. Direct physical damage by osteophytes at condylar margins is one mechanism [16]. Further, the ACL is intra-articular and so is at risk of devascularisation caused by chronic synovitis. The removal of ACL synovium in rabbit models was found to cause very similar changes to the ACL as those observed in human osteoarthritis [18].

Taken together the findings of these studies suggest that an intact ACL is necessary to confine cartilage wear to the anteromedial tibial plateau. Chronic damage to and eventual rupture of the ACL in the presence of osteoarthritis are likely caused by direct physical and vascular damage, and in turn lead to spreading of wear areas posteriorly on the medial tibial plateau and to the lateral compartment.

Anteromedial osteoarthritis has characteristic findings upon clinical assessment [14]. Pain is not necessarily localised to the medial compartment, but is present on walking, worse on standing and reduced on sitting. There is a varus deformity on knee extension of 5–15°, which is passively correctable at 20 degrees of flexion, and spontaneous correction at 90 degrees of flexion. On intra-operative inspection, both cruciate ligaments are intact. The cartilage of the anteromedial tibial plateau and inferior medial femoral condyle are eroded with bone-on-bone contact, while at the posterior aspect of both the cartilage is preserved. The articular cartilage of the lateral compartment is at full thickness. The MCL length is preserved, while the posterior capsule is shortened [14].

3.3 Unicompartmental Knee Arthroplasty

The aim of the UKA is to replace the diseased articular compartment when knee osteoarthritis is confined to a single compartment. The soft tissues and opposite compartment are preserved, allowing them to resume their physiological function.

3.3.1 History

The concept of UKA for the prevention of pain in osteoarthritis was described by Campbell in 1940 when he used vitallium plates within the medial compartment of arthritic knees [19]. McKeever and MacIntosh then trialled the use of metal inserts to replace the tibial surface of a single compartment in valgus and varus deformities. This provided pain relief but overall unsatisfactory results due to prosthesis migration [20, 21]. McKeever later added a keel to his tibial plateau prosthesis to overcome this [22]. Gunston and polycentric UKA devices were introduced in the early 1970s [22]. The St Georg sled was developed in 1969, and good results were reported at 4 year follow-up in a study of 294 patients [23]. This was a cemented polycentric metal femoral condyle articulating on flat polyethylene tibial components, as were the Mamor implants developed in 1972 [24]. These first-generation modern implants were at high risk of deformation and early wear, and so were further developed to introduce a metal-backed component [25]. Good clinical results were reported for both implant designs in single compartment disease [23, 26]. However, some groups reported poor outcomes in UKA, often due to inadequate patient selection or material failures [27, 28]. In conjunction with rapid developments and improvements in outcomes following TKA, this led to many surgeons abandoning the use of UKA altogether [22].

In 1976, Goodfellow et al. in Oxford first proposed the use of meniscal bearing knee prostheses, initially for bicompartmental tibiofemoral arthroplasty [29]. They later described its application for UKA, suggesting adverse outcomes in previous UKA to be caused by poor patient selection, inadequate prosthesis design, and surgical technique [30]. From 1982, this Oxford UKA (OUKA) was mainly used in knees with isolated medial osteoarthritis and intact ACL [30].

3.3.2 Indications

In an osteoarthritic knee where symptoms justify arthroplasty, the Oxford group describe a series of indications for the use of UKA [14].

Intact ACL is necessary for UKA. Deschamps et al. noted that the majority of knees with ACL laxity noted pre-operatively, UKA failed. Most of these failures required further surgery after a mean time of 3.5 years [31]. These findings were supported by those reported by Goodfellow et al. Their study of 301 patients up to 9 years following UKA found a 95% survival rate at for knees with intact ACL, compared with 81% in knee with damaged or absent ACL [32].

There must be full thickness preservation of the lateral tibial plateau articular cartilage to allow UKA. Wear within this compartment suggests impending failure of the ACL and is an absolute contraindication for UKA. Fibrillation and chondromalacia are often seen in the lateral compartment caused by chronic synovitis within the joint and are not of concern. Goodfellow et al. describe their use of valgus-stressed radiographs to assess lateral compartment cartilage thickness [14]. They report little or no deterioration of the lateral compartment in follow-up of over 10 years following UKA in patients pre-operatively screen with this method [33].

The Oxford group also require any varus deformity to be fully correctable in 20 degrees of flexion, and for posterior cartilage to be intact within the medial tibial plateau [14]. These two requirements are complementary; as previously discussed, intact posterior cartilage allows tensioning of the MCL on flexion of the knee, preventing contracture, and allowing correction of varus deformity without soft tissue release.

Flexion deformity is often present in anteromedial osteoarthritis of the knee. The posterior joint capsule shortens due to chronic synovitis and voluntary reduction in extension caused by pain. Osteophytes may also restrict posterior capsular ligament movement, as well as directly impinging on extension anteriorly. UKA is permissible in flexion deformity of up to 15°. This will usually correct spontaneously after surgery as soft tissue release is not required and so the posterior capsule is not required to stretch beyond its physical constraints following the procedure. Flexion deformity beyond 15° is generally indicative of ACL deficiency.

3.3.3 Other Indications

In addition to anteromedial osteoarthritis, UKA has been proposed for other indications. Focal avascular necrosis of the medial femoral condyle or tibial plateau requires evaluation with MRI. Good results have been reported with both the Marmor knee and OUKA [34, 35]. UKA has also been used for failed high tibial osteotomy with persistent symptoms. However, results have generally been poor and inferior to TKA and so this application is not recommended [36–39].

Lateral compartment osteoarthritis represents approximately 10% of all unicompartmental osteoarthritis. Lateral UKA is challenging both due to anatomical constraints and lesser prevalence and so reduced surgical experience. Reports vary with respect to suitability of lateral UKA. The Oxford group report poorer outcomes for lateral OUKA compared with medial OUKA due to high dislocation rate [40, 41]. However, a recent systematic review of the literature found no difference between medial and lateral for all UKA [9].

3.3.4 Outcomes in UKA

UKA allows preservation of bone stock and soft tissues, and the physiological impact of the pro-

cedure is less. Siman et al. reported a study of patients aged over 75 years, comparing UKA with TKA. Patients in the UKA group had shorter operative times, shorter length of stay, less intra-operative blood loss, and post-operative transfusion requirement. Their mobility also improved better and more quickly post-operatively [8]. Other studies agree, with further findings of reduced blood loss [42, 43], shorter length of stay and lower readmission rate [44], and reduced incidence of thromboembolism, infection, stroke, and myocardial infarction [45] for UKA compared with TKA.

Functional outcomes are also better for UKA. Rougraff et al. compared 81 tricompartmental knee arthroplasties with 120 UKA and found improved range of motion and ambulatory function in the UKA group. The gait is more physiological and biomechanics of the knee more completely restored [46]. UKA also preforms better than TKA when compared using outcome scores. A study of 390 knees comparing TKA with twin-peg OUKA by Lum et al. in 2016 found improved knee society scores at approximately 5 years post-operatively [47]. Another study of 101 patients aged over 75 years of age found better Knee Society, Forgotten Joint and Knee Injury Osteoarthritis Outcome Scores at last follow-up [48]. Similarly, better Forgotten Joint Scores were seen for UKA in patients one- and two-years post-operative.

Revision rates are often used as a comparative measure of success for an implant and are recorded at individual, local, regional, and national levels. For UKA 10-year survival rates of more than 90% have been reported [49, 50], with a centre which specialises in UKA reporting a 10-year survival rate of 96% in 1000 phase 3 OUKA [51]. However, revision rate of UKA has been reported as higher than those for TKA by a number of sources; according to registry data, UKA are 2.1–2.8 times more likely to be revised [45, 52, 53]. Several factors must be considered when interpreting these outcomes. Revision of UKA is technically easier. This is reflected in a lower threshold for revision: Goodfellow et al. reported that 63% of UKA implants with a post-operative Oxford knee score (OKS) of under 20 (very poor) were revised but only 12% of TKA with the same score [53]. UKA is also more likely to be used in younger, more active patients because of its better functional outcome, and these demographics are independent risk factors for revision. Additionally, there is a large difference in revision rates for UKA between high and low volume surgeons [54]. Some knee surgeons may only perform one or two UKA per year, while best results are seen in those for whom UKA makes up at least 20% of their operative caseload [55]. Despite higher revision rates, UKA remains more cost-effective than TKA especially for younger patients [56].

Outcomes and mechanism of failure vary for different types of UKA. A randomised study of 56 knees comparing fixed and mobile bearing UKAs found improved kinematics and lower incidences of radiolucencies in the mobile bearing group, but with no difference in patient reported outcome score [57]. Mobile bearing UKAs are more likely to fail with early bearing dislocation, while late polyethylene wear occurs more commonly in fixed-bearing implants [58]. Despite this difference in failure mode, a systematic review of the literature by Ko et al. found no significant difference in overall reoperation rate between the two types [59]. A systematic review of 10 papers and 1199 knees comparing cemented UKAs with cementless found no difference with respect to clinical outcome and revision and reoperation rate, but that for cementless implants, operative times were shorter and in post-operative radiographs, there was a lower incidence of radiolucent lines [60].

3.3.5 Limitations to UKA Use

Approximately 60% of patients with knee osteoarthritis have disease isolated to the medial compartment [4–7], and approximately one-third of all patients eligible for TKA are suitable for UKA [14, 61]. However, only 8–12% of arthroplasties are unicompartmental [8, 9]. The reasons for this are multifactorial. UKA is generally perceived as more challenging, and surgeons may be reluctant to perform the procedure given the need for

higher volume for better results [14]. Additionally, patient selection is controversial. Kozinn and Scott have made recommendations for the characteristics of ideal fixed-bearing UKA candidates in their 1989 paper [62]. These are often applied as eligibility criteria and are as follows: isolated medial compartment disease; aged less than 60 years; low level of physical activity; weight less than 82 kg; a cumulative angular deformity of less than 15°; both cruciate ligaments intact; a pre-operative range of flexion of 90; a flexion contracture of <5°; minimal pain at rest; no radiographic or intra-operative evidence of chondrocalcinosis or patellofemoral osteoarthritis; no inflammatory arthropathy. Applying these as strict eligibility criteria, some groups have found only 6% of patients to be eligible for UKA [63]. Others also apply additional exclusion criteria such as presence of lateral compartment and patellofemoral osteophytes and lateral compartment chondromalacia, and find even fewer to be suitable [64]. The Oxford group applies less stringent criteria, removing restrictions including those on patellofemoral arthritis, weight, and age [14]. They contend that they have applied these criteria for a number of years with excellent clinical results, and the discrepancy may be because the original criteria were for fixed-bearing UKA while the OUKA is a mobile bearing implant.

3.4 Conclusion

Unicompartmental knee arthroplasty is a potential alternative to total knee arthroplasty for selected indications, primarily isolated anteromedial osteoarthritis. There is increasing demand for knee arthroplasty, and indications are expanding. Younger, more active patients with greater physical demands and higher expectations are now undergoing joint arthroplasties. The rate of UKA is increasing, and the procedure represents an excellent option for a significant proportion of patients. The retention of other articular compartments and soft tissues provide excellent clinical outcomes and a procedure with lower rates of complications and better recovery. Revision rates for UKA remain higher than TKA, but these may be artificially inflated. Careful patient selection and adequate volume of procedures are vital for best outcomes.

Professor Pandit is a National Institute for Health Research (NIHR) Senior Investigator. The views expressed in this article are those of the author(s) and not necessarily those of the NIHR, or the Department of Health and Social Care.

References

1. Lawrence RC, Felson DT, Helmick CG, et al. Estimates of the prevalence of arthritis and other rheumatic conditions in the United States. Part II. Arthritis Rheum. 2008;58(1):26–35. https://doi.org/10.1002/art.23176.
2. Culliford D, Maskell J, Judge A, et al. Future projections of total hip and knee arthroplasty in the UK: results from the UK clinical practice research Datalink. Osteoarthr Cartil. 2015;23(4):594–600. https://doi.org/10.1016/j.joca.2014.12.022.
3. Kurtz S, Ong K, Lau E, Mowat F, Halpern M. Projections of primary and revision hip and knee arthroplasty in the United States from 2005 to 2030. J Bone Joint Surg Am. 2007;89(4):780–5. https://doi.org/10.2106/JBJS.F.00222.
4. Ledingham J, Regan M, Jones A, Doherty M. Radiographic patterns and associations of osteoarthritis of the knee in patients referred to hospital. Ann Rheum Dis. 1993;52(7):520–6.
5. Davies AP, Vince AS, Shepstone L, Donell ST, Glasgow MM. The radiologic prevalence of patellofemoral osteoarthritis. Clin Orthop Relat Res. 2002;402:206–12.
6. Ahlbäck S. Osteoarthrosis of the knee. A radiographic investigation. Acta Radiol Diagn (Stockh). 1968;Suppl 277:7–72.
7. Rout R, McDonnell S, Benson R, et al. The histological features of anteromedial gonarthrosis—the comparison of two grading systems in a human phenotype of osteoarthritis. Knee. 2011;18(3):172–6. https://doi.org/10.1016/j.knee.2010.04.010.
8. Siman H, Kamath AF, Carrillo N, Harmsen WS, Pagnano MW, Sierra RJ. Unicompartmental knee arthroplasty vs total knee arthroplasty for medial compartment arthritis in patients older than 75 years: comparable reoperation, revision, and complication rates. J Arthroplast. 2017;32(6):1792–7. https://doi.org/10.1016/j.arth.2017.01.020.
9. van der List JP, McDonald LS, Pearle AD. Systematic review of medial versus lateral survivorship in unicompartmental knee arthroplasty. Knee. 2015;22(6):454–60. https://doi.org/10.1016/j.knee.2015.09.011.
10. National Joint Registry. National Joint Registry 15th annual report. National Joint Registry; 2018.
11. Hernborg JS, Nilsson BE. The natural course of untreated osteoarthritis of the knee. Clin Orthop Relat Res. 1977;123:130–7.
12. Altman RD, Fries JF, Bloch DA, et al. Radiographic assessment of progression in osteoarthritis. Arthritis Rheum. 1987;30(11):1214–25.
13. White SH, Ludkowski PF, Goodfellow JW. Anteromedial osteoarthritis of the knee. J Bone Joint Surg Br. 1991;73(4):582–6.
14. Goodfellow JW, Pandit HG, Dodd CA, Murray DW. Unicompartmental arthroplasty with the Oxford knee. 2nd ed. Oxford: Goodfellow Publishers Limited.
15. Rout R, McDonnell S, Hulley P, et al. The pattern of cartilage damage in antero-medial osteoarthritis of the knee and its relationship to the anterior cruciate ligament. J Orthop Res. 2013;31(6):908–13. https://doi.org/10.1002/jor.22253.
16. Harman MK, Markovich GD, Banks SA, Hodge WA. Wear patterns on tibial plateaus from varus and valgus osteoarthritic knees. Clin Orthop Relat Res. 1998;352:149–58.
17. Keyes GW, Carr AJ, Miller RK, Goodfellow JW. The radiographic classification of medial gonarthrosis. Correlation with operation methods in 200 knees. Acta Orthop Scand. 1992;63(5):497–501.
18. Robinson D, Halperin N, Nevo Z. Devascularization of the anterior cruciate ligament by synovial stripping in rabbits. An experimental model. Acta Orthop Scand. 1992;63(5):502–6.
19. Campbell WC. Interposition of vitallium plates in arthroplasties of the knee. Preliminary report. By Willis C. Campbell, 1940. Clin Orthop Relat Res. 1988;226:3–5.
20. MacIntosh DL. Hemiarthroplasty of the knee using a space-occupying prosthesis for painful Varus and valgus deformities. J Bone Jt Surg. 1958;40(A):1431.
21. MacIntosh DL, Hunter GA. The use of the hemiarthroplasty prosthesis for advanced osteoarthritis and rheumatoid arthritis of the knee. J Bone Joint Surg Br. 1972;54(2):244–55.
22. Bruni D, Iacono F, Akkawi I, Gagliardi M, Zaffagnini S, Marcacci M. Unicompartmental knee replacement: a historical overview. Joints. 2013;1(2):45–7.
23. Engelbrecht E, Siegel A, Rottger J, Buchholz HW. Statistics of total knee replacement: partial and total knee replacement, design St. Georg: a review of a 4-year observation. Clin Orthop Relat Res. 1976;120:54–64.
24. Marmor L. The modular knee. Clin Orthop Relat Res. 1973;94:242–8.
25. Palmer SH, Morrison PJ, Ross AC. Early catastrophic tibial component wear after unicompartmental knee arthroplasty. Clin Orthop Relat Res. 1998;350:143–8.
26. Marmor L. Marmor modular knee in unicompartmental disease. Minimum four-year follow-up. J Bone Joint Surg Am. 1979;61(3):347–53.

27. Lindstrand A, Ryd L, Stenström A. Polyethylene failure in two total knees. Wear of thin, metal-backed PCA tibial components. Acta Orthop Scand. 1990;61(6):575–7.

28. Insall J, Aglietti P. A five to seven-year follow-up of unicondylar arthroplasty. J Bone Joint Surg Am. 1980;62(8):1329–37.

29. Campi S, Tibrewal S, Cuthbert R, Tibrewal SB. Unicompartmental knee replacement - current perspectives. J Clin Orthop Trauma. 2018;9(1):17–23. https://doi.org/10.1016/j.jcot.2017.11.013.

30. Goodfellow JW, Tibrewal SB, Sherman KP, O'Connor JJ. Unicompartmental Oxford meniscal knee arthroplasty. J Arthroplast. 1987;2(1):1–9.

31. Deschamps G, Lapeyre B. [Rupture of the anterior cruciate ligament: a frequently unrecognized cause of failure of unicompartmental knee prostheses. Apropos of a series of 79 lotus prostheses with a follow-up of more than 5 years]. Rev Chir Orthop Reparatrice Appar Mot. 1987;73(7):544–51.

32. Goodfellow J, O'Connor J. The anterior cruciate ligament in knee arthroplasty. A risk-factor with unconstrained meniscal prostheses. Clin Orthop Relat Res. 1992;(276):245–52.

33. Weale AE, Murray DW, Crawford R, et al. Does arthritis progress in the retained compartments after "Oxford" medial unicompartmental arthroplasty? A clinical and radiological study with a minimum ten-year follow-up. J Bone Joint Surg Br. 1999;81(5):783–9.

34. Marmor L. Unicompartmental arthroplasty for osteonecrosis of the knee joint. Clin Orthop Relat Res. 1993;294:247–53.

35. Langdown AJ, Pandit H, Price AJ, et al. Oxford medial unicompartmental arthroplasty for focal spontaneous osteonecrosis of the knee. Acta Orthop. 2005;76(5):688–92. https://doi.org/10.1080/17453670510041772.

36. Meding JB, Keating EM, Ritter MA, Faris PM. Total knee arthroplasty after high tibial osteotomy. A comparison study in patients who had bilateral total knee replacement. J Bone Joint Surg Am. 2000;82(9):1252–9.

37. Scott RD, Cobb AG, McQueary FG, Thornhill TS. Unicompartmental knee arthroplasty. Eight- to 12-year follow-up evaluation with survivorship analysis. Clin Orthop Relat Res. 1991;271:96–100.

38. Vorlat P, Verdonk R, Schauvlieghe H. The Oxford unicompartmental knee prosthesis: a 5-year follow-up. Knee Surg Sports Traumatol Arthrosc. 2000;8(3):154–8. https://doi.org/10.1007/s001670050206.

39. Rees JL, Price AJ, Lynskey TG, Svärd UC, Dodd CA, Murray DW. Medial unicompartmental arthroplasty after failed high tibial osteotomy. J Bone Joint Surg Br. 2001;83(7):1034–6.

40. Murray DW, Goodfellow JW, O'Connor JJ. The Oxford medial unicompartmental arthroplasty: a ten-year survival study. J Bone Joint Surg Br. 1998;80(6):983–9.

41. Weston-Simons JS, Pandit H, Kendrick BJL, et al. The mid-term outcomes of the Oxford Domed Lateral unicompartmental knee replacement. Bone Joint J. 2014;96-B(1):59–64. https://doi.org/10.1302/0301-620X.96B1.31630.

42. Schwab P-E, Lavand'homme P, Yombi JC, Thienpont E. Lower blood loss after unicompartmental than total knee arthroplasty. Knee Surg Sports Traumatol Arthrosc. 2015;23(12):3494–500. https://doi.org/10.1007/s00167-014-3188-x.

43. Price AJ, Webb J, Topf H, et al. Rapid recovery after oxford unicompartmental arthroplasty through a short incision. J Arthroplast. 2001;16(8):970–6.

44. Drager J, Hart A, Khalil JA, Zukor DJ, Bergeron SG, Antoniou J. Shorter hospital stay and lower 30-day readmission after unicondylar knee arthroplasty compared to total knee arthroplasty. J Arthroplast. 2016;31(2):356–61. https://doi.org/10.1016/j.arth.2015.09.014.

45. Liddle AD, Judge A, Pandit H, Murray DW. Adverse outcomes after total and unicompartmental knee replacement in 101 330 matched patients: a study of data from the National Joint Registry for England and Wales. Lancet. 2014;384(9952):1437–45. https://doi.org/10.1016/S0140-6736(14)60419-0.

46. Laurencin CT, Zelicof SB, Scott RD, Ewald FC. Unicompartmental versus total knee arthroplasty in the same patient. A comparative study. Clin Orthop Relat Res. 1991;273:151–6.

47. Lum ZC, Lombardi AV, Hurst JM, Morris MJ, Adams JB, Berend KR. Early outcomes of twin-peg mobile-bearing unicompartmental knee arthroplasty compared with primary total knee arthroplasty. Bone Joint J. 2016;98-B(10 Supple B):28–33. https://doi.org/10.1302/0301-620X.98B10.BJJ-2016-0414.R1.

48. Fabre-Aubrespy M, Ollivier M, Pesenti S, Parratte S, Argenson J-N. Unicompartmental knee arthroplasty in patients older than 75 results in better clinical outcomes and similar survivorship compared to total knee arthroplasty. A matched controlled study. J Arthroplasty. 2016;31(12):2668–71. https://doi.org/10.1016/j.arth.2016.06.034.

49. Parratte S, Ollivier M, Lunebourg A, Abdel MP, Argenson J-N. Long-term results of compartmental arthroplasties of the knee: long term results of partial knee arthroplasty. Bone Joint J. 2015;97-B(10 Suppl A):9–15. https://doi.org/10.1302/0301-620X.97B10.36426.

50. Mohammad HR, Strickland L, Hamilton TW, Murray DW. Long-term outcomes of over 8,000 medial Oxford phase 3 unicompartmental knees—a systematic review. Acta Orthop. 2018;89(1):101–7. https://doi.org/10.1080/17453674.2017.1367577.

51. Pandit H, Jenkins C, Gill HS, Barker K, Dodd C, a. F, Murray DW. Minimally invasive Oxford phase 3 unicompartmental knee replacement: results of 1000 cases. J Bone Joint Surg Br. 2011;93(2):198–204. https://doi.org/10.1302/0301-620X.93B2.25767.

52. Chawla H, van der List JP, Christ AB, Sobrero MR, Zuiderbaan HA, Pearle AD. Annual revision rates of partial versus total knee arthroplasty: a comparative meta-analysis. Knee. 2017;24(2):179–90. https://doi.org/10.1016/j.knee.2016.11.006.

53. Goodfellow JW, O'Connor JJ, Murray DW. A critique of revision rate as an outcome measure: re-interpretation of knee joint registry data. J Bone Joint Surg Br. 2010;92(12):1628–31. https://doi.org/10.1302/0301-620X.92B12.25193.

54. Liddle AD, Pandit H, Judge A, Murray DW. Effect of surgical caseload on revision rate following total and unicompartmental knee replacement. J Bone Joint Surg Am. 2016;98(1):1–8. https://doi.org/10.2106/JBJS.N.00487.

55. Hamilton TW, Rizkalla JM, Kontochristos L, et al. The interaction of caseload and usage in determining outcomes of unicompartmental knee arthroplasty: a meta-analysis. J Arthroplast. 2017;32(10):3228–3237.e2. https://doi.org/10.1016/j.arth.2017.04.063.

56. Ghomrawi HM, Eggman AA, Pearle AD. Effect of age on cost-effectiveness of unicompartmental knee arthroplasty compared with total knee arthroplasty in the U.S. J Bone Joint Surg Am. 2015;97(5):396–402. https://doi.org/10.2106/JBJS.N.00169.

57. Li MG, Yao F, Joss B, Ioppolo J, Nivbrant B, Wood D. Mobile vs. fixed bearing unicondylar knee arthroplasty: a randomized study on short term clinical outcomes and knee kinematics. Knee. 2006;13(5):365–70. https://doi.org/10.1016/j.knee.2006.05.003.

58. Cheng T, Chen D, Zhu C, et al. Fixed- versus mobile-bearing unicondylar knee arthroplasty: are failure modes different? Knee Surg Sports Traumatol Arthrosc. 2013;21(11):2433–41. https://doi.org/10.1007/s00167-012-2208-y.

59. Ko Y-B, Gujarathi MR, Oh K-J. Outcome of unicompartmental knee arthroplasty: a systematic review of comparative studies between fixed and mobile bearings focusing on complications. Knee Surg Relat Res. 2015;27(3):141–8. https://doi.org/10.5792/ksrr.2015.27.3.141.

60. Campi S, Pandit HG, Dodd C, Murray DW. Cementless fixation in medial unicompartmental knee arthroplasty: a systematic review. Knee Surg Sports Traumatol Arthrosc. 2017;25(3):736–45. https://doi.org/10.1007/s00167-016-4244-5.

61. Svärd UC, Price AJ. Oxford medial unicompartmental knee arthroplasty. A survival analysis of an independent series. J Bone Joint Surg Br. 2001;83(2):191–4.

62. Kozinn SC, Scott R. Unicondylar knee arthroplasty. J Bone Joint Surg Am. 1989;71(1):145–50.

63. Stern SH, Becker MW, Insall JN. Unicondylar knee arthroplasty. An evaluation of selection criteria. Clin Orthop Relat Res. 1993;286:143–8.

64. Ritter MA, Faris PM, Thong AE, Davis KE, Meding JB, Berend ME. Intra-operative findings in varus osteoarthritis of the knee. An analysis of pre-operative alignment in potential candidates for unicompartmental arthroplasty. J Bone Joint Surg Br. 2004;86(1):43–7.

Conventional Indications for Unicompartmental Knee Arthroplasty

4

Caroline Vincelot Chainard and Henri Robert

Surgical management of tibiofemoral osteoarthritis (OA) continues to be debated after more than 50 years. Three solutions are possible: high tibial or distal femoral osteotomy (HTO/DFO), total knee arthroplasty (TKA) and unicompartmental knee arthroplasty (UKA) after failure of well-conducted medical treatment (change to the patient's activities, nonsteroidal anti-inflammatory drugs or NSAIDs, chondroprotective medications, intra-articular injections, orthotics). Osteotomies were long reserved for young, active subjects, and arthroplasties tended to be preferable in older subjects who were largely inactive. Schematically, tibial osteotomies restore good anatomical alignment of the tibia when a deformity tends to be epiphyseal (constitutional varus or Lévigne's epiphysis), but require slight overcorrection (Fig. 4.1). They are indicated in unicompartmental OA, in young subjects whose knee is stable and has complete mobility. They have several limitations: nonimmediate weightbearing, long rehabilitation and lengthy sick leave. They expose patients to specific complications: neurovascular, delayed consolidation or even disunion, infection and cosmetically unpleasant result in overcorrection.

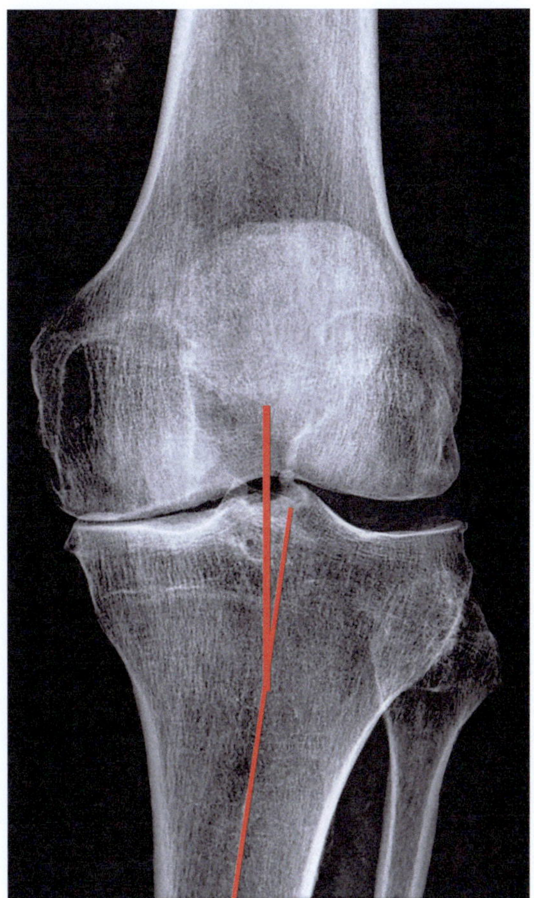

Fig. 4.1 Anterior view of a knee with epiphyseal varus deformity

C. V. Chainard
Orthopaedic Surgery Department, Angers University Hospital, Angers, France

H. Robert (✉)
Orthopaedic Surgery Department, Haut Anjou Hospital, Chateau-Gontier, France

In our experience, HTO continues to be indicated in young, athletic patients with epiphyseal varus deformity and Ahlbäck stage ≤2. Osteotomies still have unconditional defenders who, by their technical expertise and volume of activity, minimise the risks [1]. According to these authors, HTO remains possible for Ahlbäck stage OA ≥ 3 and absence of the anterior cruciate ligament (ACL). Currently, indications for HTO are declining even though UKA is increasing [2]. In France, 9500 UKA were implanted in 2011 and 12,250 in 2019, i.e. a 36% rise in 8 years (www. atih.sante.fr).

UKA has progressively developed from the 1970s under the impulsion of Leonard Marmor in the USA and Phillipe Cartier in France. Initial disappointing results with UKA, often due to technical errors or improper indications, led to restrictive indications and many contraindications. In a multicentre study, there was only 67% survival of UKA in a series by Hernigou and Deschamps [3]. These poor results have been confirmed by other authors or registers: 80% survival at 10 years for UKA in a Finnish register versus 91% to 94% for TKA, and 10% revision for UKA versus 3–10% for TKA at 10 years in the Swedish or UK register [4]. Surgical revision rates are biased because revising a UKA is considered easier than revising a TKA. Therefore, the indication for UKA revision will be established more easily and the register rates reflect this difference [5].

Considering these initial results, TKA with broad indications, a simpler technique and satisfactory results have left little place for UKA. Yet the functional results of TKA are highly variable depending on the articles (up to 20% of dissatisfied patients despite the well-established indication for TKA) and always better in publications by an experienced team than in national registers. However, we are witnessing a return to UKA in the choice of treatment [6]. The rate of UKA varies from 0% to 50% (mean 9%) in indications in the United Kingdom [7]. These rates are 5% in the USA, 7.6% in Denmark in 2010, 7.9% in Australia in 2018, 8% in Sweden since 2014, 10% in New Zealand in 2009, 12% in France and 14% in Switzerland [8]. Survival rates at 10 and 20 years have improved with better patient selection, implants and placement techniques: "Modern cemented uni-knee replacement provided durable pain relief and long-term restoration of knee function" [9]. UKA offers many advantages: near-normal kinematic, preservation of bone stock and ligaments, less invasive surgery, simpler postoperative follow-up, possible outpatient surgery, lower morbidity (pain, infection, stiffness), lower mortality (myocardial infarction, pulmonary embolism, stroke) and better function [10]. Functional scores (patients' pain, mobility and satisfaction) are better with UKA than with TKA, and current 10-year survival rates are close to those of TKA [11–14].

The objective of UKA surgery is to perform tibiofemoral resurfacing in order to correct monocompartmental wear, without restoring a normal axis in a lower limb in anteroposterior presentation. In medial UKA, overall residual varus deformity of about $2°$ (HKA $\approx 178°$) is desirable to avoid decompensation of the contralateral compartment [12] (Fig. 4.2). The persistence of this varus deformity does not expose the patient to early PE deterioration, particularly in mobile-bearing UKA [15]. UKA cannot correct a diaphyseal or metaphyseal bone defect (disunion, sequelae of osteotomy, epiphyseal varus deformity). Anteromedial tibiofemoral OA-(AMOA)- (often after meniscectomy) is the leading indication for UKA (> 90%), followed by ON (5%), the sequelae of fracture of the medial or lateral tibial plateau [8].

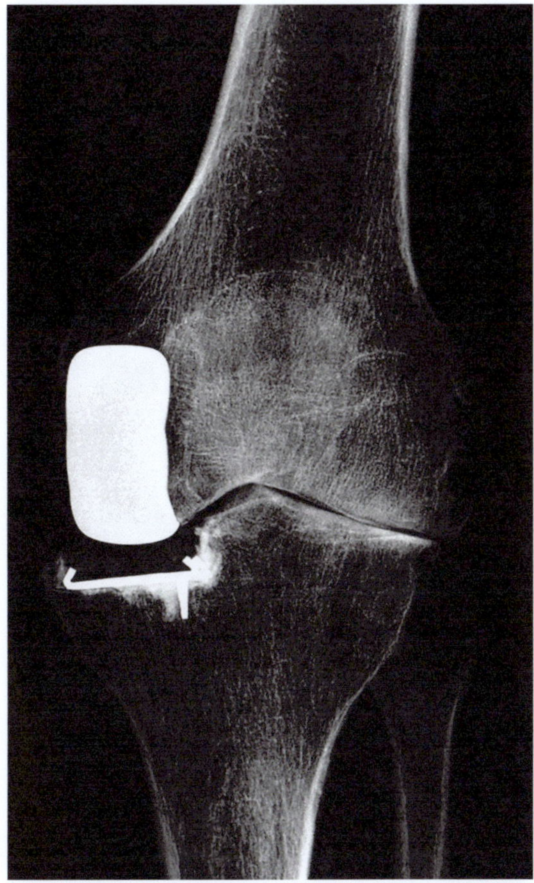

Fig. 4.2 Decompensation at 10 years postop. with valgus deformity of a medial UKA

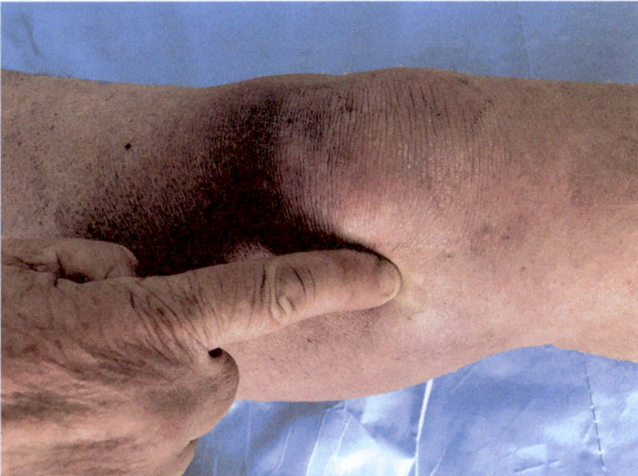

Fig. 4.3 The "finger sign", the patient's finger indicates the elective site of pain

4.1 Anteromedial Osteoarthritis (AMOA)

The clinical assessment should seek to identify the specific site of pain (the "finger sign" pointing to the MTF joint space) (Fig. 4.3) and the mechanical characteristic (pain on walking, prolonged standing). Four points of the clinical examination are important: mobility in flexion–extension, sagittal stability, patellofemoral mobility and reducibility of the varus deformity. AOMA is often accompanied by moderate flexion deformity of 10–15° and loss of complete flexion of 10–20°. Sagittal stability, evidencing competent ACL, should be sought comparatively by the Lachman test or laximetry measurements (KT-1000, Telos, GNRB®). Patellar mobility is tested: the patella is mobile, painless and there is no clash. Reducibility of

varus is assessed with the knee in 20° flexion; it can be partial or complete (Fig. 4.4 a, b). The radiological assessment includes at least: an anterior view with comparative weightbearing views (a profile view in extension with weightbearing), a patellofemoral view at 30° and the long axis with weightbearing on one foot. Narrowing of the TF joint space is graded on a weightbearing scale according to the Ahlbäck classification (four stages). Overall varus is the sum total of narrowing of the joint space and epiphyseal varus. It can be considered that the total loss of MTF cartilage (5 mm) results in varus of 5°, i.e. 1° per millimetre [16]. Testing in valgus flexion will correct the deformity in the absence of epiphyseal varus because there is no retraction of the medial collateral ligament (MCL), and this will make it possible to recognise the thickness of the cartilage in the lateral compartment. In cases of epiphyseal varus, a deformity of up to 7° can persist [13]. A preoperative deformity greater than 15° should lead distension of the convexity (lateral dislocation) to be suspected, which contraindicates UKA. An X-ray assessment can be supplemented by a forced varus image in cases of moderate MTF (narrowing of the joint space), which may be enhanced. Tibial subluxation in an anterior view with weightbearing, often worsened by an X-ray view in valgus, is a contraindication to UKA (Fig. 4.5). A profile in extension makes it possible to detect rupture of the ACL by evidencing anterior tibial translation [17] (Fig. 4.6). MRI or CT scans has no place in the standard assessment.

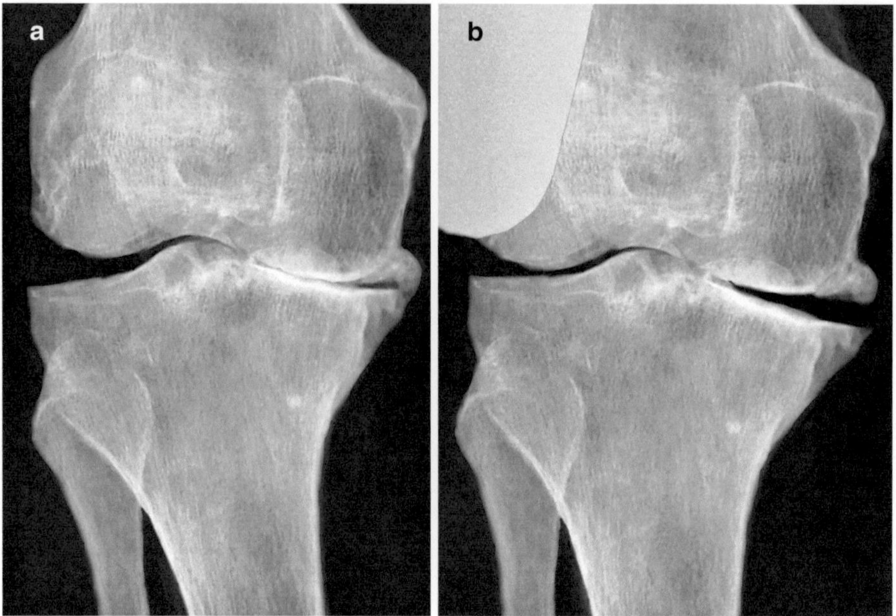

Fig. 4.4 (**a**) Varus knee deformity under load. (**b**) Complete reducibility of varus, without hypercorrection

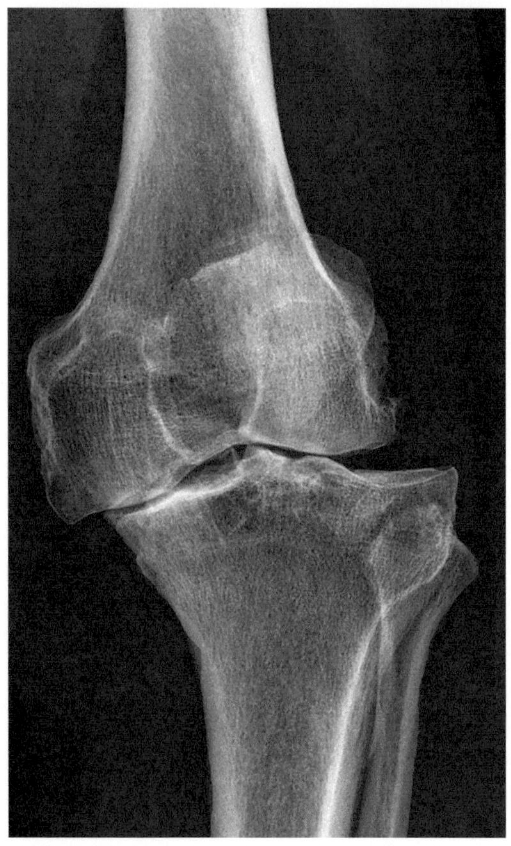

Fig. 4.5 Lateral subluxation of AMOA, which contraindicates UKA

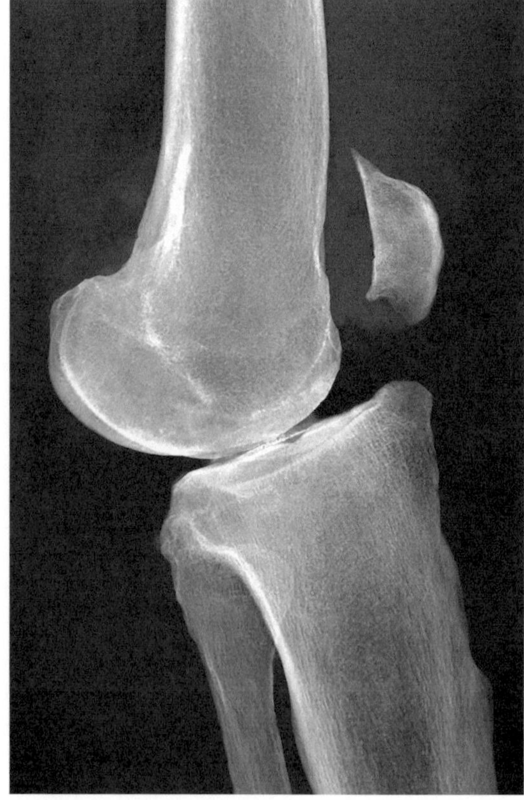

Fig. 4.6 Anterior subluxation in a sagittal view under load, which contraindicates UKA

4.2 Osteonecrosis (ON)

ON occurs following a localised vascular break in the subchondral bone with secondary chondral damage opposite and then sequestration. It can be primary and more rarely secondary (lengthy corticosteroid therapy, trauma, transplantation, chronic alcohol abuse, lupus, etc.). ON most often affects the femoral condyle in females over 50 years of age. ON is manifest by unilateral sudden-onset pain with no X-ray changes. Medical imaging makes it possible to confirm the diagnosis. X-rays underevaluate signs of aseptic osteonecrosis in the early stage. Later in progression, one or more of the following signs are observed: a subchondral radiotransparent area with/without a sclerotic border, flattening of the joint surface of the femoral condyle, free bodies in the joint interspace and a periosteal reaction; subsequently, degenerative lesions can develop. MRI detects early lesions, with sensitivity equivalent to that of scintigraphy but with better specificity. MRI is recommended in the preoperative assessment to evaluate the volume of necrotic bone to be resected.

The indications for medial or lateral UKA in ON are rare, with 3.3% of UKA implanted in the Mayo Clinic between 2002 and 2014 [18]. Transplantation of cancellous bone or cemented filler for a condylar defect can be performed. The results of UKA in ON are good with 93% survival at 10 years after UKA in primary ON, but are less optimal in secondary ON [18]. The survival rate at 12 years is 96.7% in 31 UKA according to a report by Parratte et al. [19].

4.3 Conventional Indications

Whenever a patient who has electively symptomatic severe AOMA, as seen in X-ray weightbearing views, requires joint replacement, UKA can be offered. Kozinn and Scott [20] in 1989 and then Deschamps [21] in 1998 published a number of absolute and relative contraindications for fixed medial UKA (Tables 4.1, 4.2, and 4.3).

Table 4.1 Absolute contraindications according to Kozinn and Scott [20]

Age < 60 years
Weight > 82 kg
Manual worker
Patellofemoral osteoarthritis
Frontal deformity >15°
Chondrocalcinosis

Table 4.2 Absolute contraindications according to Deschamps [21]

Bi- or tricompartmental OA
Anterior tibial translation of more than 10 mm or a soft stop in the Lachman test
Frontal laxity of the convexity
BMI > 30 kg/m^2
Rheumatic or other inflammatory disorders.

Table 4.3 Relative contraindications according to Deschamps [21]

Osteoporosis of the tibial plateau, particularly in a context of obesity
Pseudarthrosis/disunion after fracture of the tibial plateau, after proximal tibial osteotomy.

The Oxford team has published results on 1000 mobile medial UKA by comparing survival rates in the "Ideal indications" group (68%) and the "Less than ideal indications" group (32%) according to Kozinn and Scott criteria [20]. Survival rates at 10 years were 93.6% and 97%, respectively, ($p > 0.05$) [16]. Series of fixed medial UKA also have high rates of survival after 10 years' follow-up: 93% for Lecuire et al. [22] and 98% for Lustig et al. [23]. In a meta-analysis of 44 articles on 9463 knees, the revision rates were comparable in the short term between fixed versus mobile-bearing UKA [24]. Results from Parratte et al. [25] confirm this study based on 156 UKA (fixed and mobile-bearing) with at least 15 years' follow-up.

UKA use by surgeons is highly variable depending on their country, experience and, in particular, trust in this implant. For surgeons who accept the indication, UKA rates vary between 10% and over 50%. The Oxford group using mobile-bearing UKA surpasses 50% in indications for AOMA [7].

4.4 Discussion of Contraindications

We are going to analyse certain contraindications in light of the literature and our experience.

4.4.1 Age < 60 Years

Clinical and radiological results for UKA in patients >60 years of age are good [26]. In patients under 60 years of age, HTO are recommended for Ahlbäck stages ≤2, while UKA is recommended in older patients [27]. The main risk of revision in the long-term follow-up of UKA in patients <60 years is wear on the PE [27]. This risk increases with younger subjects, activity and follow-up [26]. PE wear will be manifested by mechanical-type pain, acceleration of residual varus deformity and instability under weightbearing. Argenson et al. have reported 11.4% PE wear requiring a simple change in a series of 35 UKA (Miller–Galante arthroplasty) implanted in patients 41–49 years of age [27]. In this series, a single UKA patient underwent revision surgery for loosening of the implant (at 5 years' postoperatively) and survival rate at 12 years was 80.6%. In a series by Pennington et al. [28] (Miller–Galante arthroplasty), the rate of revision surgery due to PE wear was 4.5% and survival 92% at 12 years' postoperatively. Oxford UKA in patients >60 years of age show better survival rates at 10 years (96%) than Oxford UKA in patients <60 years of age (91%).

PE with fixed-bearing UKA should be highly reticulated and has a minimum thickness of 7–8 mm [29].

Oxford UKA can have low PE thickness (meniscal bearing), but greater than 3 mm [30].

TKA in subjects <60 years of age can also yield high survival rates: 96% at 12 years according to Morgan et al. [31] and 95% for Duffy et al. [32]. The decision to perform arthroplasty (TKA and UKA) in patients <60 years of age should be motivated by intensity of pain, functional impairment and in full knowledge of specific risks (early revision) with each implant. The benefit will be that much greater when the preoperative functional score is poor. Consequently, age should not be a contraindication to UKA according to Kennedy et al.: "Earlier surgery may be preferable", but HTO remains perfectly justified in hyperactive patients [33].

4.4.2 Chondrocalcinosis

Chondrocalcinosis is characterised by deposits of calcium pyrophosphate crystals in the knee joint cartilage, meniscus or synovial membrane (prevalence of 5%). It is well identified by X-rays and confirmed by histology. It is necessary to differentiate chondrocalcinosis "disease", which is a real contraindication, from chondrocalcinosis "as an accompaniment", which is asymptomatic, nonprogressive and routinely observed during progression of osteoarthritis disease (Fig. 4.7 a, b). According to Hernigou et al., there is no deterioration of the opposite compartment or reduction in survival rates at 10 or 15 years compared to a series without chondrocalcinosis [34].

4.4.3 Patellofemoral Osteoarthritis (PFOA)

Anterior pain in the knee should be analysed to differentiate typically patellar pain from pain caused by flexion with anterior tibial osteophytes, ACL conflict in the femoral intercondylar notch or posterior capsule retraction. These causes of pain identifiable in a profile X-ray view (anterior tibial osteophyte or in the notch) are accessible with a surgical release technique (resection of osteophytes, notchplasty) (Fig. 4.8 a, b). A patella with little mobility and a painful flap, particularly with lateral PF narrowing, can be a contraindication. PFOA will progress slowly and manifest more than 10 years' postoperatively in 10% of fixed-plateau UKA cases [35]. UKA with mobile-bearing plateau seem much more "patella friendly" with PFOA. Only stage-four PFOA ("bone against bone") or fixed patellar subluxation is a contraindication (Fig. 4.9); moderate nonsymptomatic joint space narrowing present in

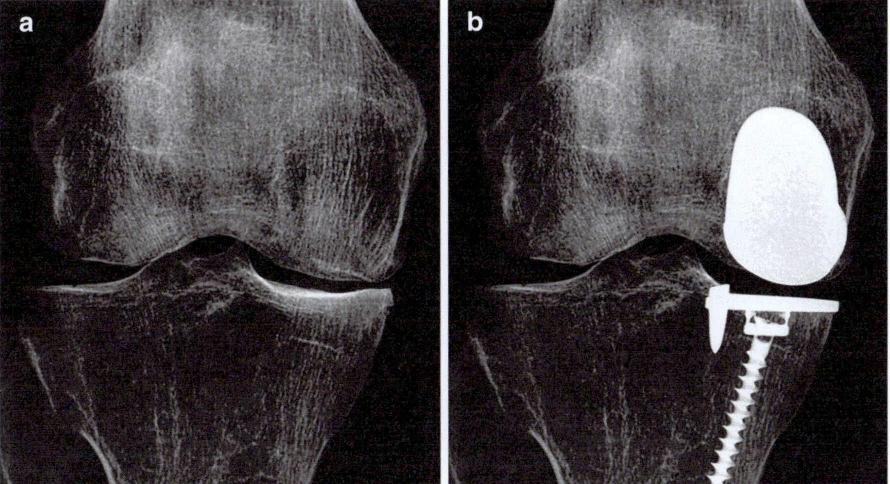

Fig. 4.7 (**a**) Bimeniscal chondrocalcinosis with AMOA. (**b**) Medial UKA with good results at seven years' follow-up

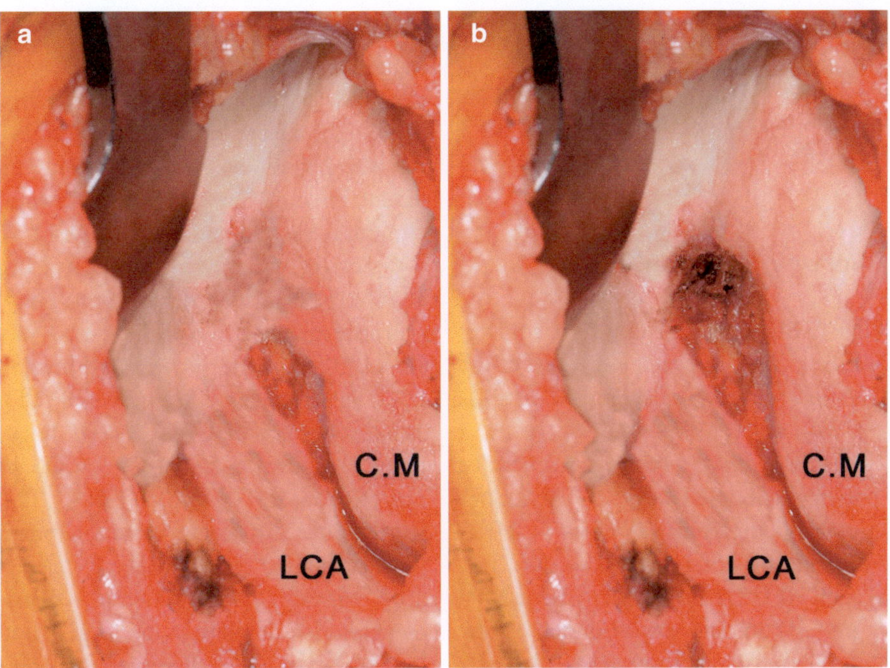

Fig. 4.8 (**a**) Bone bloc in the anterior notch at the origin of flexion's contracture. (**b**) Release of the anterior notch

54% of UKA cases in the Oxford group do not penalise long-term results [16]. Medial or lateral patellar and trochlear osteophytes in mirror image can be symptomatic (Fig. 4.10). Regularisation of osteophytes after a parapatellar approach is a prerequisite to placement of a medial or lateral UKA. The condylar implant should not be impinging forward to avoid a secondary conflict [36]. Symptomatic PFOA (without complete joint space narrowing) can be the source of pain in cases of squatting but is not an absolute contraindication to UKA [10].

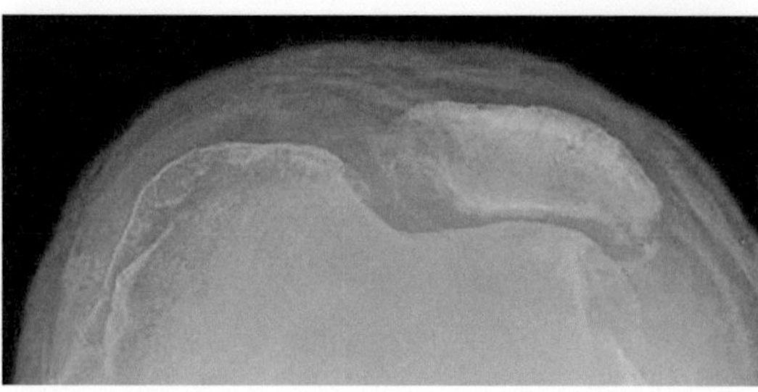

Fig. 4.9 Lateral patellofemoral arthritis and subluxation is a contraindication to UKA

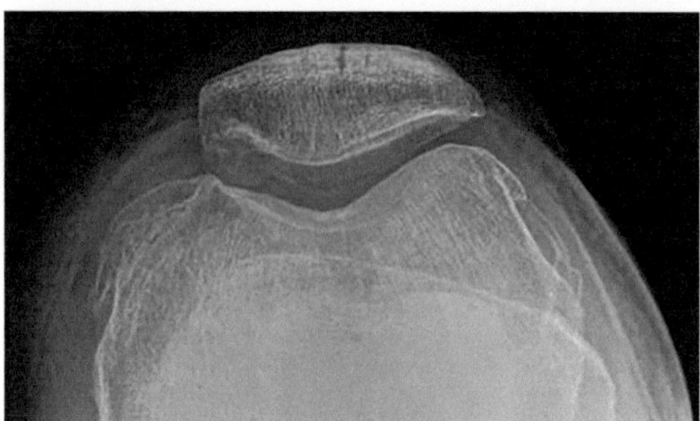

Fig. 4.10 Patellofemoral osteophytes does not contraindicate UKA

4.4.4 Overweight Patients

Excess weight (BMI > 30 kg/m^2 or weight > 82 kg) may expose the patient to premature wear of the polyethylene followed by loosening of a tibial implant [13, 20].

Many series have not shown a difference between patients with BMI < or > 30 kg/m^2. Cavaignac et al. compared 200 cases of UKA (full poly-cemented) in patients whose BMI was <30 kg/m^2 with 80 UKA in patients whose BMI was >30 kg/m^2. There was no difference in the Knee Society Score or survival rate at 12 years' mean follow-up [37]. These results are confirmed by series by Tabor et al. [38] (80% survival at 20 years' follow-up) and Xing et al. [39] (178 UKA at 2 years' follow-up). Results are also good in mobile-bearing-plateau UKA. Pandit et al. [16] studied the results of 1000 mobile-bearing-plateau UKA according to Kozinn and Scott criteria. With 10 years' follow-up, these

authors concluded: "The thresholds proposed by Kozinn and Scott using weight, age, activity, the state of the patellofemoral joint and chondrocalcinosis should not be considered to be contraindications for the use of the Oxford UKR" [16]. According to Bonutti et al., for severe obesity (BMI > 35 kg/m^2), the clinician should probably remain cautious in UKA indications [40].

4.4.5 Absence of the Anterior Cruciate Ligament (ACL)

It is necessary to differentiate previous post-traumatic rupture of the ACL, often accompanied by meniscal lesions, from "trophic" ruptures occurring progressively in a degenerative process. Such secondary types of OA in younger, active patients are characterised by asymmetrical loss of tibiofemoral substance related to anterior translation of the tibia (anterior wear on the condyle and posterior wear on the tibia). The anterior cartilage in the tibia remains intact for a long time, and an X-ray in extension can appear falsely normal; only a weightbearing view X-ray (Schuss) with 30° to 40° flexion will always be useful because the cupule is posterior. According to Deschamps, if a profile view with weightbearing in extension shows 10-mm anterior translation of the tibia, a UKA is strongly contraindicated [15]. In these cases, conduct of a UKA will be sanctioned early by anterior loosening of the implant or posterior wear (Fig. 4.11) [17, 41]. It is possible to combine UKA and simultaneous ACL surgery with good results in these cases of secondary rupture. Perioperative discovery of degenerative damage to the ACL is not a contraindication to UKA because there is no fixed anterior translation of the tibia due to capsule rigidity and posterior tibial osteophytes. Sagittal positioning of the tibial implant should not leave a sagittal slope ≥ 5° [41]. Combined one-stage surgery remains difficult with longer follow-up.

Medium-term (5-year) results of UKA with a deteriorated ACL do not differ from those of UKA with a competent ACL [42].

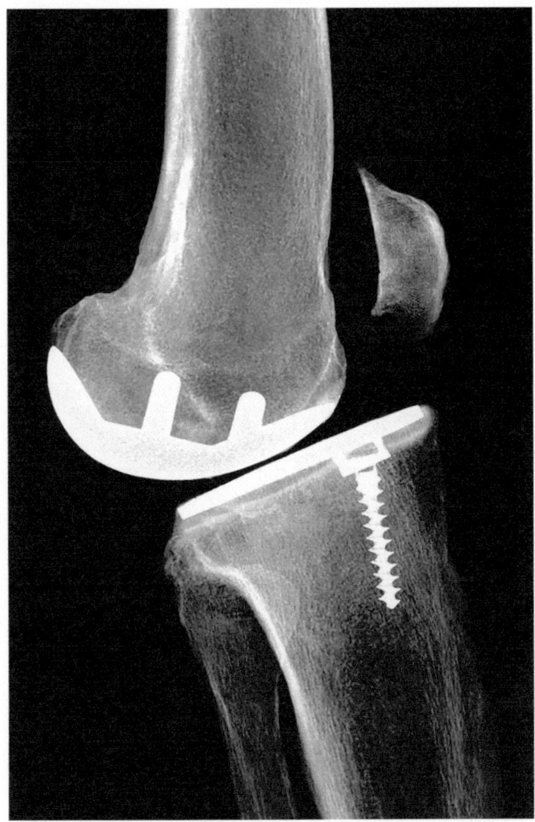

Fig. 4.11 Early failure of UKA (radiolucent line under the tibial plateau) by anterior subluxation of the tibia (previous neglected rupture of the ACL)

4.5 Conclusion

"Conventional indications" for UKA are too restrictive and should be revised. If they were applied, only 10% of AMOA would be eligible [10]. It is possible to exceed reasonably the 20% rate in AMOA. The risk of revision surgery (due to tibial malposition) of UKA is much higher when the annual number of UKA procedures performed by a surgeon is low. "With usage rates of 20% or more, patients should have all the benefits of UKA without the high revision rate" [5, 10, 11].

References

1. Lobenhoffer P. Indication for Uni knee replacement versus osteotomy around the knee. J Knee Surg. 2017;30(8):769–73.
2. Rodriguez-Merchan CR. Unicompartmental knee osteoarthritis (UKOA): unicaaaompartmental knee arthroplasty (UKA) or high tibial osteotomy (HTO)? Arch Bone J Surg. 2016;4(4):307–13.
3. Hernigou P, Deschamps G. Prothèses uni compartimentales du genou. In: Symposium SOFCOT 1995. Rev Chir Orthop. 1996:Supp 1, pp. 23–60.
4. Koskinen E, Eskelinen A, Paavolainen P, Pulkkinen P, Rernes V. Comparison of survival and cost-effectiveness between unicondylar arthroplasty and total knee arthroplasty in patients with primary osteo arthritis. Acta Orthopedica. 2008;79-4:499–07.
5. Murray DW, Liddle AD, Dodd CAF, Pandit H. UKA: is the glass half full or half empty? Bone Joint J. 2015;97-B(Suppl A):3–8.
6. Argenson JN, Flechner X. Minimally invasive UKA. Knee. 2004;11:341–7.
7. Murray DW, Parkinson RW. Usage of UKA. Bone Joint J. 2018;100-B(4):432–5.
8. Swiss Register. http://www.swissorthopaedics.ch/images/content/SIRIS/KurzfassungF.pdf.
9. Argenson JN, Blanc G, Aubaniac JM, Parratte S. Modern unicompartmental knee arthroplasty with cement: a concise FU at a mean of 20 years of a previous report. J Bone Joint Surg Am. 2013;95-A:905–9.
10. Kim TK, Mittal A, Meshram P, Kim WH, Choi SM. Evidence-based surgical technique for medial unicompartmental knee arthroplasty. Knee Surg Related Res. 2021;33:2. Online 2021 Jan 7.
11. Liddle AD, Pandit H, Judge A, Murray DW. Patient report outcomes following total and uni knee replacement: a study of 14076 matched patients from NJR for England and Wales. Bone Joint J. 2015;97-B:793–801.
12. Newman J, Pydisetty RV, Ackroyd C. Unicompartmental or total knee replacement. The 15 years results of a prospective randomized controlled trial. J Bone Joint Surg Am. 2009;91(1):52–7.
13. Deschamps G, Chol C. Fixed bearing uni knee arthroplasty. Patient selection and operative technique. Orthop Trauma Surg Res. 2011;97:648–61.
14. Deng M, Hu Y, Zhang Z, Zhang H, Qu Y, Shao G. Unicondylar knee replacement versus total knee replacement for the treatment of medial knee osteoarthritis: a systematic review and meta analysis. Arch Orthop Trauma Surg. 2021;141:1361–72.
15. Gulati A, Pandit H, Jenkins C, Chau R, Dodd CA, Murray DW. The effect of leg alignment on the outcome of uni knee replacement. J Bone Joint Surg Br. 2009;91-B:469–74.

16. Pandit H, Jenkins C, Gill HS, Price AJ, Murray DW. Unnecessary contraindications for mobile-bearing UKA. J Bone Joint Surg Br. 2011;93-B:622–8.
17. Deschamps G, Lapeyre B. Rupture of the ACL is frequently unrecognised cause of failure of UKA. Rev Chir Orthop Reparatrice Appar Mot. 1987;1:323–30.
18. Chalmers BP, Mehrotra KG. Reliable outcomes and survivorship of unicompartmental knee arthroplasty for isolated compartment osteonecrosis. Bone Joint J. 2018;100-B(4):450–4.
19. Parratte S, Argenson JN, Dumas J, Aubaniac JM. Unicompartmental knee arthroplasty for avascular osteonecrosis. Clin Orthop Relat Res. 2007;464:37–42.
20. Kozinn SC, Scott R. Unicondylar knee arthroplasty. J Bone Joint Surg Am. 1989;71-A:145–50.
21. Deschamps G, Cartier P, Epinette JA, Hernigou P. Indications et limites des prothèses Unicompartimentales. Cahiers d'enseignement de la SOFCOT. 1998;65:287–96.
22. Lecuire F, Berard JB, Martres S. Minimum 10-year follow-up results of ALPINA cementless hydroxyapatite-coated anatomic unicompartmental knee arthroplasty. Eur J Orthop Surg Traumatol. 2014;24(3):385–94.
23. Lustig S, Elguindy A, Servien E. 5- to 16- year follow-up of 54 consecutive lateral unicondylar knee arthroplasties with a fixed-all polyethylene bearing. J Arthroplasty. 2011;26(8):1318–25.
24. Peersman G, Stuyts B, Vanderlangenbergh T, Cartier P, Fennema P. Fixed- versus mobile-bearing UKA: a systematic review and meta-analysis. Knee Surg Sports Traumatol Arthrosc. 2015;23(11):3296–305.
25. Parratte S, Pauly V, Aubaniac JM, Argenson JN. No long-term difference between fixed and mobile medial unicompartmental arthroplasty. Clin Orthop Relat Res. 2012;470:61.
26. Berger RA, Meneghini RM, Jacobs JJ. Results of unicompartmental knee arthroplasty at a minimum of ten years of follow-up. J Bone Joint Surg Am. 2005;87(5):999–1006.
27. Argenson JN, Parratte S, Bertani A. The new arthritic patient and arthroplasty treatment options. J Bone Joint Surg Am. 2009;91(Suppl 5):43–8.
28. Pennington DW, Swienchowski JJ, Camargo M. Unicompartmental knee arthroplasty in patients sixty years of age or younger. J Bone Joint Surg Am. 2003;85-A(10):1968–73.
29. Hernigou P, Poignard A, Filippini P, Zilber S. Retrieved unicompartmental implants with full PE tibial components: the effects of knee alignment and polyethylene thickness on creep and wear. Open Orthop J. 2008;11(2):51–6.
30. Pandit H, Kendtick B, Bottomley N, Price A, Murray D, Dodd C. The implications of damage to the lateral femoral condyle on medial unicompartmental knee replacement. J Bone Joint Surg Br. 2010;92(3):374–9.
31. Morgan M, Brooks S, Nelson RA. Total knee arthroplasty in young active patients using a highly congruent fully mobile prosthesis. J Arthroplasty. 2007;22(4):525–30.
32. Duffy GP, Trousdale RT, Stuart MJ. Total knee arthroplasty in patients ≤ 55 years. Clin Orthop Relat Res. 1998;356:22–7.
33. Kennedy LG, Newman JH, Ackroyd CE, Dieppe PA. When should we do knee replacements? Knee. 2003;10:161–6.
34. Hernigou P, Pascale W, Pascale V, Homma Y. La chondrocalcinose primaire ou secondaire influence-t-elle la survie à long terme d'une arthroplastie unicompartimentale ? Clin Orthop Relat Res. 2012;470:973–9.
35. Berger RA, Meneghini RM. The progression of patellofemoral arthrosis after medial unicompartmental replacement: results at 11 to 15 years. Clin Orthop Relat Res. 2004;428:92–9.
36. Hernigou P, Deschamps G. Patellar impingement following UKA. J Bone Joint Surg Am. 2002;84-A:1132–7.
37. Cavaignac E, Lafontan V, Reina N. Obesity has no adverse effect on the outcome of unicompartmental knee replacement at a minimum follow-up of seven years. Bone Joint J. 2013;95-B(8):1064–8.
38. Tabor OB Jr, Tabor OB, Bernard M, Wan JY. Unicompartmental knee arthroplasty: long-term success in middle-age and obese patients. J Surg Orthop Adv. 2005;14(2):59–63.
39. Xing Z, Katz J, Jiranek W. Unicompartmental knee arthroplasty: factors influencing the outcome. J Knee Surg. 2012;25(5):369–73.
40. Bonutti PM, Goddard MS, Zywiel MG. Outcomes of unicompartmental knee arthroplasty stratified by body mass index. J Arthroplasty. 2011;26(8):1149–53.
41. Hernigou P, Deschamps G. Posterior slope of the tibial implant and the outcome of UKA. J Bone Joint Surg Am. 2004;86-A:506–11.
42. Boissonneault A, Pandit H. No difference in survivorship after unicompartmental knee arthroplasty with or without an intact anterior cruciate ligament. Knee Surg Sports Traumatol Arthrosc. 2013;21(11):2480–6.

The Modern Indications for Medial UKA the "Oxford Philosophy" Deciphered

5

T. Gicquel, J. C. Lambotte, F. X. Gunepin, and Arnaud Clavé

Since the first unicompartmental knee arthroplasties (UKA) in the 1950s, the implants' design, surgical technique and patient selection criteria have evolved with the early failures and successes, improving satisfaction, functional results, and implant survival.

Progressively, the indications have been refined and the list of contraindications lengthened. In 1989, Kozinn and Scott published in the American JBJS a *Current Concept Review* referring to and proposing the characteristics of the ideal candidate to undergo UKA (Table 5.1) [1]. In the international literature, proposals have since been revised and sometimes changed in order to be formulated into absolute selection criteria under the term "Kozinn and Scott criteria" or "traditional criteria". In reality, most publications using "Kozinn and Scott criteria" refer to stricter selection criteria than those initially published. According to regularly published criteria, only 2–6% of knee replacement surgery patients would be eligible for UKA.

In contrast, the Oxford team of John Goodfellow and John O'Connor, designer of the Oxford Unicompartmental Knee Arthroplasty (OUKA), has in the last three decades validated broader patient selection criteria [2, 3] that can currently be considered "modern". In particular, they have demonstrated that the rate of revision surgery for UKA decreases when the number of arthroplasties performed by the surgeon increases (Table 5.2 and Figs. 5.1 and 5.2). This phenomenon seems to relate to significant differences in the level of technical control, patient selection quality, and threshold for early revision surgery between surgeons with high and low numbers of arthroplasties performed [6].

The latter data has led to awareness that if the technical benefit for patients is to be sustained, it is important to increase the number of replacement surgeries. Yet this increase can only be made uniformly by redefining the selection criteria, i.e. increasing the indications and/or ignoring any unnecessary contraindications.

The widening of the selection criteria, nevertheless, should be scientifically validated for application with complete patient safety.

Therefore, this postulate raises questions that we will attempt to answer:

T. Gicquel · F. X. Gunepin
Clinique Mutualiste de la Porte de L'Orient, Lorient, France

Rennes University Teaching Hospital. Orthopaedic and Traumatology Surgery Department, Rennes, France

J. C. Lambotte
Rennes University Teaching Hospital. Orthopaedic and Traumatologie Surgery Department, Rennes, France

A. Clavé (✉)
Orthopaedic and Traumatology Surgery Department, Saint-George Private Hospital, Nice, France

LaTIM, UMR 1101 INSERM-UBO, Brest, France

A. Clavé, F. Dubrana (eds.), *Unicompartmental Knee Arthroplasty*,
https://doi.org/10.1007/978-3-031-48332-5_5

Table 5.1 Profile of the ideal candidate to undergo medial unicompartmental arthroplasty (UKA) according to the original Kozinn and Scott text published in 1989 [1]

Age	Greater than 60 years and low functional demand. But cementless implants can be indicated in younger patients who meet the other criteria.
Weight	Less than 82 kg.
Level of activity	The patient should not be physically extremely active or perform overly strenuous work.
Pain	Should not be painful at rest because this may be the sign of an inflammatory component. The procedure better relieves pain produced by weightbearing and walking.
Joint mobility	Flexion arc greater than 90°. Permanent flexion deformity less than 5°.
Deformity	Varus deformity less than 10°. The deformity should be suitable for perioperative correction after removal of the osteophytes.
Perioperative considerations	The final decision should be made after arthrotomy. Very small cartilaginous lesions in the non-weightbearing area of the lateral compartment are not contraindications to UKA. Patellofemoral pain is a relative contraindication. Asymptomatic patellar chondromalacia is not a contraindication. In cases of patellar subchondral exposure or in a weightbearing area of the lateral compartment, total knee arthroplasty is recommended. The two cruciate ligaments should be intact. UKA is an effective treatment of avascular necrosis localised in a single compartment. Patients with inflammatory disorders such as rheumatoid arthritis are not good candidates for UKA. Radiological chondrocalcinosis is a relative contraindication.

Table 5.2 Relationship between the number of unicompartmental arthroplasties (UKA) performed each year by a surgeon and the revision rate based on figures from the UK National Joint Registry, according to Liddle et al. [4]

Number of UKA implanted annually	Annual revision rate (%)
Between 1 and 2	4
10	2
30	1

Fig. 5.1 From Liddle et al. [5]

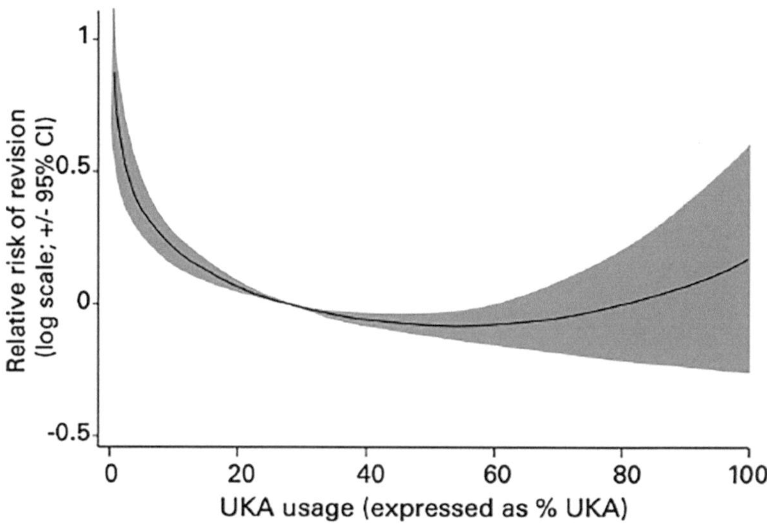

Fractional polynomial graph demonstrating the effect of increasing unicondylar knee arthroplasty (UKA) usage on the relative risk of revision (multivariable model). The vertical axis represents the relative risk of revision and is expressed on a logarithmic scale from -1 to 1. CI, confidence interval.

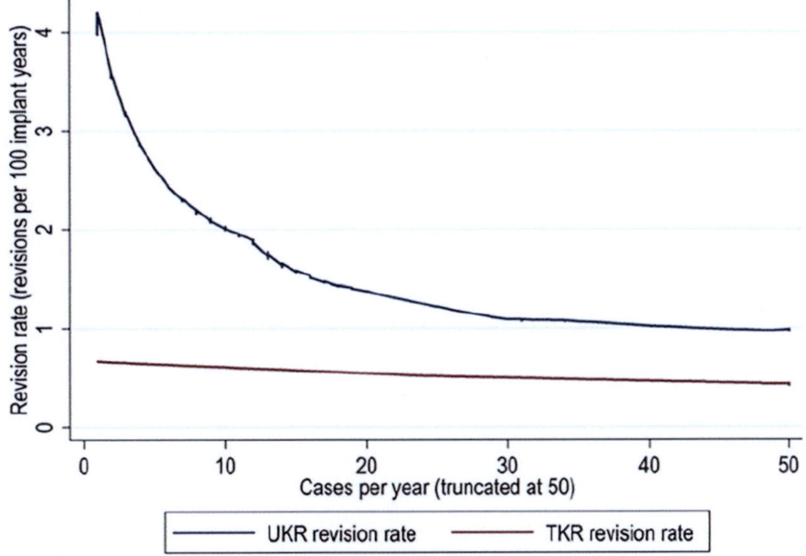

LOWESS curve demonstrating the effect of increasing caseload on revision rates following UKR and TKR (up to fifty cases).

Fig. 5.2 From Liddle [5]

Is it possible to increase the annual number of UKA by widening the indications?

Is it possible to increase the annual volume of replacement procedures by ignoring certain "traditional" contraindications?

Particular case of ACL: What strategy should be adopted in patients with medial tibiofemoral OA and a nonfunctional or ruptured ACL?

5.1   Can the Annual Number of Arthroplasties Be Increased by Widening the Indications?

The main indication chosen by the authors and generally in the literature is tibiofemoral anteromedial OA (AMOA) [7, 8]. This is a nosological concept that has been proposed and then validated by the Oxford team since the 1980s [7, 8] and corresponds to medial tibiofemoral knee OA with a competent anterior cruciate ligament and for which simple, reproducible diagnostic criteria have been established [9].

5.1.1   Anteromedial Osteoarthritis (AMOA) [10]

Tibiofemoral anteromedial osteoarthritis (AMOA) corresponds to a nosological entity resulting in relatively isolated wear on the internal tibiofemoral compartment in the anteromedial aspect with a functional anterior cruciate ligament. It is the main indication for UKA.

The clinical and radiological physical diagnosis is explained by several pathophysiological characteristics:

1. Tibial wear (on the cupula) is anterior because the anterior cruciate ligament is functional.

   In complete extension, the knee has a varus deformity. The posterior condylar shell is partially retracted or in conflict on osteophytes, preventing correction of the varus deformity (Fig. 5.3b) and contributing to permanent flexion deformity of the knee (Fig. 5.3a). Moreover, postoperatively, its progressive stretching will make it possible to see this flexion deformity correct itself until relatively late progression.

2. Since the posterior parts of the tibial plateau and femoral condyle are not worn out, when the knee is bent 90° the point of tibiofemoral contact is made in an area of preserved cartilage. The height of the joint space is restored (Fig. 5.3c) and the varus deformity spontaneously reduced with the patient in the seated position (Fig. 5.3d).

3. As a result of continuous flexion–extension movements during the day, the medial collateral ligament (MCL) is stretched during each flexion, which prevents its retraction. Therefore, the deformity is reducible during a forced valgus movement at 20°, making it possible to relax the posterior condylar shell (Fig. 5.3e and f).

Fig. 5.3 Pathophysiology of anteromedial wear of the knee. (**a** and **b**) in maximum extension, the retracted condylar shell limits extension and prevents reduction of the varus deformity. (**c** and **d**) in flexion at 90°, the unworn part of the joint surface is in contact, making it possible to reduce varus wear and prevent retraction of the medial collateral ligament. (**e** and **f**) unlocked knee (20° flexion), the relaxed condylar shell makes it possible to reduce varus wear

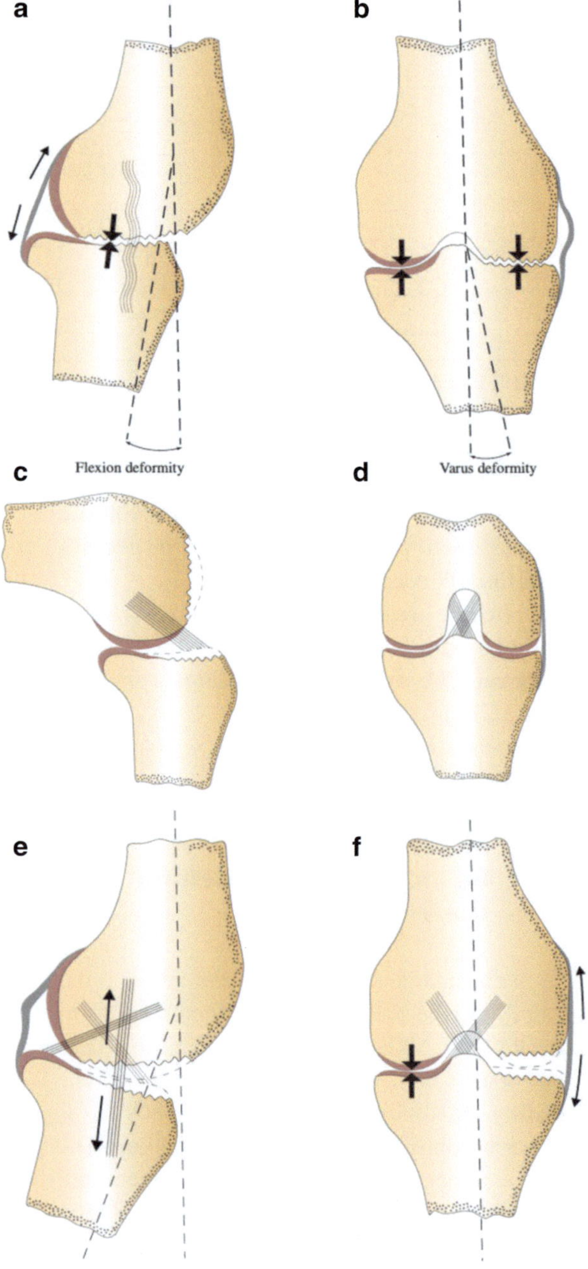

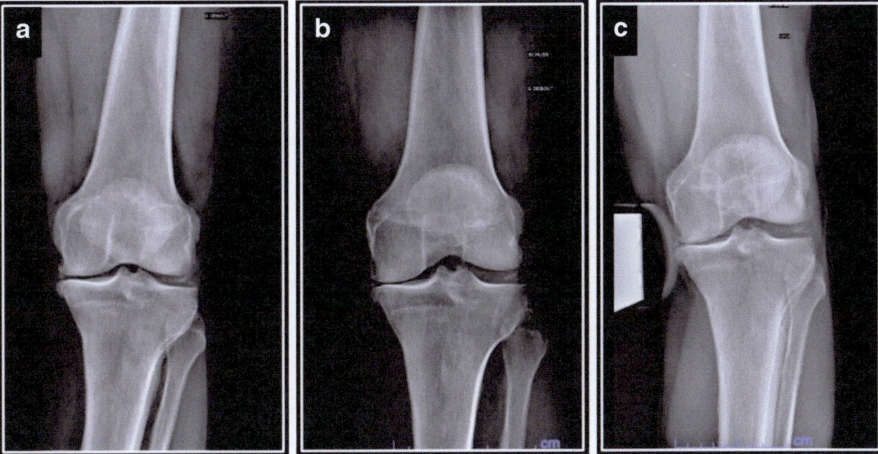

Fig. 5.4 X-rays of the same knee: anterior view with weightbearing (**a**) showing incomplete wear (Ahlbäck 2) increasing in weightbearing view (**b**) and in forced varus (**c**), which reveal Ahlbäck 3 bone-on-bone contact

5.1.1.1 Clinically

Assessment of functional impact is the main factor making it possible to establish the indication for prosthetic surgery (TKR or UKA). In an AMOA presentation, in our view, the location of pain does not appear to be a decisive factor between TKR and UKA. Therefore, although patients describe medial pain (the "finger sign") in most cases, this is not essential because in a third of cases pain may not be solely medial and may also be anterior, posterior, and more rarely lateral, which does not affect the outcome [11].

Ligament testing should find reducibility of varus (either by forced valgus at 20° flexion or in seated position), confirming that the MCL is not retracted and suggesting that we are indeed in the AMOA setting. Assessment of the ACL by the Lachman–Trillat test or anterior "drawer test", which has poor sensitivity in this context, is not considered sufficient to predict the condition of the ACL [12, 13].

5.1.1.2 Radiologically

A radiographic assessment is sufficient but certain X-ray views are essential:

1. An anteroposterior view with weightbearing should reveal complete wear of the tibiofemoral compartment with bone-on-bone contact (Ahlbäck >3). If this is not visible on a stan-dard X-ray film, a film in schuss (weightbearing) position (Rosenberg view) or a forced varus view may be necessary (Fig. 5.4).

To propose UKA, *complete wear with exposure of subchondral bone is essential.* A UKA procedure in cases of incomplete wear exposes the patient to a high risk of residual pain, a poor functional result with 25% of patients not being improved, and an implant revision rate increased sixfold [14–16].

2. A profile X-ray view (Fig. 5.5) makes it possible to locate the tibial cup and ensure that the anterior cruciate ligament is indeed functional [9]. In fact, without a functional ACL, the biomechanics of the knee are altered and the internal compartment no longer plays its role of a stable medial pivot during flexion–extension, which is the source of wear on the anterior cupula. The internal femoral condyle will have greater sagittal travel and move back into the tibia, ultimately resulting in wear of the posterior part of the tibial plateau. For some authors, however, this assessment is not always easy to do [17] and therefore raises the potential perioperative risk of the procedure being converted into TKR. MRI in this case could make it possible to conclude with greater certainty [13].

3. An X-ray view in forced valgus should make it possible to assess the status of the lateral

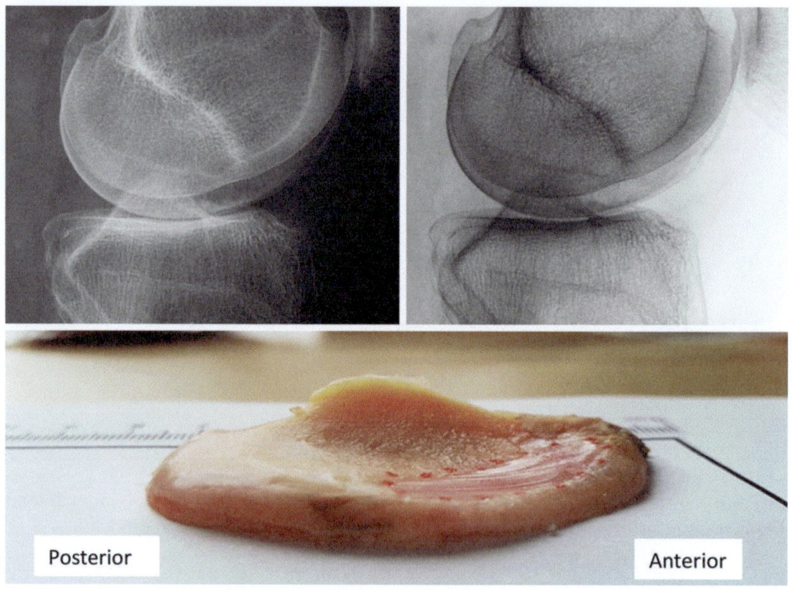

Fig. 5.5 Anterior wear in a profile X-ray view and presentation of tibial wear perioperatively

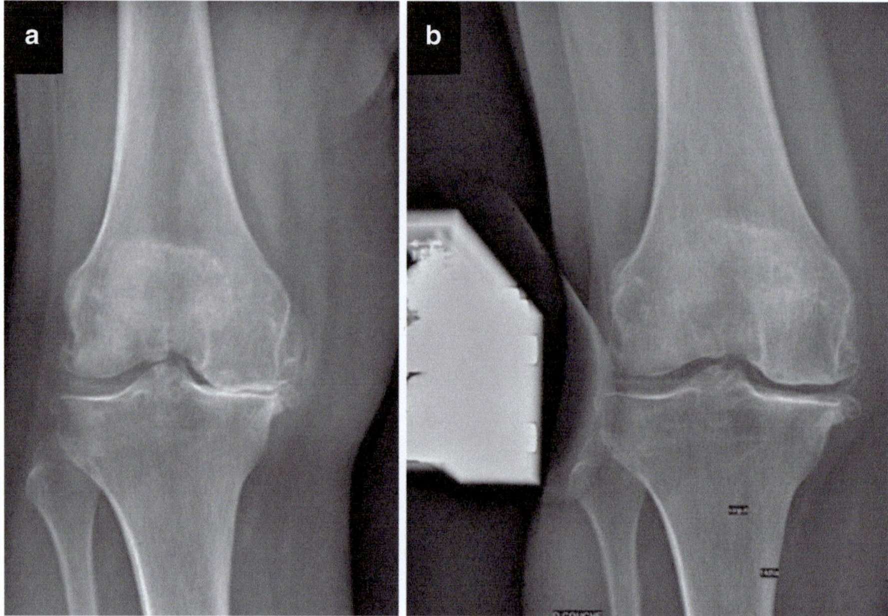

Fig. 5.6 Tibiofemoral knee OA, weightbearing view (**a**) and in forced valgus (**b**), making it possible to confirm the reducibility of varus wear deformity and conservation of the cartilage height of the lateral tibiofemoral compartment despite the presence of lateral osteophytosis and meniscal calcinosis

tibiofemoral compartment and its conservation. The presence of lateral osteophytes is not a contraindication to medial UKA [18], but a loss of lateral cartilage height should exclude medial UKA [19]. Moreover, it confirms that the MCL is not retracted and retains its physiological characteristics (Fig. 5.6).

4. A patellofemoral X-ray series (Skyline view) making it possible to assess this joint. See below.

Hamilton and Clavé [9] have validated a decision-making checklist: the Oxford Radiological Decision Aid (https://www.oxfordpartialknee.net/content/dam/zb-minisites/oxford-partial-knee-hcp/documents/oxford-decision-aid-flyer.pdf).

5.1.2 Aseptic Osteonecrosis

It is possible to propose UKA in the setting of femoral osteonecrosis. This has been demonstrated for many years by a number of authors [20, 21] and survival in this indication reaches 92% at 15 years [22–26]. In a series limited to five knees, however, Chalmers et al. recommend vigilance in light of the enhanced risk of infection and loosening of the prosthesis found in cases of osteonecrosis secondary to numerous local injections of corticosteroids [27].

Although this disorder is much rarer [28], osteonecrosis of the medial tibial plateau is also accessible by UKA [29, 30].

In all cases, preoperative MRI is necessary to confirm the diagnosis and assess the extent of necrosis. The use of a cemented implant may be necessary, and its availability in the operating room should be verified if the operator does not usually perform a cemented procedure, particularly a femoral implant (Fig. 5.7).

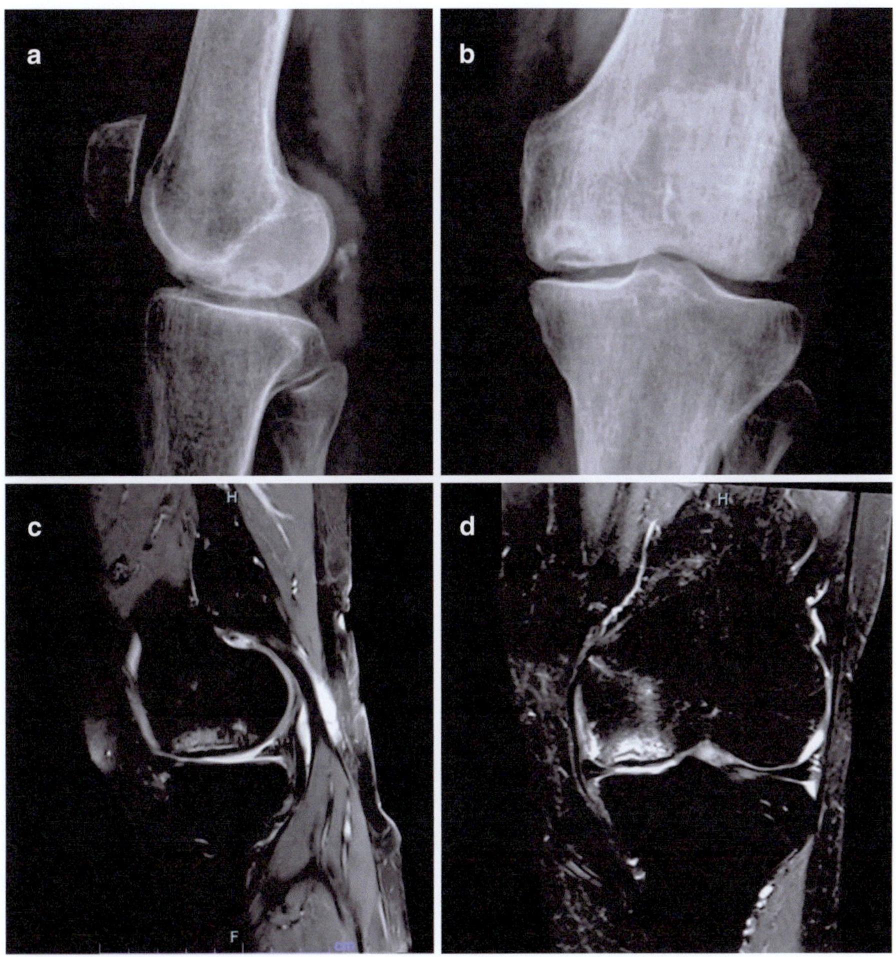

Fig. 5.7 Radiographic (**a** and **b**) and MRI (**c** and **d**) presentation of aseptic osteonecrosis of the medial femoral condyle

5.1.3 Medial Tibiofemoral OA After Tibial Osteotomy (HTO)

Prior HTO is not a systematic obstacle to the conduct of UKA [31]. Nevertheless, this indication is complex and has been little studied. Limits should be determined both in terms of ligament status and alignment of the lower limb or bone structure (mechanical medial proximal tibial angle, mMPTA) [32, 33].

The ideal situation is a lower limb in residual varus, without hypercorrection of tibial varus (mMPTA $\leq 90°$). Preoperative MRI makes it possible to ensure a satisfactory lateral compartment.

Use of fixed-plateau UKA and navigation ensures that the operator has not produced excessive intra-articular correction [34] (Fig. 5.8).

5.1.4 Bicompartmental UKA

Two circumstances can lead to the placement of two unicompartmental arthroplasties (including one medial UKA) in the same knee:

- Either at the outset, in the same surgical stage in cases of bicompartmental wear, particularly involving the medial tibiofemoral compartment. This proposal is not promoted, mainly as a precautionary measure by the Oxford team [10], but many experienced authors offer it.
- or at an interval after an initial UKA in cases of secondary deterioration of another knee compartment. In this chapter, we will only discuss the use of medial UKA to treat deterioration of the medial tibiofemoral compartment sometime after a patellofemoral or lateral tibiofemoral UKA.

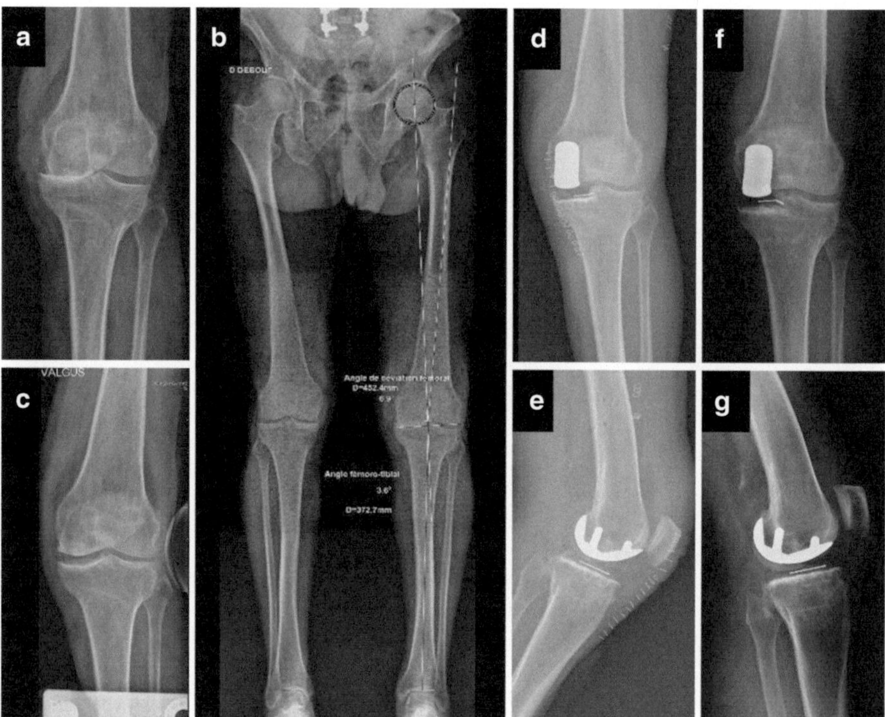

Fig. 5.8 AMOA 22 years after an HTO (**a**). The preoperative assessment revealed reducible residual varus of 4° (**b**) and conservation of the height of the lateral tibiofemoral compartment in an X-ray view in forced valgus (**c**). (**d** and **e**) Immediate postoperative X-ray views. (**f** and **g**) X-ray views with 7 years' postoperative follow-up

5.1.4.1 Medial Unicompartmental Arthroplasty and Simultaneous Patellofemoral Arthroplasty

The status of the patellofemoral compartment is seldom a contraindication to UKA (see the following chapter) and therefore indications for combined medial UKA and patellofemoral UKA are rare [12].

5.1.4.2 Simultaneous Medial and Lateral Unicompartmental Arthroplasty

It is useful to remember that initially the OUKA designed in 1976 was implanted solely as a Bi-UKA until 1982, the year when the indication for medial UKA and the AMOA concept prevailed [10].

A recent review of the literature [35] suggests that this combination can be proposed to patients presenting with bicompartmental tibiofemoral OA, with a nonsymptomatic patellofemoral joint, an intact anterior cruciate ligament, a reducible deformity, and conserved joint mobility.

Few results are reported in the literature and it is not possible for the time being to recommend this strategy. Its utility may lie primarily in preservation of the joint biomechanics and proprioception provided by preservation of the cruciate ligaments [36].

5.1.4.3 Medial Unicompartmental Arthroplasty at an Interval After Another Unicompartmental Arthroplasty

In the setting of deterioration of the medial tibiofemoral compartment after an initial procedure, UKA seems to be an attractive alternative to TKR to treat deterioration of the medial compartment after lateral UKA [37]. In this case, the first UKA should have enabled significant relief during a certain period of time and deterioration of the medial compartment secondarily until bone-on-bone contact in order to propose medial UKA.

5.1.5 OA After Fracture

Indications for medial UKA after a fracture are very rare. There are no series in the literature. Particular vigilance should be paid to possible ligament lesions concomitant to fracture, particularly MCL, which can contraindicate placement of UKA.

5.1.6 Joint Deterioration in Inflammatory Disorders

Joint deteriorations related to active systemic inflammatory disease of the knee joint are not indications for UKA. No recent publication has reported the use of unicompartmental implants in this context.

Take-Home Messages
1. Tibiofemoral knee anteromedial OA (AMOA) and aseptic osteonecrosis of the femoral condyle are the main indications for unicompartmental arthroplasty.
2. It is possible to perform UKA in other types of mechanical deterioration of the knee, but there are few such indications and results are unpredictable.
3. Joint deteriorations in systemic inflammatory diseases are not indications for UKA.

5.2 Can the Annual Number of Procedures Be Increased by Limiting the Current Contraindications?

Although it is not possible to increase the number of procedures by widening the indications, it does appear important to examine the validity of the "traditional" contraindications. When Kozinn and Scott criteria are strictly applied, less than 10% of surgical treatments of knee OA are eligible for UKA [38]. Yet under 10%, the annual revision rate is greater than 2% [39]. When the UKA usage rate increases and reaches a level of between 40% and 60%, the revision rate decreases and is not then significantly different from that of TKR (Fig. 5.2) [5, 39]. These rates can only be reached by reducing the list of "traditional" contraindications. High body weight, young age, major physical activity, radiological chondrocalcinosis, clinical and radiological evidence of patellofemoral damage, medial subluxation of the tibia, and osteophytes in the lateral plateau should no longer be considered as formal contraindications to the conduct of UKA. For Pandit and Hamilton, patients presenting with these criteria, deemed "contraindications" by Kozinn and Scott, have a UKA result that is at least as good in both function and survival as patients who present with "ideal" criteria according to Kozinn and Scott [40, 41].

5.2.1 Body Weight

Obese patients have similar implant survival and similar or even better functional improvement to patients in other BMI classes [42–46]. Moreover, survival seems independent of BMI [38].

In comparison with TKR [47], UKA in obese patients may be useful with better postoperative joint mobility, lower risk of infection (0% vs. 0.5%), and decreased need for mobilisation during general anaesthesia (3.7% versus 9.2%).

Therefore, body weight is not a contraindication to UKA which, if we use the Kozinn and Scott restrictive criteria, would prevent its conduct in half of patients [40] (Fig. 5.9).

5.2.2 Age and Physical Activity

Although younger patients (≤ 50 years, ≤ 55 years or ≤ 60 years of age, according to studies) in cohort studies have results (functional, quality of life, and implant survival) that are as good as in older subjects [48–52], data from registers often show evidence of an unfavourable effect of younger age on implant survival [53, 54].

In comparison with TKR [55], UKA in younger patients may enable better mobility without significantly improving functional scores.

Viewpoint

Treatment of knee OA in younger patients is complex. Although all of them suffer intensely from knee symptoms, this population is relatively heterogeneous in terms of physical activity, occupational activity, and intra-articular lesions.

Surgeons faced with increasing demand from their patients should not propose UKA if the indication is not clearly established. It is imperative that joint space narrowing is complete. Although this was proposed for a time, perhaps wrongly, through the concept of transient UKA [56], UKA should not be seen as a *simpler* alternative to TKR that is avoided because the patient is too young and/or the joint is not worn out enough.

In surgical registers, the overall number of UKA is relatively high but a large proportion of the implants are inserted by surgeons who individually perform few procedures [4]. The hypothesis can reasonably be formulated that if such procedures involve younger patients, the indication is not or seldom mastered, explaining in part the poor results in registers on these patients.

In patients with a high level of activity preoperatively, implant survival and function are at least as good as in patients with a lower level of activity. Therefore, the level of physical activity should not be considered as a contraindication to UKA [57, 58].

On the other hand, patients over the age of 75 years present results that are at least as good as in younger patients or those who undergo TKR

Fig. 5.9 (**a**) Post, preoperative, and delta Oxford knee score according to BMI; (**b**) survival over time depending on BMI. From Murray et al. [42]

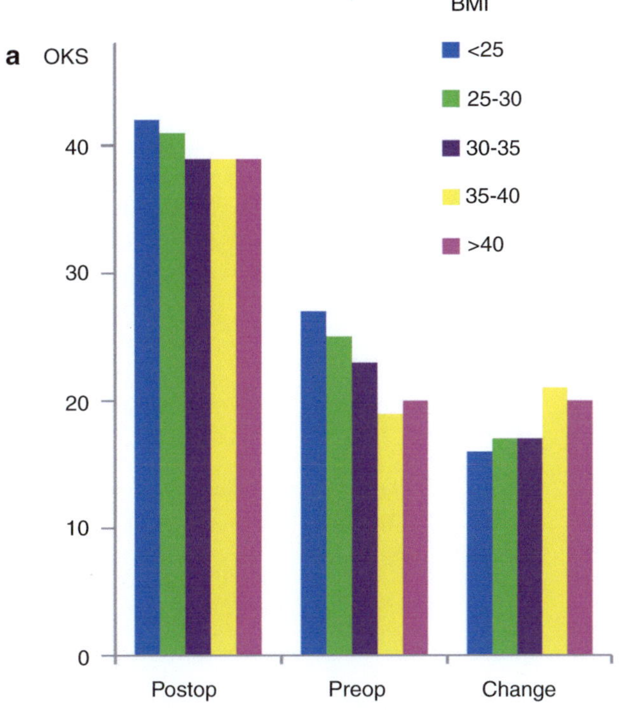

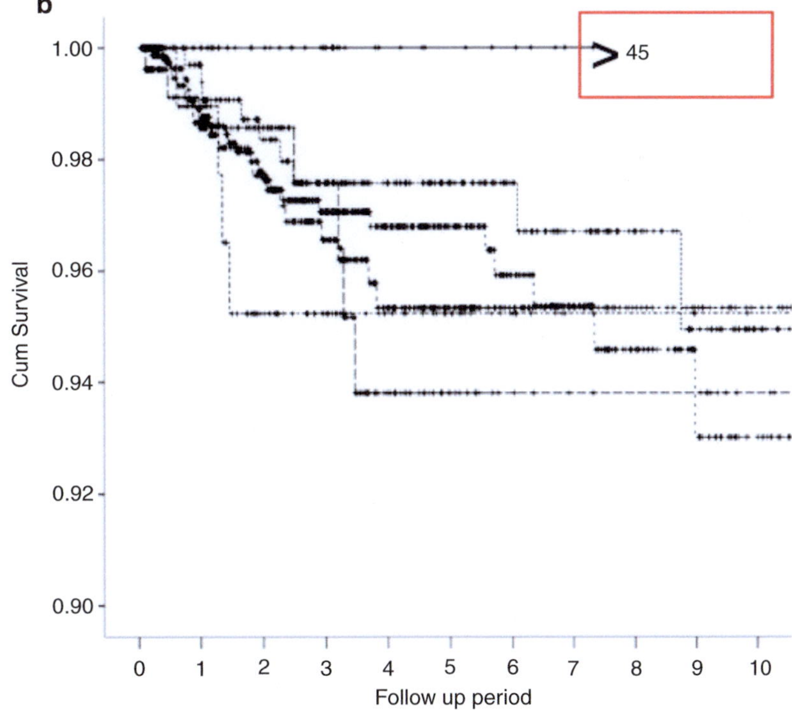

[59]. In older and more fragile patients, the choice of UKA over TKR seems logical to avoid the more serious complications with TKR [60–62].

Because of the many external factors influencing the choice, the decision between TKR, HTO (high tibial osteotomy), and UKA in younger patients has not been fully determined, but age and physical activity should not be deemed absolute contraindications at the risk of needlessly excluding 24% and 10% of patients from UKA, respectively [40] (Fig. 5.10).

5.2.3 Flexion Deformity

Up to 15°, flexion deformity is not a contraindication to UKA. Intra-articular procedures, particularly release of the intercondylar notch and removal of osteophytes (at the foot of the ACL, behind the medial condyle and medial tibial plateau), make it possible to correct a major part of the flexion deformity. If all these procedures for release have been correctly performed, a possible postoperative minor flexion deformity will correct itself over the year after surgery by progressive stretching of the periarticular structures.

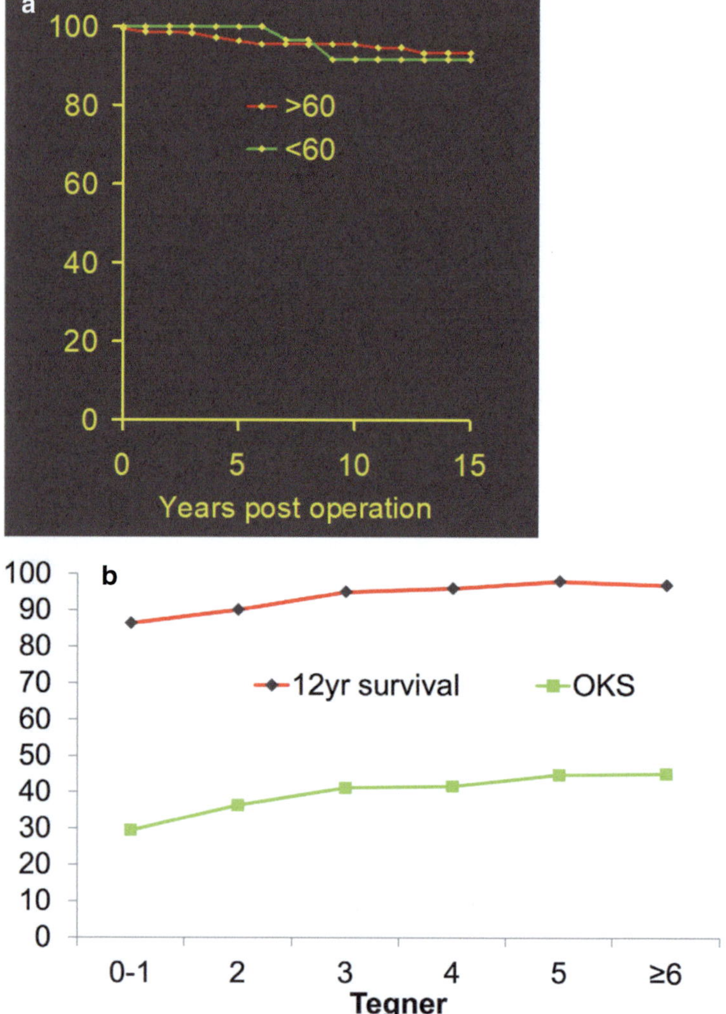

Fig. 5.10 (a) survival over time according to age (> or < at 60 years); (b) survival at 12 years and Oxford knee score based on Tegner activity score [57] and Murray et al. The London Knee Meeting 2014

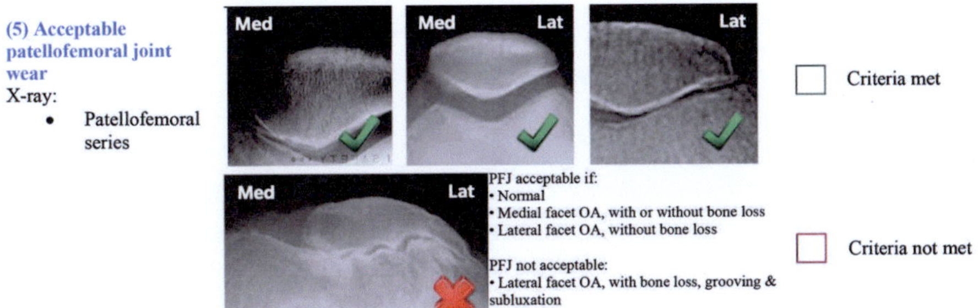

Fig. 5.11 Radiographic criteria for patellofemoral wear adapted from the *Oxford Decision Aid* [9]. If any criteria are "met", the status of the patellofemoral compartment is not a contraindication to UKA (https://www.oxfordpar- tialknee.net/content/dam/zb-minisites/oxford-partial- knee-hcp/documents/oxford-decision-aid-flyer.pdf) (courtesy of Zimmer-Biomet)

Beyond 15°, the status of the ACL and the causes of flexion deformity must be correctly assessed. In fact, flexion of more than 15° is frequently related to a deficient or absent ACL and/ or major deterioration of the other knee compartments.

5.2.4 Patellofemoral Joint

The status of the patellofemoral joint has always been the source of tension and debate. Currently, it continues to be an area of concern and uncertainty for many surgeons, often leading as a precautionary measure to preferring TKR.

In most cases, however, the condition of the patellofemoral joint does not represent a contraindication to the conduct of medial UKA.

Clinically, the presence of anterior pain is not a factor for dissatisfaction or failure [63, 64]. The existence of an authentic patellofemoral pain syndrome [65] has never been studied in the literature and would merit further investigation.

Radiologically, whenever the patella remains centred or the wear is solely medial, this does not have any consequences [63, 66–69]. In contrast, it is necessary to be vigilant in cases of lateral subluxation or lateral wear [70] and to consider this as a potential contraindication. Nevertheless,

in the absence of severe lateral wear, a defective patellofemoral radiological alignment does not affect the functional result of UKA according to some authors [71].

The presence of cartilage lesions, perhaps discovered perioperatively, should not needlessly worry the surgeon. Even when loss of substance is total (Fig. 5.11), including from the bottom of the trochlea, the result of UKA is unaffected if this cartilage loss does not involve the lateral facet of the patella [64, 68, 72–74]. Therefore, there is no need to change the indication perioperatively, but patients must be informed that anterior pain can take time to disappear and that residual discomfort on climbing stairs can persist [75] (Fig. 5.12).

5.2.5 Chondrocalcinosis

Although meniscal chondrocalcinosis (meniscal calcinosis) is not always associated with histological chondrocalcinosis and reciprocally, it seems that patients who have histological chondrocalcinosis are at greater risk of having decreased implant survival [76].

The presence of radiological signs of chondrocalcinosis (meniscal calcifications) is not a contraindication to the conduct of UKA [76, 77].

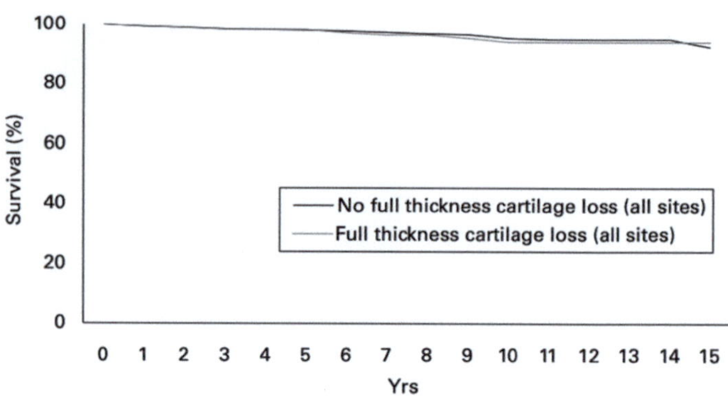

Fig. 5.12 According to Hamilton [64], survival of medial UKA with and without full-thickness cartilage loss in the patellofemoral joint

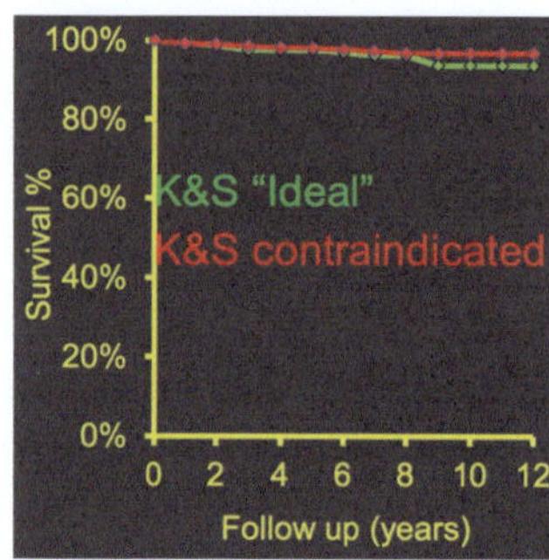

Fig. 5.13 Survival over time according to compliance with Kozinn and Scott criteria. From Pandit et al. [40]

Take-Home Messages

1. If the surgical indication is correctly established (tibiofemoral knee antero-medial OA), the patient's age and physical activity are not absolute contraindications to medial UKA.
2. Analysis of the patellofemoral joint's condition is difficult. Patellofemoral contraindications to UKA are marginal and mainly related to extreme wear of the joint's lateral facet. Anterior pain does not predict an unfavourable result of UKA.
3. Unjustified contraindications are responsible for limiting the use of UKA by surgeons in the treatment of knee anteromedial OA (AMOA) (Fig. 5.13).

5.3 Specific Case: What Strategy Should Be Adopted in Patients with Medial Tibiofemoral OA and a Nonfunctional or Ruptured ACL?

The question of the possibility of performing unicompartmental arthroplasty on a knee that presents with a nonfunctional anterior cruciate ligament is delicate. The absence of a functional anterior cruciate ligament has long been considered as an absolute contraindication due to more frequent tibial loosening of the implant and premature polyethylene wear [2, 78, 79], probably explained by biomechanical changes such as the pushing back of the tibiofemoral contact point [80] and sliding rather than rolling of the femoral condyle [81] (soaping phenomenon).

However, the good functional results of UKA in younger patients with high functional demand [57, 58] and the procedure's low morbidity in fragile elderly patients [60] have encouraged some teams to use these implants even in patients with a nonfunctional ACL.

The population of patients with a nonfunctional ACL in medial tibiofemoral OA is heterogeneous and it is possible to differentiate the three different nosological entities described below.

5.3.1 Advanced Anteromedial OA (Advanced AMOA)

This occurs in generally elderly patients, over 70 years of age, who initially have tibiofemoral knee anteromedial OA, but progression of the disorder and, in particular, of osteophytes of the intercondylar notch has gradually led to loss of functioning due to erosion of the ACL.

Patients rarely complain of knee instability because loss of ACL function is progressive and the knee is stabilised by the osteoarthritic ankylosis.

As an alternative to TKR, UKA without reconstruction of the ACL can be considered, taking care to decrease the tibial slope in comparison to either the native slope of the medial tibial plateau or the implant's usual slope [82–85]. In return, implant survival and functional result do not seem to be different from that of UKA with a functional ACL in a population of the same age [84, 86, 87]. Nevertheless, it is necessary to be cautious during surgery because balancing such implants is made difficult by the imperative to reduce the slope, possible retraction of the ACL, and posterior progression of wear.

5.3.2 Posteromedial OA (PMOA)

This affects younger patients, generally under 60 years of age. Rupture of the ACL is traumatic, longstanding and sometimes ignored by patients, and wear on the tibial plateau is immediately posterior by anterior tibial translation and wear on the posterior segment of the medial meniscus.

Patients have not always complained of instability or have changed their physical activities to avoid it.

This corresponds to *Postero Medial Osteo Arthritis* (PMOA) as opposed to *Antero Medial Osteo Arthritis* (AMOA), although the term is not used in the literature.

As an alternative to TKR, it appears possible to propose UKA together with ligamentoplasty of the ACL. Initial functional results are very satisfactory and likely meet these younger patients' expectations [88–93]. Nevertheless, long-term survival remains little documented and requires more extensive studies [92, 94]. In addition, the combination of these two procedures makes them more complex and should be reserved for surgeons who are experienced in both.

5.3.3 Post-Ligamentoplasty Tibiofemoral Knee Anteromedial OA (Post-Ligamentoplasty AMOA)

This nosological entity is probably the most complex of all because it necessitates assessing the functional aspect of the ligamentoplasty (Table 5.3). This form of OA affects younger or even very young patients (sometimes under 50 years of age) who often have high to very high functional demand and whose knee has already "benefitted" from several ligament surgeries.

The conduct of TKR is clearly the simplest and most proven solution. Tibial valgus osteotomy also retains all of its utility when wear is

Table 5.3 Factors for or against the functional aspect of a ligamentoplasty in a patient with medial tibiofemoral knee OA and a history of reconstruction of the anterior cruciate ligament

	Factors supporting functional ligamentoplasty	Factors supporting nonfunctional ligamentoplasty
Aetiology of deterioration	Iatrogenic after meniscectomy in a pronounced varus knee deformity	Residual laxity responsible for meniscus/cartilage deterioration
History	Only one reconstruction	Repeated ligamentoplasty
Time aspect	Recent ligamentoplasty	Previous ligamentoplasty
Symptoms	Stable	Unstable
Laxity[a]	No laxity	Laxity

aLaxity is difficult to judge because ligamentoplasty can be relaxed by loss of cartilage height in the medial compartment; the conduct of a UKA can sometimes retighten a ligamentoplasty that initially appears lax in testing moderate. Discussing the conduct of UKA is possible, but a precise analysis of the functional aspect of a ligamentoplasty is essential even if it is complex.

Therefore, in cases of satisfactory ligamentoplasty (Table 5.3), UKA may be considered. In other cases, the combination of UKA with revision of a ligamentoplasty, although theoretically feasible in our opinion, does not seem appropriate due to the many technical difficulties in both the choice of the type of graft and placement of the tibial tunnel.

The case of a Lemaire-type extra-articular ligamentoplasty raises a different problem: the joint that is naive for prior ligamentoplasty encourages the conduct of UKA + ligamentoplasty, but it is important to assess the lateral compartment correctly and to be mindful of deterioration of the lateral tibiofemoral compartment, particularly with older surgeries [95, 96].

5.3.4 Take-Home Message (Table 5.4)

Table 5.4 Summary of various nosological categories in relation to medial tibiofemoral OA with a native nonfunctional anterior cruciate ligament

	1. Advanced AMOA	2. PMOA	3. Post-ligamentoplasty AMOA
Patient's age	"Elderly"	"Young"	"Young"
Pathophysiology	Initial anteromedial OA Progressive erosion of the ACL	Previous rupture of the ACL Initial posterior wear of the tibial plateau	To be determined in order to define the therapeutic project
Stability	Stable	+/− stable	+/− stable
Therapeutic	UKA (or TKR)	ACL + UKA (or TKR)	UKA or TKR according to the condition of the ligamentoplasty

5.4 Conclusion

Widening the selection criteria for UKA-eligible patients is necessary in order to reach a number and rate of UKA which can limit the rate of revision surgery. Widening the selection criteria essentially involves reviewing the limitation of contraindications. However, it is not appropriate to seek to widen the indication of UKA at the risk of running into technical difficulties in its conduct and exposing the patient to an uncertain result.

Tibiofemoral knee anteromedial OA (AMOA) is the prime indication for medial UKA and, if reasonable contraindications are followed, makes it possible to reach a UKA rate of 30% to 40% in the clinical practice of this chapter's authors.

5.5 Final Take-Home Messages

Question 1: Is it possible to increase the annual number of UKA by widening the indications?

The main indication retained by the Oxford team is tibiofemoral anteromedial OA (AMOA) [7, 8]. It is a nosological concept that they have proposed and then validated since the 1980s [7, 8], corresponding to medial tibiofemoral knee OA with a competent anterior cruciate ligament and for which simple, reproducible diagnostic criteria have been established [9].

Other indications of UKA exist, such as osteonecrosis (femoral and tibial), bicompartmental OA (bi-UKA), failure of tibial valgus osteotomy (TVO), post-traumatic OA, etc., but these are much rarer [7, 8]. Although widely validated in femoral osteonecrosis, the use of UKA in other indications remains marginal and the volume of publications is low.

AMOA is the main indication, representing over 95% of UKA procedures for the Oxford team. Good knowledge of it is therefore essential in the identification of patients potentially eligible for this surgery.

Widening the indications to marginal indications (less than 5%) is not a good method of increasing the volume of such procedures.

Furthermore, these cases are often complex with an uncertain result.

Question 2: Is it possible to increase the annual number of procedures by ignoring certain "traditional" contraindications?

Although it is not possible to increase the number of procedures by widening the indications, it does appear important to examine the validity of the "traditional" contraindications. When the Kozinn and Scott criteria are strictly applied, less than 10% of surgical types of knee OA are eligible for UKA [38]. Yet under 10%, the annual revision rate is greater than 2% [39]. When the rate of UKA use increases and reaches a value of between 40% and 60%, the rate of revision surgery decreases and is not then significantly different from that of TKR (Fig. 5.2) [5, 39]. These rates can be reached by reducing the list of "traditional" contraindications. High weight, young age, major physical activity, radiological chondrocalcinosis, clinical and radiological patellofemoral damage, medial subluxation of the tibia, and osteophytes in the lateral plateau should not be seen as formal contraindications to the conduct of UKA. Patients presenting with criteria considered as "contraindications" under Kozinn and Scott criteria have, according to Pandit and Hamilton, a UKA result at least as good in functional aspect and survival as patients presenting with "ideal" Kozinn and Scott criteria [40, 41].

Avoiding unnecessary contraindications makes it possible to increase the rate of use and annual volume of UKA in a safe manner and consequently to decrease the implant revision rate.

Question 3: Specific case: What strategy should be adopted in patients with medial tibiofemoral OA and a nonfunctional or ruptured ACL?

The absence of an anterior cruciate ligament is a contraindication to UKA, whether according to "Kozinn and Scott" criteria or to the designers of the OUKA system. Despite this, many surgeons continue to show interest in the topic and scientific publications are becoming more numerous. UKA is then conceived as an alternative to TKR either to optimise the functional result in younger patients or as a result of its lower morbidity in the elderly.

Nevertheless, a precise but difficult analysis of the nosological category is essential since the treatments proposed will not be the same between elderly patients presenting with progressive erosion of the ACL in advanced AMOA, younger patients presenting with posteromedial OA or younger patients presenting with post-ligamentoplasty medial tibiofemoral OA. Not all of these patients will be eligible for UKA, and for those who are the conduct of combined ligamentoplasty must be discussed.

References

1. Kozinn SC, Scott R. Unicondylar knee arthroplasty. J Bone Joint Surg Am. 1989;71:145–50.
2. Goodfellow JW, Kershaw CJ, Benson MK, O'Connor JJ. The Oxford knee for unicompartmental osteoarthritis. The first 103 cases. J Bone Joint Surg Br. 1988;70:692–701.
3. Carr A, Keyes G, Miller R, et al. Medial unicompartmental arthroplasty. A survival study of the Oxford meniscal knee. Clin Orthop Relat Res. 1993;295:205–13.
4. Liddle AD, Pandit H, Judge A, Murray DW. Effect of surgical caseload on revision rate following total and unicompartmental knee replacement. J Bone Joint Surg Am. 2016;98:1–8. https://doi.org/10.2106/JBJS.N.00487.
5. Liddle AD, Pandit H, Judge A, Murray DW. Optimal usage of unicompartmental knee arthroplasty: a study of 41,986 cases from the National Joint Registry for England and Wales. Bone Joint J. 2015;97-B:1506–11. https://doi.org/10.1302/0301-620X.97B11.35551.
6. Liddle AD. CORR insights®: no differences in outcomes scores or survivorship of unicompartmental knee arthroplasty between patients younger or older than 55 years of age at minimum 10-year followup. Clin Orthop Relat Res. 2019;477:1447–9. https://doi.org/10.1097/CORR.0000000000000797.
7. Goodfellow JW, Tibrewal SB, Sherman KP, O'Connor JJ. Unicompartmental Oxford Meniscal knee arthroplasty. J Arthroplast. 1987;2:1–9. https://doi.org/10.1016/s0883-5403(87)80025-6.
8. White SH, Ludkowski PF, Goodfellow JW. Anteromedial osteoarthritis of the knee. J Bone Joint Surg Br. 1991;73:582–6.
9. Hamilton TW, Pandit HG, Lombardi AV, et al. Radiological Decision Aid to determine suitability for medial unicompartmental knee arthroplasty: development and preliminary validation. Bone Joint J. 2016;98-B:3–10. https://doi.org/10.1302/0301-620X.98B10.BJJ-2016-0432.R1.
10. Goodfellow J, O'Connor J, Pandit H, et al. Unicompartmental arthroplasty with the Oxford knee. 2nd ed. Goodfellow Publishers Limited; 2015.
11. Liddle AD, Pandit H, Jenkins C, et al. Preoperative pain location is a poor predictor of outcome after Oxford unicompartmental knee arthroplasty at 1 and 5 years. Knee Surg Sports Traumatol Arthrosc. 2013;21:2421–6. https://doi.org/10.1007/s00167-012-2211-3.
12. Scott CEH, Holland G, Krahelski O, et al. Patterns of cartilage loss and anterior cruciate ligament status in end-stage osteoarthritis of the knee. Bone Joint J. 2020;102-B:716–26. https://doi.org/10.1302/0301-620X.102B6.BJJ-2019-1434.R1.
13. Johnson AJ, Howell SM, Costa CR, Mont MA. The ACL in the arthritic knee: how often is it present and can preoperative tests predict its presence? Clin Orthop Relat Res. 2013;471:181–8. https://doi.org/10.1007/s11999-012-2505-2.
14. Hamilton TW, Pandit HG, Inabathula A, et al. Unsatisfactory outcomes following unicompartmental knee arthroplasty in patients with partial thickness cartilage loss: a medium-term follow-up. Bone Joint J. 2017;99-B:475–82. https://doi.org/10.1302/0301-620X.99B4.BJJ-2016-1061.R1.
15. Niinimäki TT, Murray DW, Partanen J, et al. Unicompartmental knee arthroplasties implanted for osteoarthritis with partial loss of joint space have high re-operation rates. Knee. 2011;18:432–5. https://doi.org/10.1016/j.knee.2010.08.004.
16. Pandit H, Gulati A, Jenkins C, et al. Unicompartmental knee replacement for patients with partial thickness cartilage loss in the affected compartment. Knee. 2011;18:168–71. https://doi.org/10.1016/j.knee.2010.05.003.
17. Heurtin T. Evaluation radiographique pré opératoire de la gonarthrose femoro-tibiale médiale: reproductibilité, fiabilité et corrélation avec les atteintes ligamentaires: étude prospective. 2018.
18. Hamilton TW, Choudhary R, Jenkins C, et al. Lateral osteophytes do not represent a contraindication to medial unicompartmental knee arthroplasty: a 15-year follow-up. Knee Surg Sports Traumatol Arthrosc. 2017;25:652–9. https://doi.org/10.1007/s00167-016-4313-9.
19. Pandit H, Spiegelberg B, Clavé A, et al. Aetiology of lateral progression of arthritis following Oxford medial unicompartmental knee replacement: a case-control study. Musculoskelet Surg. 2016;100:97–102. https://doi.org/10.1007/s12306-015-0394-8.
20. Cartier P, Gaggiotti G, Jully JL. [*primary osteonecrosis of the medial femoral condyle. Unicompartmental or total replacement?]. Int Orthop. 1988;12:229–35. https://doi.org/10.1007/BF00547168.
21. Marmor L. Unicompartmental arthroplasty for osteonecrosis of the knee joint. Clin Orthop Relat Res. 1993;294:247–53.
22. Ollivier M, Jacquet C, Lucet A, et al. Long-term results of medial unicompartmental knee arthroplasty for

knee avascular necrosis. J Arthroplast. 2019;34:465–8. https://doi.org/10.1016/j.arth.2018.11.010.

23. Bruni D, Iacono F, Raspugli G, et al. Is unicompartmental arthroplasty an acceptable option for spontaneous osteonecrosis of the knee? Clin Orthop Relat Res. 2012;470:1442–51. https://doi.org/10.1007/s11999-012-2246-2.

24. Fukuoka S, Fukunaga K, Taniura K, et al. Medium-term clinical results of unicompartmental knee arthroplasty for the treatment for spontaneous osteonecrosis of the knee with four to 15 years of follow-up. Knee. 2019;26:1111–6. https://doi.org/10.1016/j.knee.2019.06.007.

25. Langdown AJ, Pandit H, Price AJ, et al. Oxford medial unicompartmental arthroplasty for focal spontaneous osteonecrosis of the knee. Acta Orthop. 2005;76:688–92. https://doi.org/10.1080/17453670510041772.

26. Yoon C, Chang MJ, Chang CB, et al. Does unicompartmental knee arthroplasty have worse outcomes in spontaneous osteonecrosis of the knee than in medial compartment osteoarthritis? A systematic review and meta-analysis. Arch Orthop Trauma Surg. 2019;139:393–403. https://doi.org/10.1007/s00402-019-03125-7.

27. Chalmers BP, Mehrotra KG, Sierra RJ, et al. Reliable outcomes and survivorship of unicompartmental knee arthroplasty for isolated compartment osteonecrosis. Bone Joint J. 2018;100-B:450–4. https://doi.org/10.1302/0301-620X.100B4.BJJ-2017-1041.R2.

28. Carpintero P, Leon F, Zafra M, et al. Spontaneous collapse of the tibial plateau: radiological staging. Skelet Radiol. 2005;34:399–404. https://doi.org/10.1007/s00256-005-0926-7.

29. Kamenaga T, Hiranaka T, Hida Y, et al. Unicompartmental knee arthroplasty for spontaneous osteonecrosis of the medial tibial plateau. Knee. 2018;25:715–21. https://doi.org/10.1016/j.knee.2018.04.006.

30. Yang W-M, Zhao C-Q, Lu Z-Y, et al. Clinical characteristics and treatment of spontaneous osteonecrosis of medial tibial plateau: a retrospective case study. Chin Med J. 2018;131:2544–50. https://doi.org/10.4103/0366-6999.244113.

31. Valenzuela GA, Jacobson NA, Buzas D, et al. Unicompartmental knee replacement after high tibial osteotomy: invalidating a contraindication. Bone Joint J. 2013;95-B:1348–53. https://doi.org/10.1302/0301-620X.95B10.30541.

32. Schlumberger M, Oremek D, Brielmaier M, et al. Prior high tibial osteotomy is not a contraindication for medial unicompartmental knee arthroplasty. Knee Surg Sports Traumatol Arthrosc. 2020;29(10):3279. https://doi.org/10.1007/s00167-020-06149-4.

33. Jones GG, Clarke S, Jaere M, Cobb JP. Failed high tibial osteotomy: a joint preserving alternative to total knee arthroplasty. Orthop Traumatol Surg Res. 2019;105:85–8. https://doi.org/10.1016/j.otsr.2018.11.004.

34. Gicquel T, Lambotte JC, Polard JL, et al. Is tibial cut navigation alone sufficient in medial unicompartmental knee arthroplasty? Continuous series of fifty nine procedures. Int Orthop. 2016;40:2511–8. https://doi.org/10.1007/s00264-016-3241-0.

35. Wada K, Price A, Gromov K, et al. Clinical outcome of bi-unicompartmental knee arthroplasty for both medial and lateral femorotibial arthritis: a systematic review-is there proof of concept? Arch Orthop Trauma Surg. 2020. https://doi.org/10.1007/s00402-020-03492-6.

36. Fuchs S, Tibesku CO, Genkinger M, et al. Proprioception with bicondylar sledge prostheses retaining cruciate ligaments. Clin Orthop Relat Res. 2003;406:148–54. https://doi.org/10.1097/01.blo.0000038053.29678.a5.

37. Lustig S, Lording T, Frank F, et al. Progression of medial osteoarthritis and long-term results of lateral unicompartmental arthroplasty: 10 to 18 year follow-up of 54 consecutive implants. Knee. 2014;21(Suppl 1):S26–32. https://doi.org/10.1016/S0968-0160(14)50006-3.

38. Stern SH, Becker MW, Insall JN. Unicondylar knee arthroplasty. An evaluation of selection criteria. Clin Orthop Relat Res. 1993;286:143–8.

39. Murray DW, Liddle AD, Liddle A, et al. Unicompartmental knee arthroplasty: is the glass half full or half empty? Bone Joint J. 2015;97-B:3–8. https://doi.org/10.1302/0301-620X.97B10.36542.

40. Pandit H, Jenkins C, Gill HS, et al. Unnecessary contraindications for mobile-bearing unicompartmental knee replacement. J Bone Joint Surg Br. 2011;93:622–8. https://doi.org/10.1302/0301-620X.93B5.26214.

41. Hamilton TW, Pandit HG, Jenkins C, et al. Evidence-based indications for mobile-bearing unicompartmental knee arthroplasty in a consecutive cohort of thousand knees. J Arthroplast. 2017;32:1779–85. https://doi.org/10.1016/j.arth.2016.12.036.

42. Murray DW, Pandit H, Weston-Simons JS, et al. Does body mass index affect the outcome of unicompartmental knee replacement? Knee. 2013;20:461–5. https://doi.org/10.1016/j.knee.2012.09.017.

43. Cavaignac E, Lafontan V, Reina N, et al. Obesity has no adverse effect on the outcome of unicompartmental knee replacement at a minimum follow-up of seven years. Bone Joint J. 2013;95-B:1064–8. https://doi.org/10.1302/0301-620X.95B8.31370.

44. Plate JF, Augart MA, Seyler TM, et al. Obesity has no effect on outcomes following unicompartmental knee arthroplasty. Knee Surg Sports Traumatol Arthrosc. 2017;25:645–51. https://doi.org/10.1007/s00167-015-3597-5.

45. Affatato S, Caputo D, Bordini B. Does the body mass index influence the long-term survival of unicompartmental knee prostheses? A retrospective multi-centre study. Int Orthop. 2019;43:1365–70. https://doi.org/10.1007/s00264-018-4217-z.

46. Molloy J, Kennedy J, Jenkins C, et al. Obesity should not be considered a contraindication to medial Oxford UKA: long-term patient-reported outcomes and implant survival in 1000 knees. Knee Surg Sports

Traumatol Arthrosc. 2019;27:2259–65. https://doi.org/10.1007/s00167-018-5218-6.

47. Lum ZC, Crawford DA, Lombardi AV, et al. Early comparative outcomes of unicompartmental and total knee arthroplasty in severely obese patients. Knee. 2018;25:161–6. https://doi.org/10.1016/j.knee.2017.10.006.

48. Lee M, Chen J, Shi LC, et al. No differences in outcomes scores or survivorship of unicompartmental knee arthroplasty between patients younger or older than 55 years of age at minimum 10-year followup. Clin Orthop Relat Res. 2019;477:1434–46. https://doi.org/10.1097/CORR.0000000000000737.

49. Felts E, Parratte S, Pauly V, et al. Function and quality of life following medial unicompartmental knee arthroplasty in patients 60 years of age or younger. Orthop Traumatol Surg Res. 2010;96:861–7. https://doi.org/10.1016/j.otsr.2010.05.012.

50. Greco NJ, Lombardi AV, Price AJ, et al. Medial mobile-bearing unicompartmental knee arthroplasty in young patients aged less than or equal to 50 years. J Arthroplast. 2018;33:2435–9. https://doi.org/10.1016/j.arth.2018.03.069.

51. Heyse TJ, Khefacha A, Peersman G, Cartier P. Survivorship of UKA in the middle-aged. Knee. 2012;19:585–91. https://doi.org/10.1016/j.knee.2011.09.002.

52. Swienckowski JJ, Pennington DW. Unicompartmental knee arthroplasty in patients sixty years of age or younger. J Bone Joint Surg Am. 2004;86-A(Suppl 1):131–42. https://doi.org/10.2106/00004623-200409001-00004.

53. Jeschke E, Gehrke T, Günster C, et al. Five-year survival of 20,946 unicondylar knee replacements and patient risk factors for failure: an analysis of German insurance data. J Bone Joint Surg Am. 2016;98:1691–8. https://doi.org/10.2106/JBJS.15.01060.

54. Liddle AD, Judge A, Pandit H, Murray DW. Determinants of revision and functional outcome following unicompartmental knee replacement. Osteoarthr Cartil. 2014;22:1241–50. https://doi.org/10.1016/j.joca.2014.07.006.

55. Goh GS-H, Bin Abd Razak HR, Tay DK-J, et al. Unicompartmental knee arthroplasty achieves greater flexion with no difference in functional outcome, quality of life, and satisfaction vs total knee arthroplasty in patients younger than 55 years. A propensity score-matched cohort analysis. J Arthroplast. 2018;33:355–61. https://doi.org/10.1016/j.arth.2017.09.022.

56. Engh GA. Orthopaedic crossfire—can we justify unicondylar arthroplasty as a temporizing procedure? In the affirmative. J Arthroplast. 2002;17:54–5. https://doi.org/10.1054/arth.2002.32448.

57. Ali AM, Pandit H, Liddle AD, et al. Does activity affect the outcome of the Oxford unicompartmental knee replacement? Knee. 2016;23:327–30. https://doi.org/10.1016/j.knee.2015.08.001.

58. Crawford DA, Adams JB, Lombardi AV, Berend KR. Activity level does not affect survivorship of unicondylar knee arthroplasty at 5-year minimum follow-up. J Arthroplast. 2019;34:1364–8. https://doi.org/10.1016/j.arth.2019.03.038.

59. Fabre-Aubrespy M, Ollivier M, Pesenti S, et al. Unicompartmental knee arthroplasty in patients older than 75 results in better clinical outcomes and similar survivorship compared to total knee arthroplasty. A matched controlled study. J Arthroplasty. 2016;31:2668–71. https://doi.org/10.1016/j.arth.2016.06.034.

60. Liddle AD, Judge A, Pandit H, Murray DW. Adverse outcomes after total and unicompartmental knee replacement in 101330 matched patients: a study of data from the National Joint Registry for England and Wales. Lancet. 2014. https://doi.org/10.1016/S0140-6736(14)60419-0.

61. Hunt LP, Ben-Shlomo Y, Clark EM, et al. 45-day mortality after 467,779 knee replacements for osteoarthritis from the National Joint Registry for England and Wales: an observational study. Lancet. 2014;384:1429–36. https://doi.org/10.1016/S0140-6736(14)60540-7.

62. Brown NM, Sheth NP, Davis K, et al. Total knee arthroplasty has higher postoperative morbidity than unicompartmental knee arthroplasty: a multicenter analysis. J Arthroplast. 2012;27:86–90. https://doi.org/10.1016/j.arth.2012.03.022.

63. Beard DJ, Pandit H, Ostlere S, et al. Pre-operative clinical and radiological assessment of the patellofemoral joint in unicompartmental knee replacement and its influence on outcome. J Bone Joint Surg Br. 2007;89:1602–7. https://doi.org/10.1302/0301-620X.89B12.19260.

64. Hamilton TW, Pandit HG, Maurer DG, et al. Anterior knee pain and evidence of osteoarthritis of the patellofemoral joint should not be considered contra-indications to mobile-bearing unicompartmental knee arthroplasty: a 15-year follow-up. Bone Joint J. 2017;99-B:632–9. https://doi.org/10.1302/0301-620X.99B5.BJJ-2016-0695.R2.

65. Cook C, Mabry L, Reiman MP, Hegedus EJ. Best tests/clinical findings for screening and diagnosis of patellofemoral pain syndrome: a systematic review. Physiotherapy. 2012;98:93–100. https://doi.org/10.1016/j.physio.2011.09.001.

66. Kang SN, Smith TO, Sprenger De Rover WB, Walton NP. Pre-operative patellofemoral degenerative changes do not affect the outcome after medial Oxford unicompartmental knee replacement: a report from an independent centre. J Bone Joint Surg Br. 2011;93:476–8. https://doi.org/10.1302/0301-620X.93B4.25562.

67. Lim JW-A, Chen JY, Chong HC, et al. Pre-existing patellofemoral disease does not affect 10-year survivorship in fixed bearing unicompartmental knee arthroplasty. Knee Surg Sports Traumatol Arthrosc. 2019;27:2030–6. https://doi.org/10.1007/s00167-018-5169-y.

68. Deckard ER, Jansen K, Ziemba-Davis M, et al. Does patellofemoral disease affect outcomes in con-

temporary medial fixed-bearing unicompartmental knee arthroplasty? J Arthroplast. 2020. https://doi.org/10.1016/j.arth.2020.03.007.

69. Berend KR, Lombardi AV, Morris MJ, et al. Does preoperative patellofemoral joint state affect medial unicompartmental arthroplasty survival? Orthopedics. 2011;34:e494–6. https://doi.org/10.3928/01477447-20110714-39.

70. Munk S, Odgaard A, Madsen F, et al. Preoperative lateral subluxation of the patella is a predictor of poor early outcome of Oxford phase-III medial unicompartmental knee arthroplasty. Acta Orthop. 2011;82:582–8. https://doi.org/10.3109/17453674.2011.618915.

71. Burger JA, Kleeblad LJ, Laas N, Pearle AD. The influence of preoperative radiographic patellofemoral degenerative changes and malalignment on patellofemoral-specific outcome scores following fixed-bearing medial unicompartmental knee arthroplasty. J Bone Joint Surg Am. 2019;101:1662–9. https://doi.org/10.2106/JBJS.18.01385.

72. Beard DJ, Pandit H, Gill HS, et al. The influence of the presence and severity of pre-existing patellofemoral degenerative changes on the outcome of the Oxford medial unicompartmental knee replacement. J Bone Joint Surg Br. 2007;89:1597–601. https://doi.org/10.1302/0301-620X.89B12.19259.

73. Adams AJ, Kazarian GS, Lonner JH. Preoperative patellofemoral chondromalacia is not a contraindication for fixed-bearing medial unicompartmental knee arthroplasty. J Arthroplast. 2017;32:1786–91. https://doi.org/10.1016/j.arth.2017.01.002.

74. Berger Y, Ftaita S, Thienpont E. Does medial patellofemoral osteoarthritis influence outcome scores and risk of revision after fixed-bearing unicompartmental knee arthroplasty? Clin Orthop Relat Res. 2019;477:2041–7. https://doi.org/10.1097/CORR.0000000000000738.

75. Konan S, Haddad FS. Does location of patellofemoral chondral lesion influence outcome after Oxford medial compartmental knee arthroplasty? Bone Joint J. 2016;98-B:11–5. https://doi.org/10.1302/0301-620X.98B10.BJJ-2016-0403.R1.

76. Kumar V, Pandit HG, Liddle AD, et al. Comparison of outcomes after UKA in patients with and without chondrocalcinosis: a matched cohort study. Knee Surg Sports Traumatol Arthrosc. 2017;25:319–24. https://doi.org/10.1007/s00167-015-3578-8.

77. Hernigou P, Pascale W, Pascale V, et al. Does primary or secondary chondrocalcinosis influence long-term survivorship of unicompartmental arthroplasty? Clin Orthop Relat Res. 2012;470:1973–9. https://doi.org/10.1007/s11999-011-2211-5.

78. Goodfellow J, O'Connor J. The anterior cruciate ligament in knee arthroplasty. A risk-factor with unconstrained meniscal prostheses. Clin Orthop Relat Res. 1992;276:245–52.

79. Deschamps G, Lapeyre B. [Rupture of the anterior cruciate ligament: a frequently unrecognized cause of failure of unicompartmental knee prostheses. Apropos of a series of 79 Lotus prostheses with a follow-up of more than 5 years]. Rev Chir Orthop Reparatrice Appar Mot. 1987;73:544–51.

80. Suggs JF, Li G, Park SE, et al. Knee biomechanics after UKA and its relation to the ACL—a robotic investigation. J Orthop Res. 2006;24:588–94. https://doi.org/10.1002/jor.20082.

81. Blunn GW, Walker PS, Joshi A, Hardinge K. The dominance of cyclic sliding in producing wear in total knee replacements. Clin Orthop Relat Res. 1991;273:253–60.

82. Adulkasem N, Rojanasthien S, Siripocaratana N, Limmahakhun S. Posterior tibial slope modification in osteoarthritis knees with different ACL conditions: cadaveric study of fixed-bearing UKA. J Orthop Surg (Hong Kong). 2019;27:2309499019836286. https://doi.org/10.1177/2309499019836286.

83. Zumbrunn T, Schütz P, von Knoch F, et al. Medial unicompartmental knee arthroplasty in ACL-deficient knees is a viable treatment option: in vivo kinematic evaluation using a moving fluoroscope. Knee Surg Sports Traumatol Arthrosc. 2020;28:1765–73. https://doi.org/10.1007/s00167-019-05594-0.

84. Hernigou P, Deschamps G. Posterior slope of the tibial implant and the outcome of unicompartmental knee arthroplasty. J Bone Joint Surg Am. 2004;86-A:506–11.

85. Suero EM, Citak M, Cross MB, et al. Effects of tibial slope changes in the stability of fixed bearing medial unicompartmental arthroplasty in anterior cruciate ligament deficient knees. Knee. 2012;19:365–9. https://doi.org/10.1016/j.knee.2011.07.004.

86. Engh GA, Ammeen DJ. Unicondylar arthroplasty in knees with deficient anterior cruciate ligaments. Clin Orthop Relat Res. 2014;472:73–7. https://doi.org/10.1007/s11999-013-2982-y.

87. Boissonneault A, Pandit H, Pegg E, et al. No difference in survivorship after unicompartmental knee arthroplasty with or without an intact anterior cruciate ligament. Knee Surg Sports Traumatol Arthrosc. 2013;21:2480–6. https://doi.org/10.1007/s00167-012-2101-8.

88. Pandit H, Beard DJ, Jenkins C, et al. Combined anterior cruciate reconstruction and Oxford unicompartmental knee arthroplasty. J Bone Joint Surg Br. 2006;88:887–92. https://doi.org/10.1302/0301-620X.88B7.17847.

89. Tinius M, Hepp P, Becker R. Combined unicompartmental knee arthroplasty and anterior cruciate ligament reconstruction. Knee Surg Sports Traumatol Arthrosc. 2012;20:81–7. https://doi.org/10.1007/s00167-011-1528-7.

90. Volpin A, Kini SG, Meuffels DE. Satisfactory outcomes following combined unicompartmental knee replacement and anterior cruciate ligament reconstruction. Knee Surg Sports Traumatol Arthrosc. 2018;26:2594–601. https://doi.org/10.1007/s00167-017-4536-4.

91. Tecame A, Savica R, Rosa MA, Adravanti P. Anterior cruciate ligament reconstruction in association with

medial unicompartmental knee replacement: a retrospective study comparing clinical and radiological outcomes of two different implant design. Int Orthop. 2019;43:2731–7. https://doi.org/10.1007/s00264-019-04341-x.

92. Ventura A, Legnani C, Terzaghi C, et al. Unicompartmental knee replacement combined to anterior cruciate ligament reconstruction: mid-term results. J Knee Surg. 2019. https://doi.org/10.1055/s-0039-1692647.

93. Tian S, Wang B, Wang Y, et al. Combined unicompartmental knee arthroplasty and anterior cruciate ligament reconstruction in knees with osteoarthritis and deficient anterior cruciate ligament. BMC Musculoskelet Disord. 2016;17:327. https://doi.org/10.1186/s12891-016-1186-5.

94. Iriberri I, Suau S, Payán L, Aragón JF. Long-term deterioration after one-stage unicompartmental knee arthroplasty and anterior cruciate ligament reconstruction. Musculoskelet Surg. 2019;103:251–6. https://doi.org/10.1007/s12306-018-0582-4.

95. Castoldi M, Magnussen RA, Gunst S, et al. A randomized controlled trial of bone-patellar tendon-bone anterior cruciate ligament reconstruction with and without lateral extra-articular tenodesis: 19-year clinical and radiological follow-up. Am J Sports Med. 2020;48:1665–72. https://doi.org/10.1177/0363546520914936.

96. Saithna A, Thaunat M, Delaloye JR, et al. Combined ACL and anterolateral ligament reconstruction. JBJS Essent Surg Tech. 2018;8:e2. https://doi.org/10.2106/JBJS.ST.17.00045.

How to Deal with a Fixed-Bearing Medial Unicompartmental Knee Arthroplasty Implant? **6**

Camille Steltzlen and Nicolas Pujol

The concept of unicompartmental knee arthroplasty was proposed by McKeever and MacIntosh in the USA in the 1950s [1]. It was then developed by Marmor [2], who introduced the concept of modular resurfacing arthroplasty. In France, Philippe Cartier, Philippe Hernigou, and Gérard Deschamps were the first to popularise this procedure. At the SOFCOT symposium in 1996, they established solid foundations for its indications and surgical technique [3, 4].

The surgical indication and preoperative planning are key factors to the procedure's success. A precise, reliable, and reproducible surgical technique will make it possible to obtain a satisfactory functional result, as well as prolonged lifespan of the implant. In order to achieve precise and reproducible placement quality, it appears that an orthopaedic surgeon would need to perform about 40 knee arthroplasties per year [5–7]. An orthopaedic knee surgeon should know how to establish the indication and perform unicompartmental arthroplasty correctly; to do so, s/he will need to follow a learning curve and acquire experience. In this chapter, we will describe the principles for placement of metal-backed fixed-bearing unicompartmental knee arthroplasties [8]. The choice of a full-polyethylene tibial implant only or metal-backed tibial implant remains debated; results are divergent. Nevertheless, it seems that the latest clinical results support metal-backed tibial implants [7, 9, 10]. In contrast, studies on the fixation of cemented or cementless implants have not shown any significant difference [11, 12]. Based on Gérard Deschamps's arguments, we also prefer an implant based on cuts rather than a resurfacing one. Since wear is mainly tibial, the use of resurfacing arthroplasty may risk lowering the articulation by an increase in femoral displacement [13].

This chapter is divided into two parts. In the first part, we will detail the preoperative planning based on analysis of the radiological assessment and in the second part, we will discuss the surgical technique.

6.1 Preoperative Planning

The objective is to reproduce the articulation's orientation in both the frontal and sagittal planes. Changes have been made in the last few years with the adoption of the concept of anatomical implants whose technique makes it possible to reproduce the initial knee deformity prior to wear progression. Therefore, it must be tailored to each patient's anatomy.

C. Steltzlen (✉) · N. Pujol
Service de Chirurgie Orthopédique et Traumatologique, Centre Hospitalier de Versailles, Le Chesnay, France
e-mail: csteltzlen@ch-versailles.fr

6.1.1 Tibial and Femoral Bone Cuts

The different bone cuts, particularly tibial cut, must have been planned based on the imaging assessment. The assessment should consist of an AP, sagittal views and weightbearing X-rays. A skyline view (at 30° flexion) is also necessary, even though the presence of osteophyte is not a contraindication to UKA if the joint is asymptomatic [14, 15]. Full-length lower limb X-ray is the key investigation in preoperative planning. It will assess the overall deformity of the lower limb. The objective is to determine the origin of the deformity, constitutional or acquired, in order to correct wear only. Some authors recommend dynamic X-rays to verify reducibility of the deformity. We do not use them.

6.1.1.1 Coronal Plane

One factor often emphasised is the notion of postoperative undercorrection. In our opinion, restoration of the anatomy is more relevant. The goal is not to take a fixed value as the postoperative objective, but to restore the initial deformity by correcting wear only [16–19]. Nevertheless, a postoperative deformity should remain limited. It may be located between 7° and 10° of the overall deformity [17]. The persistence of a major postoperative deformity can carry a risk of increasing the rate of early implant failure [20–22]. In order to assess the resection height, it is first necessary to determine an objective for the final deformity. For example, if the initial deformity is 9° varus and the targeted final deformity is 3° varus, the axis would need to be corrected by 6°. In arthroplasties with dependent cuts, the axis is corrected by a single tibial cut. In order to correct the axis by 6° using a tibial implant with a minimal thickness of 8 mm, it is necessary to resect 2 mm of bone on the tibial side. After assessing the resection height, it is necessary to assess the angle of inclination in the tibial section plane (Figs. 6.1 and 6.2) [23]. This incline should also be fol-

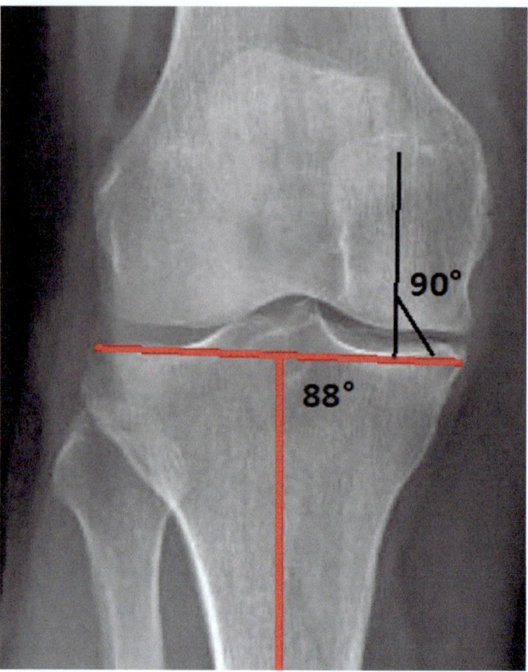

Fig. 6.1 Angle of the tibial cut, which in this example is at 88°

lowed during the conduct of femoral distal and posterior cuts. They should be parallel to the tibial cut to avoid positioning on the femoral implant's edges in flexion and extension.

6.1.1.2 Sagittal Plane

The tibial slope should also be assessed preoperatively and restored at the end of the procedure (Figs. 6.3 and 6.4). A decrease would have the effect of closing the space for flexion, limiting flexion movements, and increasing stress on the posterior part of the tibial plateau with an increased risk of implant loosening. An excessive increase would multiply the tension on the anterior cruciate ligament at the risk of rupture and decreasing the space in extension, and therefore limiting extension movements [24]. Then between 4° and 8° of postoperative posterior slope is recommended [25].

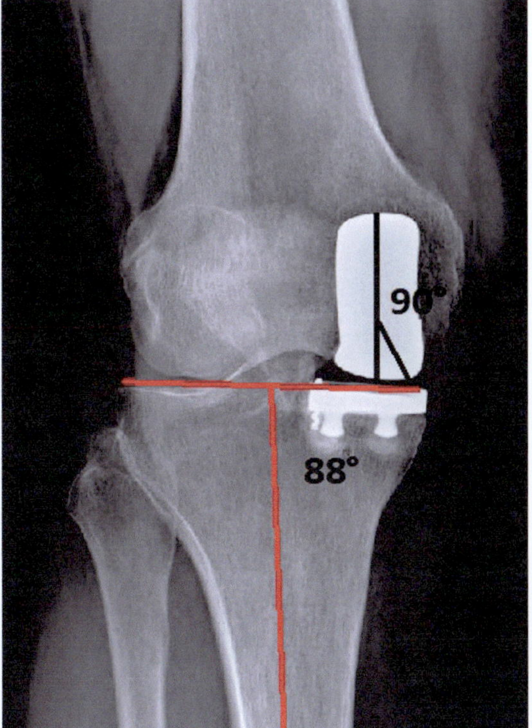

Fig. 6.2 Postoperative restoration of the tibial coronal plane inclination

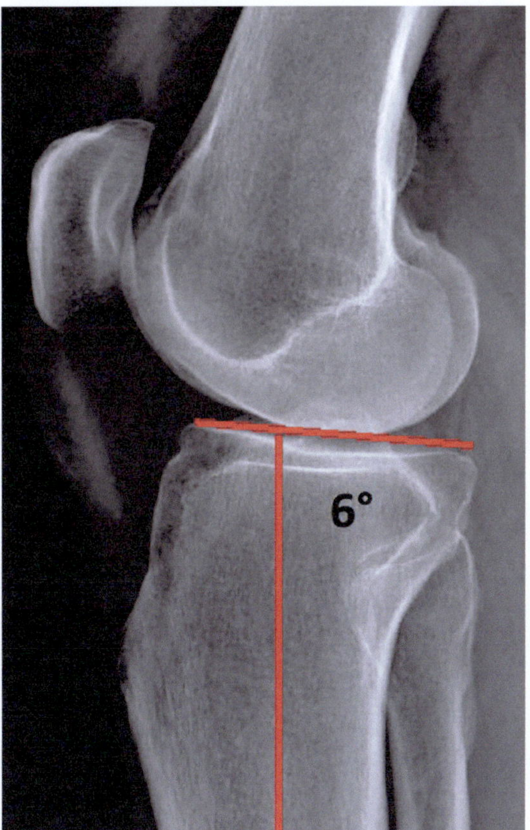

Fig. 6.3 Preoperative assessment of the tibial slope

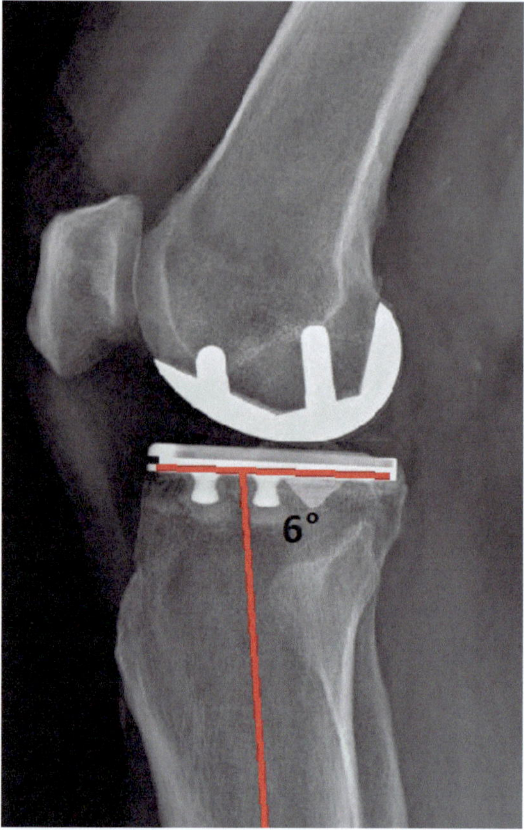

Fig. 6.4 Postoperative restoration of the tibial slope

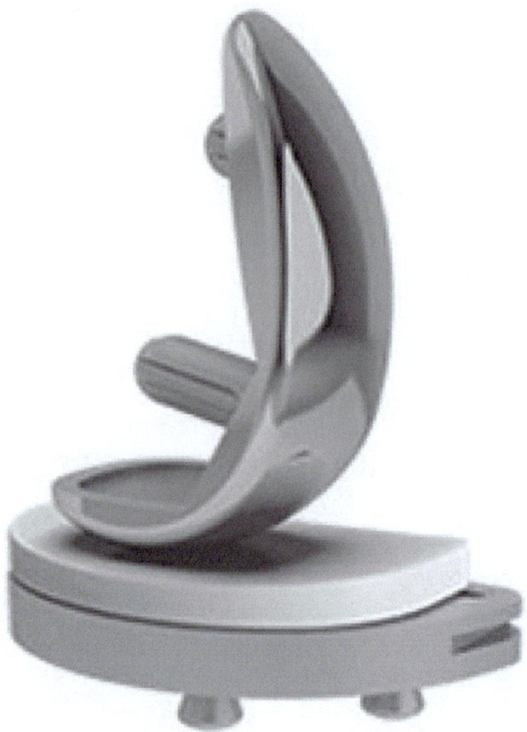

Fig. 6.5 Physica ZUK Lima Corporate® insert (courtesy of LIMA)

6.2 Surgical Technique

In this section, we will describe a surgical technique for dependent cuts arthroplasty derived from the Miller–Galante arthroplasty technique (Fig. 6.5).

6.2.1 Approach

A medial parapatellar approach is used. The incision starts at the upper border of the patella and extends up to the ATT (anterior tibial tuberosity) (Fig. 6.6). It is performed through the medial patellar flange. It can sometimes be necessary to increase the size of the approach by going through fibres of the vastus medialis over about 1 cm in order to dislocate the patella more easily. In a second phase, it is necessary to expose the medial tibial plateau without releasing the medial collat-

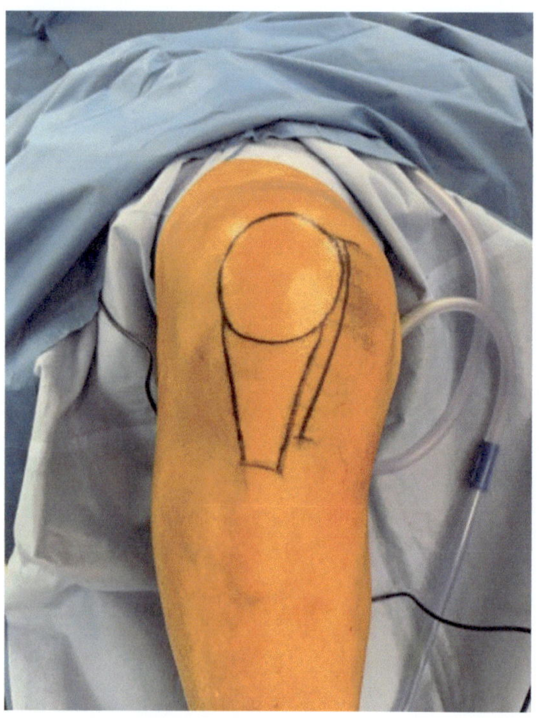

Fig. 6.6 Parapatellar approach

eral ligament, which could result in a tendency to overcorrect the deformity by increasing the polyethylene in response to the ligament laxity induced by its release. For that, a double-bend retractor is inserted just under the collar of the tibial osteophytes, without prior release, and this is amply sufficient to expose it. Osteophytes in the tibia and femur are removed. This stage is important to facilitate correction of the acquired deformity and enable good implant positioning in the frontal plane. The femoral implant should be positioned close to the intercondylar notch so that it is opposite the tibial implant. Excision of osteophytes from the intercondylar notch may also correct a slight preoperative flexion deformity.

6.2.2 Tibial Resection

Cuts are dependent.

First, tibial resection is performed. It is necessary to calculate preoperatively the targeted final postoperative deformity. Thus, we should be able to determine the height of tibia cut, which alone prefigures the amount of correction when using dependent cuts implants.

6.2.2.1 In the Coronal Plane

The surgeon starts by placing the extramedullary cutting guide with the knee in 90° flexion. At this stage, it is necessary that the resection plane reproduces the physiological tibial coronal angle (Fig. 6.2). To reproduce this angle in moderate deformities, the surgeon can align the ancillary material with the tibial crest by modulating adjustment at the level of the malleolar clamp (Fig. 6.7). A probe is then introduced into the section guide and the bottom of the bone cup, which will enable bone resection of the height planned preoperatively (Fig. 6.8).

6.2.2.2 In the Sagittal Plane

Assessment of the tibial slope is an important stage. The objective is to reproduce the physi-

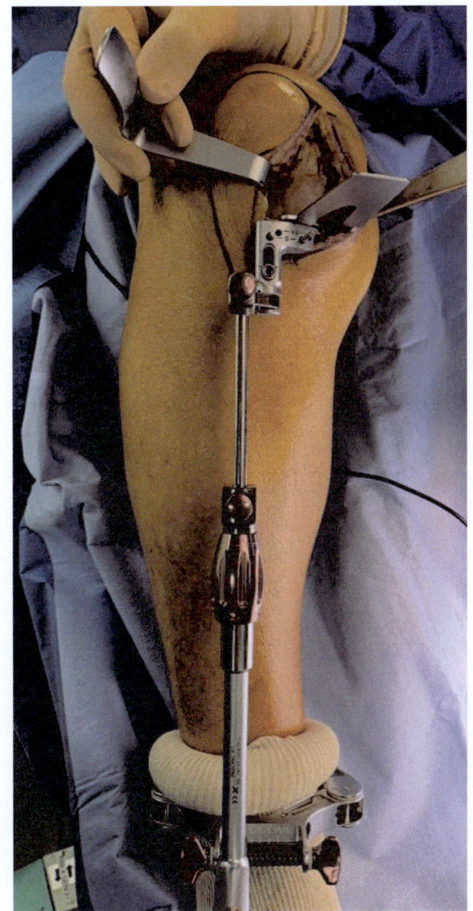

Fig. 6.7 Extramedullary viewfinder aligned on the tibial crest

ological slope. After assessing the level of resection, a pin is introduced into the section guide to verify its sagittal axis and check that it follows the native tibial slope (Fig. 6.9). Vertical cut is then performed, first using a sagittal saw. It should leave the tibial spine intact, particularly insertion of the anterior cruciate ligament. The axis of this section should follow the axis of the lateral wall of the medial condyle.

The tibial plateau is removed with the knee in slight flexion. The quantity removed should not be greater posteriorly. It reflects the future tibial slope of the implant.

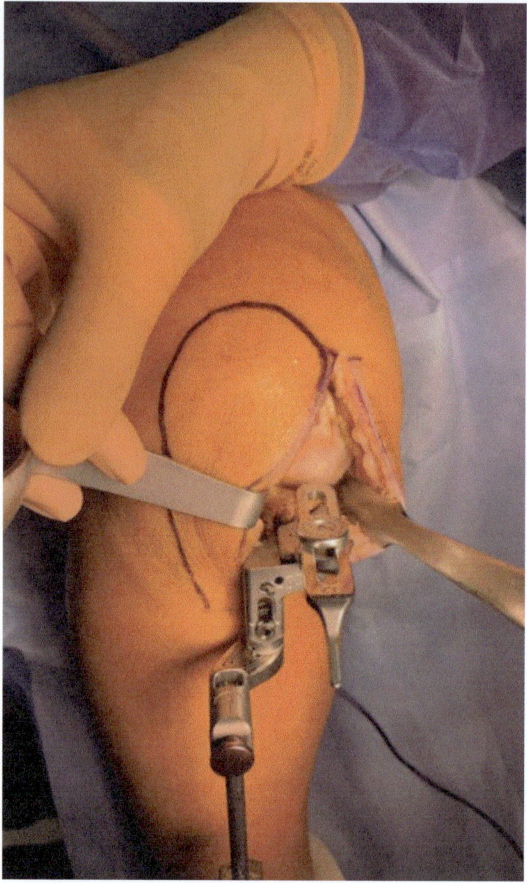

Fig. 6.8 Stylus used to evaluate the cut level

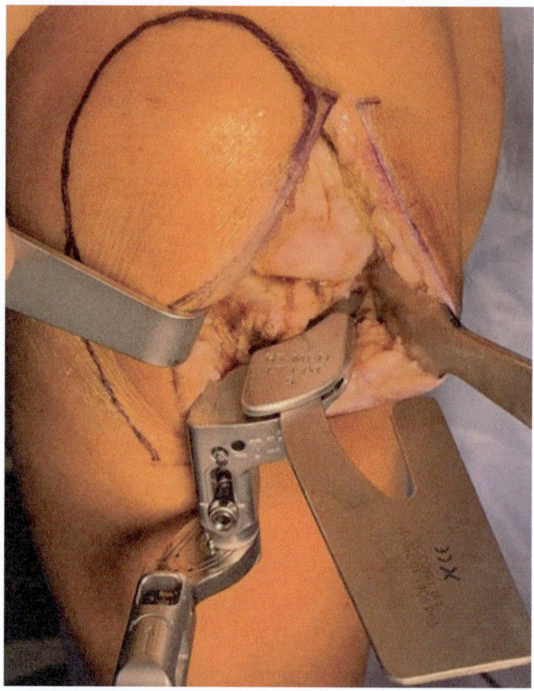

Fig. 6.9 Control of the cut height and tibial slope

6.2.3 Femoral Cuts

6.2.3.1 Distal Femoral Cut

In the frontal plane, both the distal femoral and the tibial cut are dependent on each other. It is performed with the knee in complete extension to avoid creating a flexion or recurvatum deformity in the cut (Fig. 6.10). Its height is defined by the instrumentation; it corresponds to the thickness of the femoral implant. The distal femoral cutting guide is fixed on an adjustable height spacer (Fig. 6.11). It starts at 8 mm, which is the minimum implant thickness. At this stage, it is possible to assess the final deformity and residual ligament laxity. If the space is deemed too tight, it is necessary to cut the tibia again. If excessive laxity is found, the thickness can be increased using a 1-mm increments spacer. In cases of major residual laxity with excess wear on the

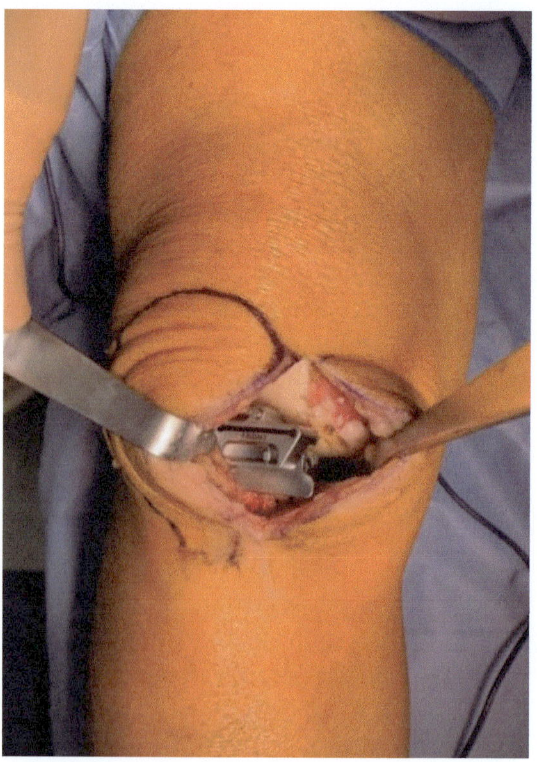

Fig. 6.10 Distal femoral cut with the knee in extension

6.2.3.2 Posterior Femoral Cut

After removing the distal femoral cut, the size of the femoral implant is assessed. The implant should not overflow the anterior border of the distal cut (Fig. 6.12). After determining its size, the section guide is placed with the knee in 90° flexion. The implant should be positioned in the coronal plane near the (intercondylar) notch so that the femoral component will be in the middle of the tibial component (Fig. 6.13). The posterior cut should be parallel to the tibial cut to avoid edge loading of the femoral component in flexion.

6.2.4 Finalisation of the Tibia and Testing

After evaluating the size of the tibia, anchoring points are made in the tibial bone.

We recommend verifying the anteroposterior position of the tibial implant. It should be positioned on the anterior cortex of the tibia to avoid subsequent sinking of the implant. Such tibial sinking is possible, particularly in cases of osteoporotic bone, and this generally occurs in its anterior part. Trial implants are then inserted into the tibia and femur. It is necessary to place the tibial insert on the tibial baseplate at a height defined with the tibial spacer used during the distal femoral cut. This height starts at 8 mm and increases by 1-mm increments. After inserting the implants, the existence of physiological laxity must be verified. In fact, there has not been any ligament release in this approach and the implant only corrects wear (which is the purpose of this type of implant and technique); there is no residual laxity and the knee has a near-normal ligament kinematic presentation. The positioning of the implants is also checked. The femoral implant should be parallel to the tibial implant in extension and flexion and should be in the middle of the tibia (Figs. 6.14 and 6.15).

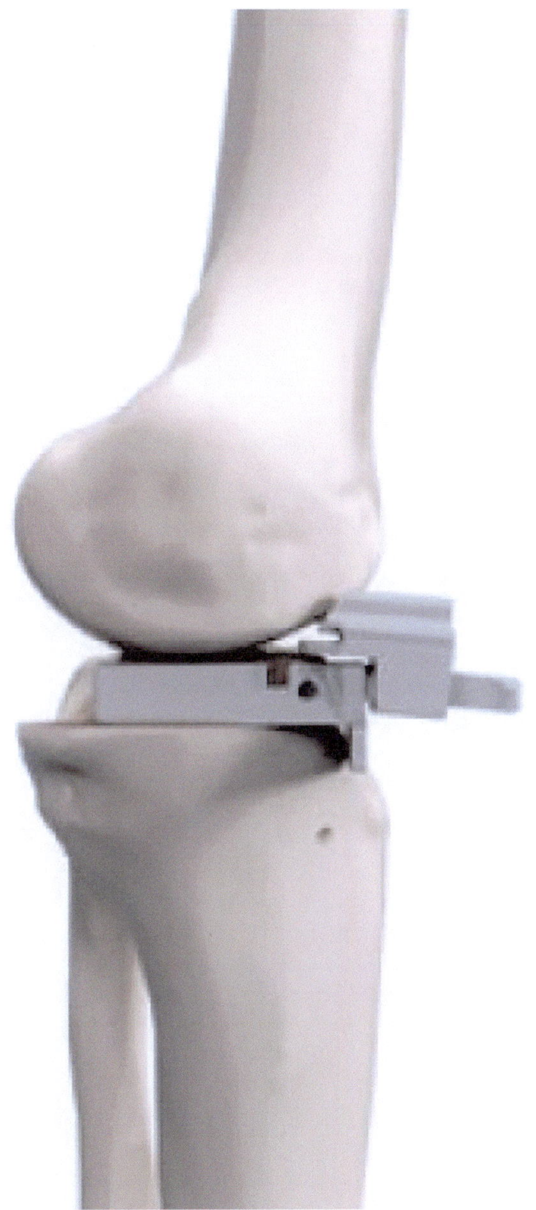

Fig. 6.11 Distal femoral cut spacer (courtesy of LIMA)

femur, it is possible to use 1- or 2-mm femoral blocks. Using these blocks will have the effect of decreasing femoral cut to distalize the femoral implant without raising the joint line, which would occur if the tibial spacer was increased.

Fig. 6.12 Control of the size of femoral implant (courtesy of LIMA)

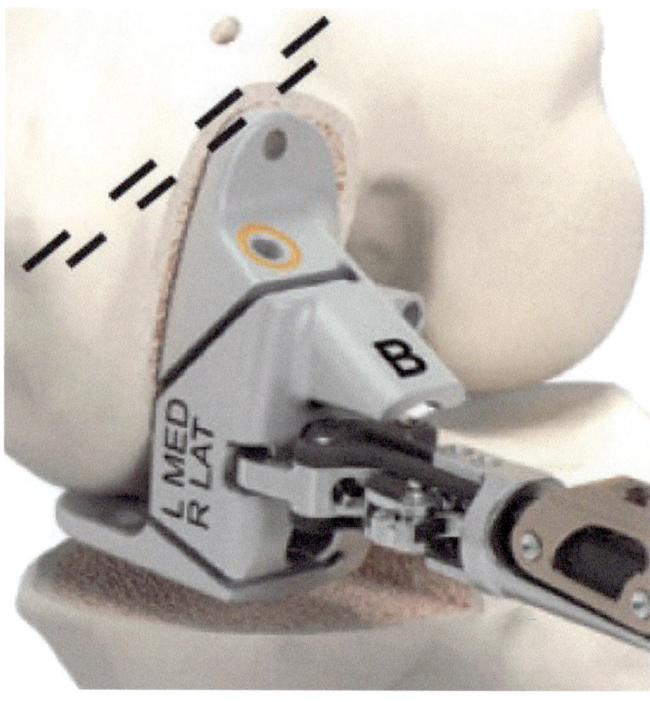

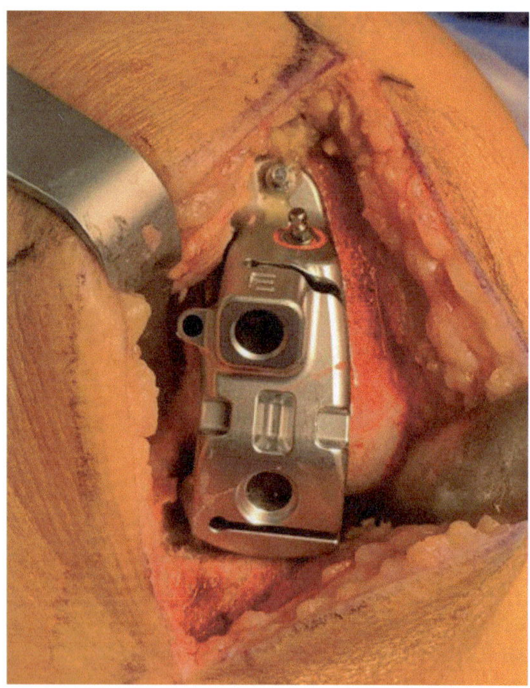

Fig. 6.13 Positioning close to the notch in the femoral cut guide

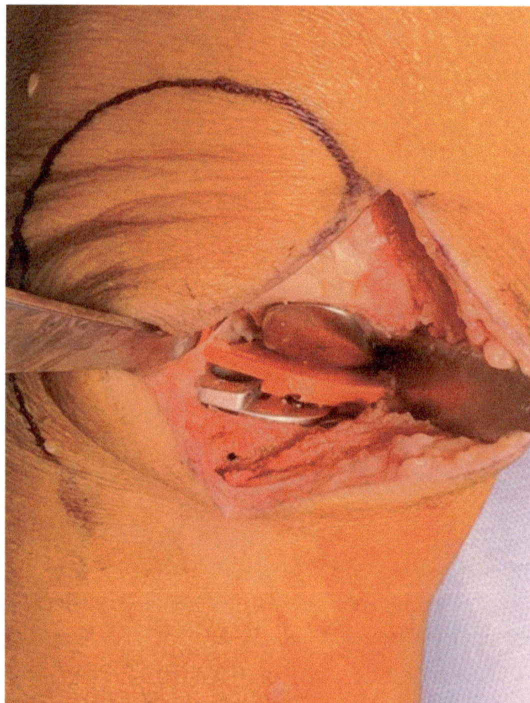

Fig. 6.14 Trial in extension

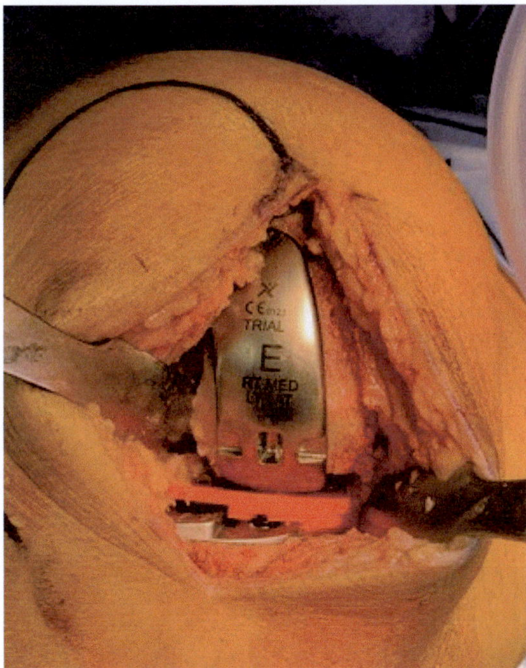

Fig. 6.15 Trial in flexion

6.3 Conclusion

A good surgical indication, precise preoperative planning, and reliable placement technique are the three essential factors to obtain good reproducible results in the medium and long terms [26–30]. Twenty percent of our indications for knee replacements are unicompartmental knee arthroplasties. It is also possible to perform this procedure at the same time on both knees with morbidity equivalent to total knee arthroplasty in a single knee [31].

References

1. Johal S, Nakano N, Baxter M, Hujazi I, Pandit H, Khanduja V. Unicompartmental knee arthroplasty: the past, current controversies, and future perspectives. J Knee Surg. 2018;31(10):992–8.
2. Marmor L. Marmor modular knee in unicompartmental disease. Minimum four-year follow-up. J Bone Joint Surg Am. 1979;61(3):347–53.
3. Cartier P, Cheaib S. Unicondylar knee arthroplasty. 2–10 years of follow-up evaluation. J Arthroplast. 1987;2(2):157–62.
4. Hernigou P, Deschamps G. Les prothéses unicompartimentales du genou. Symposium 70° Reunion annuelle de la SOFCOT. Rev Chir Orthop Reparatrice Appar Mot. 1996;82(1 Suppl):23–60.
5. Badawy M, Fenstad AM, Bartz-Johannessen CA, Indrekvam K, Havelin LI, Robertsson O, et al. Hospital volume and the risk of revision in Oxford unicompartmental knee arthroplasty in the Nordic countries –an observational study of 14,496 cases. BMC Musculoskelet Disord. 2017;18(1):388.
6. Badawy M, Espehaug B, Indrekvam K, Havelin LI, Furnes O. Higher revision risk for unicompartmental knee arthroplasty in low-volume hospitals. Acta Orthop. 2014;85(4):342–7.
7. Zambianchi F, Digennaro V, Giorgini A, Grandi G, Fiacchi F, Mugnai R, et al. Surgeon's experience influences UKA survivorship: a comparative study between all-poly and metal back designs. Knee Surg Sports Traumatol Arthrosc. 2015;23(7):2074–80.
8. Baur J, Zwicky L, Hirschmann MT, Ilchmann T, Clauss M. Metal backed fixed-bearing unicondylar knee arthroplasties using minimal invasive surgery: a promising outcome analysis of 132 cases. BMC Musculoskelet Disord. 2015;16(1):177.
9. Hutt JRB, Farhadnia P, Massé V, LaVigne M, Vendittoli P-A. A randomised trial of all-polyethylene and metal-backed tibial components in unicompartmental arthroplasty of the knee. Bone Joint J. 2015;97-B(6):786–92.
10. Koh IJ, Suhl KH, Kim MW, Kim MS, Choi KY, In Y. Use of all-polyethylene tibial components in unicompartmental knee arthroplasty increases the risk of early failure. J Knee Surg. 2017;30(8):807–15.
11. Kerens B, Schotanus MGM, Boonen B, Boog P, Emans PJ, Lacroix H, et al. Cementless versus cemented Oxford unicompartmental knee arthroplasty: early results of a non-designer user group. Knee Surg Sports Traumatol Arthrosc. 2017;25(3):703–9.
12. Campi S, Pandit HG, Dodd C, Murray DW. Cementless fixation in medial unicompartmental knee arthroplasty: a systematic review. Knee Surg Sports Traumatol Arthrosc. 2017;25(3):736–45.
13. Deschamps G, Chol C. Fixed-bearing unicompartmental knee arthroplasty. Patients' selection and operative technique. Orthop Traumatol Surg Res. 2011;97(6):648–61.
14. Adams AJ, Kazarian GS, Lonner JH. Preoperative patellofemoral chondromalacia is not a contraindication for fixed-bearing medial unicompartmental knee arthroplasty. J Arthroplast. 2017;32(6):1786–91.
15. Lim JW-A, Chen JY, Chong HC, Pang HN, Tay DKJ, Chia S-L, et al. Pre-existing patellofemoral disease does not affect 10-year survivorship in fixed bearing unicompartmental knee arthroplasty. Knee Surg Sports Traumatol Arthrosc. 2019;27(6):2030–6.

16. Zuiderbaan HA, van der List JP, Chawla H, Khamaisy S, Thein R, Pearle AD. Predictors of subjective outcome after medial unicompartmental knee arthroplasty. J Arthroplast. 2016;31(7):1453–8.
17. Hernigou P, Deschamps G. Alignment influences wear in the knee after medial unicompartmental arthroplasty. Clin Orthop. 2004;423:161–5.
18. Kim KT, Lee S, Kim TW, Lee JS, Boo KH. The influence of postoperative tibiofemoral alignment on the clinical results of unicompartmental knee arthroplasty. Knee Surg Relat Res. 2012;24(2):85–90.
19. Perkins TR, Gunckle W. Unicompartmental knee arthroplasty: 3- to 10-year results in a community hospital setting. J Arthroplast. 2002;17(3):293–7.
20. Vasso M, Del Regno C, D'Amelio A, Viggiano D, Corona K, Schiavone PA. Minor varus alignment provides better results than neutral alignment in medial UKA. Knee. 2015;22(2):117–21.
21. Gulati A, Pandit H, Jenkins C, Chau R, Dodd C, Murray DW. The effect of leg alignment on the outcome of unicompartmental knee replacement. J Bone Joint Surg Br. 2009;91(4):469–74.
22. Gulati A, Chau R, Simpson DJ, Dodd C, Gill HS, Murray DW. Influence of component alignment on outcome for unicompartmental knee replacement. Knee. 2009;16(3):196–9.
23. Asada S, Inoue S, Tsukamoto I, Mori S, Akagi M. Obliquity of tibial component after unicompartmental knee arthroplasty. Knee. 2019;26(2):410–5.
24. Takayama K, Matsumoto T, Muratsu H, Ishida K, Araki D, Matsushita T, et al. The influence of posterior tibial slope changes on joint gap and range of motion in unicompartmental knee arthroplasty. Knee. 2016;23(3):517–22.
25. Weber P, Schröder C, Schwiesau J, Utzschneider S, Steinbrück A, Pietschmann MF, et al. Increase in the tibial slope reduces wear after medial unicompartmental fixed-bearing arthroplasty of the knee. Biomed Res Int. 2015;2015:736826.
26. Biswal S, Brighton RW. Results of unicompartmental knee arthroplasty with cemented, fixed-bearing prosthesis using minimally invasive surgery. J Arthroplast. 2010;25(5):721–7.
27. Winnock de Grave P, Barbier J, Luyckx T, Ryckaert A, Gunst P, Van den Daelen L. Outcomes of a fixed-bearing, medial, cemented unicondylar knee arthroplasty design: survival analysis and functional score of 460 cases. J Arthroplasty. 2018;33(9):2792–9.
28. Argenson J-NA, Blanc G, Aubaniac J-M, Parratte S. Modern unicompartmental knee arthroplasty with cement: a concise follow-up, at a mean of twenty years, of a previous report. J Bone Joint Surg Am. 2013;95(10):905–9.
29. Parratte S, Ollivier M, Lunebourg A, Abdel MP, Argenson J-N. Long-term results of compartmental arthroplasties of the knee: long term results of partial knee arthroplasty. Bone Joint J. 2015;97-B(10 Suppl A):9–15.
30. Kim KT, Lee S, Lee JS, Kang MS, Koo KH. Long-term clinical results of unicompartmental knee arthroplasty in patients younger than 60 years of age: minimum 10-year follow-up. Knee Surg Relat Res. 2018;30(1):28–33.
31. Siedlecki C, Beaufils P, Lemaire B, Pujol N. Complications and cost of single-stage vs. two-stage bilateral unicompartmental knee arthroplasty: a case-control study. Orthop Traumatol Surg Res. 2018;104(7):949–53.

Principles of the Oxford® (Zimmer Biomet) Unicompartmental Knee Arthroplasty (OUKA)

François Hardeman and Arnaud Clavé

7.1 Introduction

This chapter describes the principles relating to placement of the Oxford® (Zimmer Biomet) unicompartmental knee replacement. The technique and philosophy described here are based on the instrumentation and fourth-generation implants known as Microplasty®.

The Oxford® knee arthroplasty is unique in design and philosophy. It enables rolling/sliding biomechanics via its mobile polyethylene (PE) insert, which has a dual articulation: its flat surface articulates with the flat tibial implant (metal back) on the one side and its concave upper part articulates fully congruently with the spherical femoral component (Fig. 7.1) on the other. When

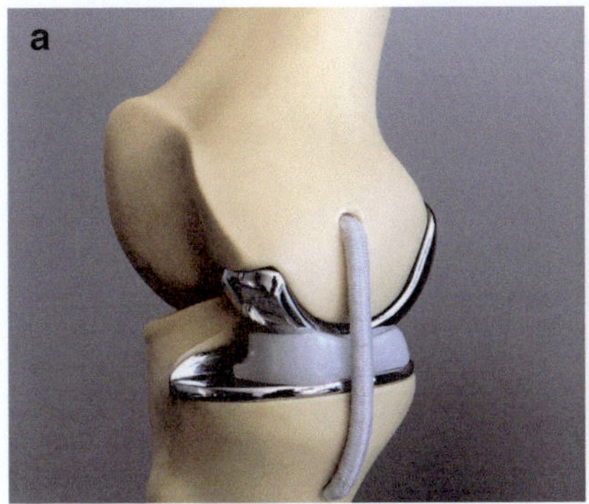

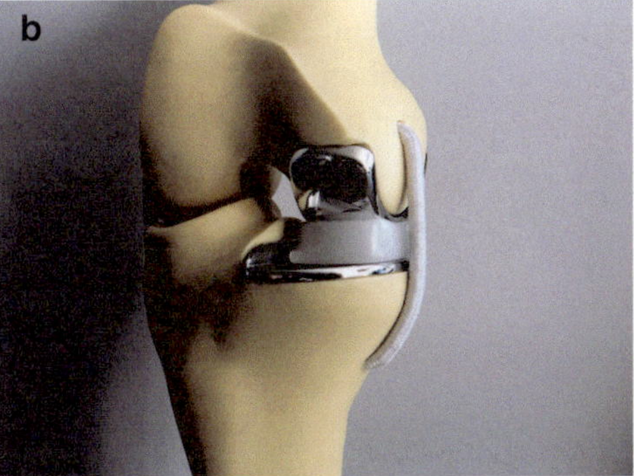

Fig. 7.1 Oxford® unicompartmental knee arthroplasty with mobile bearing (**a**) 3/ view of an Oxford® unicompartmental knee in a bone model (**b**) frontal view of an Oxford® unicompartmental knee in a bone model

F. Hardeman
Department of Orthopaedic Surgery and
Traumatology, Jan Ypermanziekenhuis,
Ypres, Belgium

A. Clavé (✉)
Department of Orthopaedic Surgery and
Traumatology, Saint George Private Hospital,
Nice, France

LaTIM, INSERM-UBO UMR 1101, Brest, France

© The Author(s), under exclusive license to Springer Nature Switzerland AG 2024
A. Clavé, F. Dubrana (eds.), *Unicompartmental Knee Arthroplasty*,
https://doi.org/10.1007/978-3-031-48332-5_7

the components are positioned correctly, therefore, this concept limits wear of the polyethylene mobile insert.

The implant was designed and developed following a meeting with Prof. John O'Connor (Engineer) and John Goodfellow (Orthopaedic Surgeon) in Oxford in 1966.

The first knee replacements were performed in 1976, but as bi/unicompartmental (medial/lateral) procedures in indications for three-compartment knee OA as an alternative to TKR. The first Oxford knee replacement done as a medial UKA was performed by John Goodfellow in 1982!

In its latest version (implant and instrumentation material) dating from 2011, called Microplasty®, the Oxford knee replacement comes in cemented and cementless versions, each including five sizes of femoral components and seven sizes of anatomical tibial components. The mobile PE has thicknesses ranging from 3 to 9 mm, and there is a range based on the size of the femoral component.

Worldwide, the most common surgical treatment for knee OA (independently of degeneration type) is total knee arthroplasty, which often requires so-called independent bone resections and ligament releases. The philosophy of Oxford unicompartmental replacement is completely different because it essentially involves a procedure designed to restore wear, which is based on balancing the ligaments in order to obtain the correct position. Therefore, it should not be considered as a bone procedure, but rather as a soft tissue procedure. Its purpose is to restore normal ligament tension. The technique is based on tension at rest on the medial collateral ligament (MCL). Since the MCL is isometric in the entire range of knee joint amplitude, it constitutes a very reliable guide to reconstructing the joint space height in the medial compartment [1].

The indication for Oxford knee replacement is based on anterointernal knee OA (osteoarthritis). This is characterised by the presence of a functionally intact ACL (anterior cruciate ligament) and the existence of conserved cartilage thickness at the posterior part of the medial tibial plateau and in the posterior medial femoral condyle. Therefore, when the knee is placed in flexion, the MCL is taut, avoiding with the passage of time retraction of the periarticular soft tissue including the MCL and posterior capsule (Fig. 7.2). Tension on the MCL will make it possible to determine the position of the components for the purpose of recreating physiological native alignment, mobility, and stability.

Fig. 7.2 Anteromedial osteoarthritis (**a** and **b**) Slack MCL due to cartilage wear and AMOA; (**c** and **d**) Tension of the MCL in flexion due to the physiological femoral roll-back thanks to a preserved ACL. The joint line level is also preserved as there is no wear at the back of the tibia and on the posterior part of the femoral condyle; (**e** and **f**) Correction of varus deformity caused by the wear. Premorbid state obtained due to the physiological behaviour of the MCL and ACL

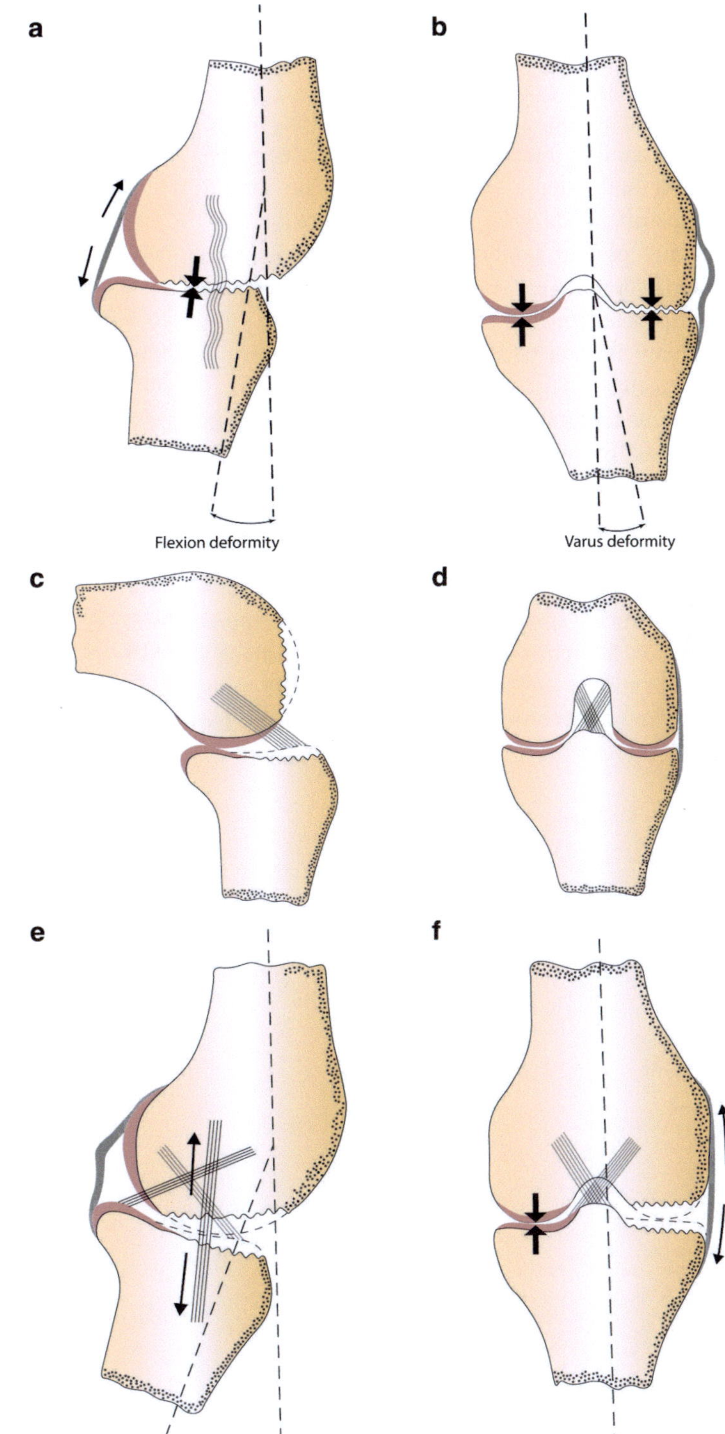

7.2 Role of the Collateral Ligaments

In a normal knee that has not undergone wear, biomechanical behaviour differs between the medial and lateral compartments. The lateral compartment has a larger opening in flexion, evidencing greater laxity of the LCL in flexion, while in the internal compartment, due to the isometric behaviour of the MCL, the 2-mm joint opening is constant throughout the arch of movement.

Permanent flexion, which among other things is caused by retraction of the posterior capsule on osteophytes, is a process frequently observed in knee OA. In AMOA, this permanent flexion generally does not exceed 15° so long as the ACL is functionally intact. Consequently, in a knee suffering from anteromedial OA with more than 20° flexion, the medial compartment can open in such a way as to regain premorbid joint space height because this opening is dictated by physiological tension of the MCL and cruciate ligaments, which are normal and efficient (Fig. 7.3).

Balancing the ligaments in independent TKR techniques with resection almost necessarily involves releasing the medial (or lateral) structures to recreate the rectangular spaces that are balanced in flexion and extension. In the setting of Oxford UKA, ligament release should never be performed. Integrity of the MCL is imperative and makes it possible to conserve joint mobility, stability, and physiological hip-knee alignment (HKA), as well as an optimal / physiological kinematic behaviour of the mobile polyethylene insert during the entire range of motion of the knee. Appropriate tension on the MCL is critical throughout the procedure, and therefore it is necessary to be careful to protect it at all times and never release or damage it. The proper balance between flexion and extension is created by removing bone from the distal femur and not by performing ligament releases.

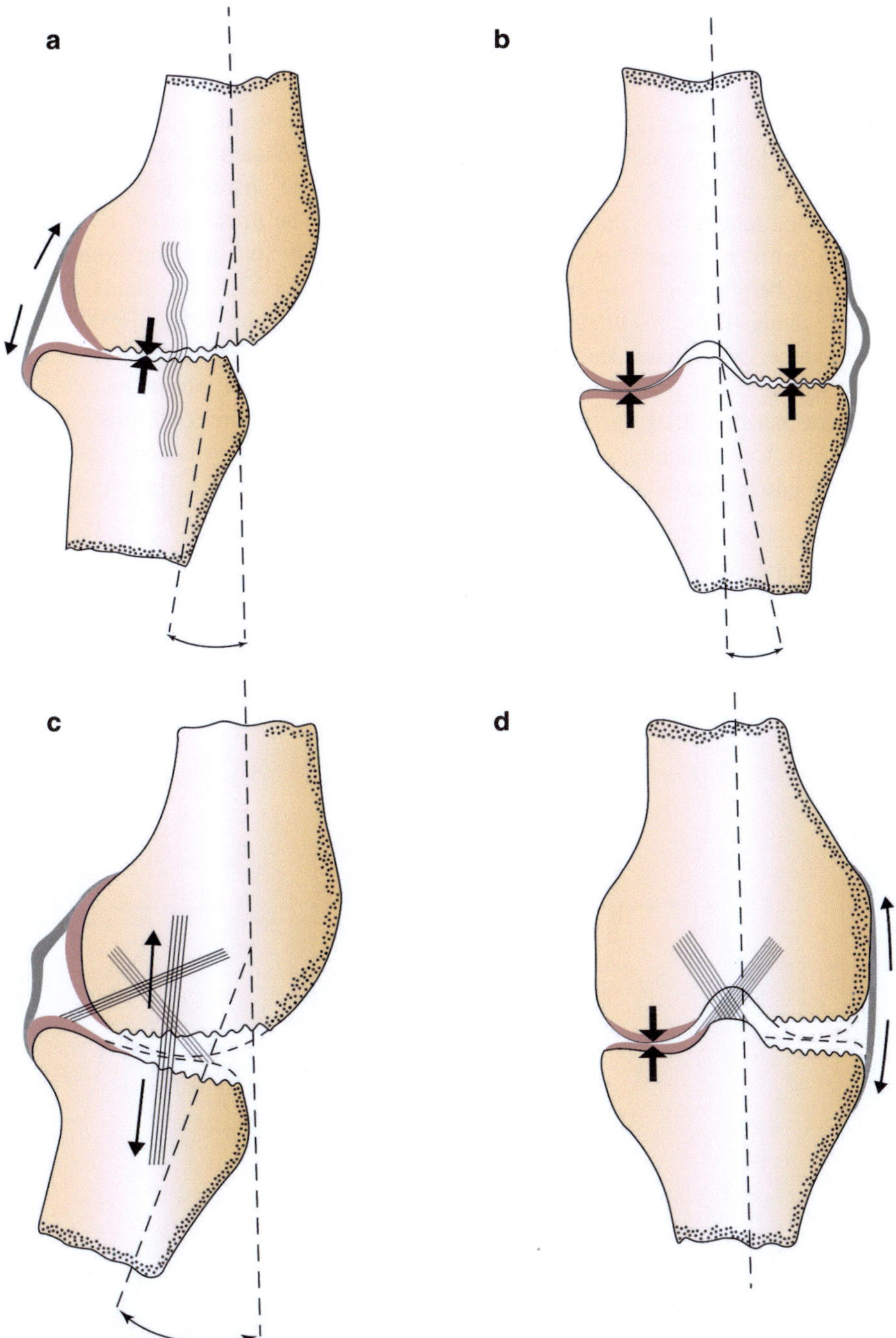

Fig. 7.3 (**a** and **b**) Tension of the MCL in flexion due to the physiological femoral roll-back thanks to a preserved ACL. The joint line level is preserved as there is no wear at the back of the tibia and on the posterior part of the femoral condyle; (**c** and **d**) Correction of varus deformity caused by the wear. Premorbid state obtained due to the physiological behaviour of the MCL and ACL

7.3 Restoring the Joint Space Height

In the medial condyle, the knee flexes and extends around a centre of rotation that coincides with the femoral insertion of the femoral MCL. As the MCL has a constant length throughout the entire joint amplitude, it is necessary to restore the correct joint level height (Fig. 7.4). If the joint space height is changed, the resulting centre of rotation will change, which can decrease MCL tension in midflexion and increase it in hyperflexion. Thus, causing pain or dislocation of the mobile polyethylene insert. Consequently, it is important to reconstruct the correct/native joint line.

In anteromedial knee OA, the cartilage remains conserved in the posterior condyle. Therefore, posterior femoral resection will aim to remove the same quantity of bone and cartilage as will be replaced by the femoral component, reconstructing native joint offset in flexion (Fig. 7.5). The thickness of the femoral component varies by size, ranging from 5.5 mm for XS to 7.45 mm for XL components.

In contrast, there is significant wear in the distal femur. This makes the distal femur unreliable to restore the joint space in extension. In the Oxford concept, the joint space in extension is reconstructed by copying the space in flexion to the space in extension. Therefore, the concept of

Fig. 7.4 Physiological tension of the MCL allows to restore the joint line level and to respect the centre of rotation of the medial femoral condyle

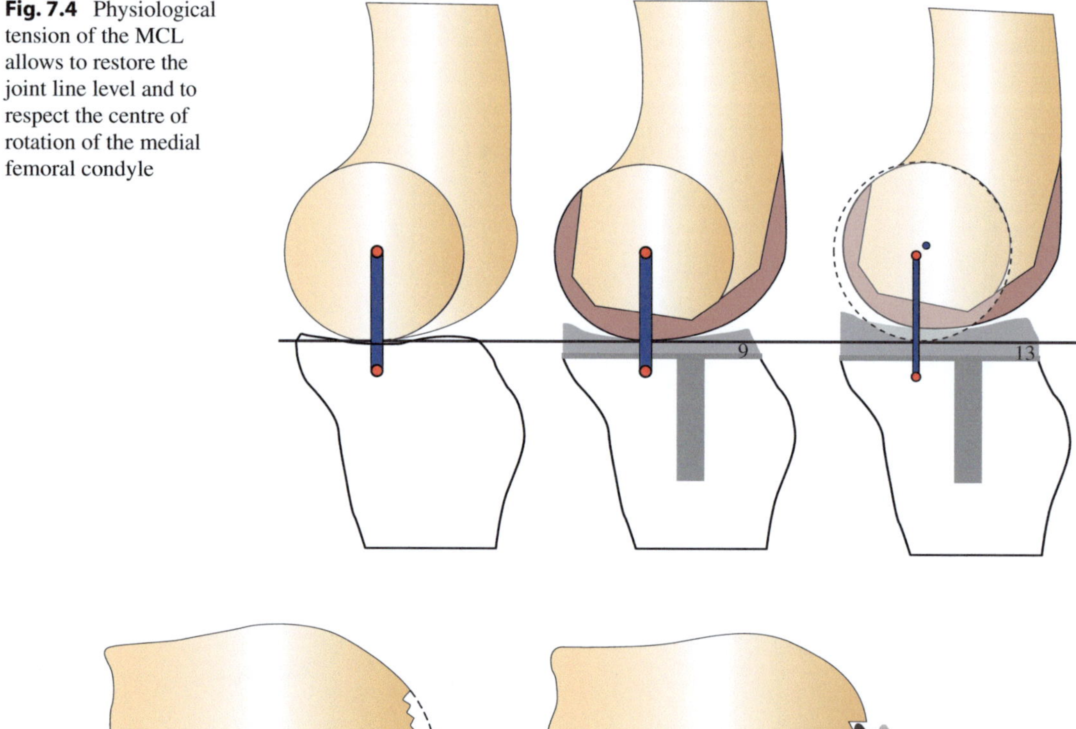

Fig. 7.5 The posterior femoral cut aims to resect an amount of bone and cartilage equal to the thickness of the femoral component. Thus it will reproduce the native joint offset in flexion

a single radius implant used by Oxford and the isometric characteristic of the MCL make this recession logical and reliable.

The height of tibial cut has little importance for restoration of the joint space. However, care should be taken not to resect too much bone on the tibia in order to avoid damaging the distal insertion of the MCL or placing the implant in a more fragile and smaller area of bone. Yet a minimum quantity of bone must be removed in order to create a sufficient space to accommodate the knee replacement components. The tibial metal-back insert has a constant thickness of 3 mm irrespective of the implant size. The minimum thickness of the polyethylene mobile insert is 3 mm. In flexion, therefore, after performing tibial resection and before performing femoral posterior cut, the space should be at least 6 mm. If more bone has been resected on the tibia, this can be corrected by increasing the thickness of the PE without theoretically affecting the joint space height.

7.4 Execution of the Procedure

7.4.1 Tibial Cut and Positioning of the Tibial Implant

The level of tibial cut height is ensured with the aid of instrumentation parts called calibration spoons and a G-clamp. The spoons are inserted with the knee at about 90° flexion and fit the femoral condyle (Fig. 7.6). They are available in different sizes matching the sizes of the femoral components (from XS to XL). In most cases, a medium size can be used. Once inserted, the anterior part of the spoon must be located at the level of placement of the premorbid cartilaginous surface of the distal condyle, i.e. about 2 to 3 mm in front of the area of eburnated bone in the distal femur. The size of the spoon in itself is unimportant because it will not determine the choice of final implant. However, it can provide relatively simply an approximation of the size of femoral compo-

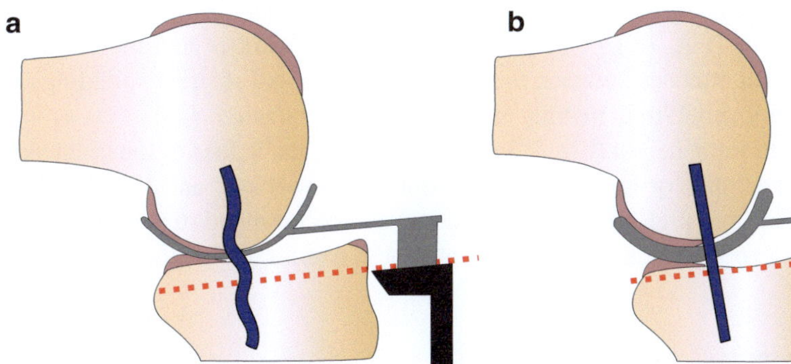

Fig. 7.6 G-Clamp and sizing spoon used to defined the height of the tibial cut. (**a**) The spoon has to be inserted in the joint and then as a spacer will stretch the MCL. If you can twist it (up to 90°) easily, it means that the MCL is not stretch enough. (**b**) A thicker spoon will compensate more cartilage and bone loss. This will put more tension on the MCL. A thicker spoon will remove less bone on the tibial side

nent to use. Nevertheless, an abacus exists which, depending on the size and sex of the patient, indicates the theoretical sizes of the femoral and tibial component to use.

Female			Male		
Size (cm)	Femur	Tibia	Size (cm)	Femur	Tibia
<153	X-small	A or B	<160	Small	A, B or C
153–165	Small	A, B or C	160–175	Medium	C or D
165–175	Medium	C or D	170–185	Large	E or F
>175	Large	E	>185	X-large	F

Spoons are available in three different thicknesses: 1, 2, and 3 mm. The thickness of the spoon makes it possible to adjust the resection height. Using a 3-mm spoon will remove 1 mm less in the tibia than a 2-mm spoon. In our experience, a spoon of 1 mm thickness is appropriate in 80% of cases. In cases of greater tibial bone loss and if excessive laxity of the MCL persists, however, a 2- or 3-mm spoon can be indicated. If the spoon can be pivoted to 90° when inserted between the tibia and femur, this indicates a defect in MCL tension; therefore, the joint space is not restored/refilled and it is necessary to repeat the test with a thicker spoon (Fig. 7.6).

A G-clamp is a part that attaches between the spoon and extramedullary guide/rod, making it possible to adjust its positioning height (Fig. 7.7). It is available in two sizes: three or four depending on the thickness of the preferred mobile insert. Similarly, in our experience, a G-clamp 4 can be chosen in most cases. Therefore, by using a 4 G-clamp that aims for a 4-mm insert, this gives us the possibility of using a higher or lower insert thickness. It is only in short (and low-weight) patients that using in a 3-mm PE is specified. However, this has the disadvantage that it is impossible to choose a lower insert thickness if necessary since the minimum thickness of polyethylene inserts is 3 mm. The advantage in seeking to use a 3-mm insert in short patients is to reduce the height of the tibial cut and therefore limit bone resection. Indeed, it is known that the greater the tibial resection, the smaller the weightbearing surface and the weaker the bone, increasing the risk of stress shielding and fracture of the tibial plateau.

Physiological values of the tibial slope are traditionally between 0° and 15°. The Oxford team does not recommend trying to reproduce the patient's natural physiological slope, with the

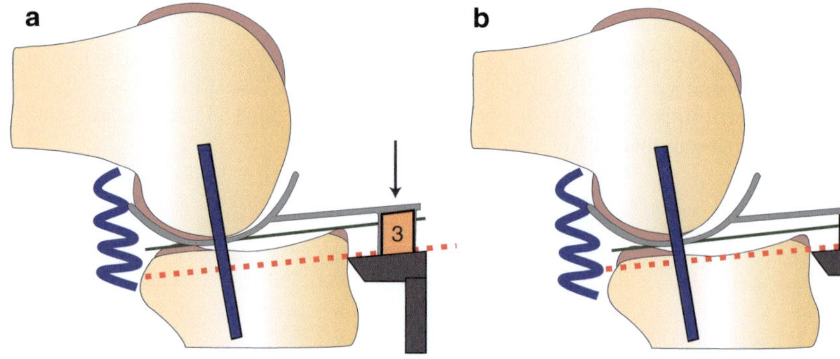

Fig. 7.7 G-Clamp and sizing spoon (**a**) A 3 G-Clamp usually leads to a 6 mm height cut for a 3 mm mobile PE (3 mm metal back and 3 mm PE); (**b**) A 4 G-Clamp usually leads to a 7 mm height cut for a 4 mm mobile PE (3 mm metal back and 4 mm PE)

objective for them and in all cases being a tibial slope of 7°. All studies reporting good results and excellent survival have been conducted in a large range of patients for whom the tibial slope had been defined as 7° posterior [2].

The tibial extramedullary guide/rod makes it possible to perform tibial sectioning perpendicular to the anatomical axis of the tibia and without considering the orientation of the joint space. In Oxford UKA and contrary to TKR, postoperative alignment of the lower limb is not determined by positioning the metal-back tibial implant in varus/valgus. Besides this, the concept of a completely congruent mobile insert makes it possible to tolerate a certain difference in angulation between the tibial plateau and femoral component, without loss of congruence. A 5° error in positioning the tibial implant in varus or valgus is considered acceptable [3].

The *sagittal tibial cut* is done flush with the tibial insertion of the ACL and aims to include a small part of the medial tibial spine. Certain median fibres of the tibial ACL insertion must occasionally be removed for better exposure of the intercondylar notch and the direction of the sagittal resection. Traditionally, the reciprocating saw is placed just on the inside of the apex of the medial tibial spine and is aimed at the homolateral anterosuperior iliac spine. The sagittal direction of the cut is in the flexion/extension axis of the tibia. This plane can be determined by moving the tibia into flexion and extension. Another aiming point is the ipsilateral anterosuperior iliac spine. It is important to avoid excessive external rotation of the cut: posteriorly the cut must be close to the insertion of the posterior cruciate ligament. The operator must be careful not to raise his/her hand (and the powerdrive, allowing the blade to plunge) and cut the posterior part of the tibia too deeply to avoid damaging the posterior tibial cortex. Damaging it drastically increases the risk of fracture. If the sagittal resection is done in too medial a position, the result will be a smaller metal-back tibial implant size, resulting in less optimal distribution of mechanical load and increasing the risk of fracture or stress-shielding pain. This can also lead to insufficient tibial coverage and conflict of the

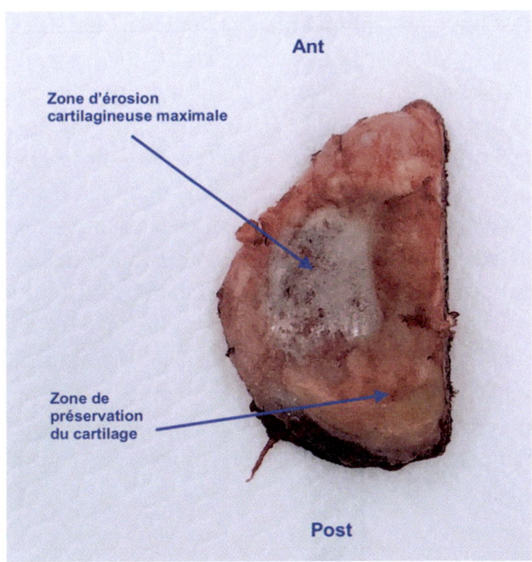

Fig. 7.8 Top view of the tibial biscuit

mobile insert against the vertical wall of the tibial component or between a metal-back medial overlap and the MCL.

When the tibial biscuit is removed, it can be inspected to confirm the diagnosis of anteromedial knee OA. Standard wear shows complete loss of cartilage in the anteromedial part, and normal cartilage thickness remains in the posterior part of the tibial slice (Fig. 7.8). At this stage, the flexion space can be determined. Therefore, if a 4 G-clamp has been used, the space obtained in flexion should be 7 mm, corresponding to a 3-mm metal-back thickness (invariable irrespective of the size of tibial implant) plus the 4 mm sought for the mobile insert. From that point, the space in flexion is defined and will not change throughout the procedure. To determine whether enough space has been created the femoral resection guide set at 4 can be inserted. When the feeling is tight 1 mm of cartilage from the posterior femoral condyle should be removed, thus proximalising the joint line with 1 mm. A recut on the tibia to remove an extra 2 mm of bone is not recommended.

The size of the tibial component can be determined (seven different sizes exist) by seeking optimal coverage between the upturned tibial resection specimen placed against a contralateral test implant. Optimal tibial coverage is necessary to prevent the risk of complications such as pain, loosening of the insert, subsidence, or fracture. Components should be balanced against the posterior and medial tibial cortices and not overlap anteriorly. Medial overlap can be tolerated if less than or equal to 2 mm [4]. In the event of overlap of more than 2 mm, it is recommended to perform a sagittal cut in a more lateral position by resecting a 2-mm slice flush or at the level of the medial tibial spine. The metal-back tibial implant must rest on the posterior cortex because the mobile insert may, in deep flexion, slide beyond the posterior border of the metal back and risk its dislocation.

7.5 Femoral Sections, Positioning of the Femoral Implant and Balancing of the Spaces

Given that the femoral component and polyethylene mobile insert are fully congruent, the mobile insert will follow the femoral component all along the area of flexion–extension with no change to the area of contact between the two parts.

A centromedullary rod will be introduced into the femoral shaft in the direction of the homolateral anterosuperior iliac spine, with its point of entry located about 10 mm directly above the lateral wall of the medial femoral condyle. This is slightly medial to the standard rod insertion for TKA. It will be connected to a positioning guide available in five sizes (corresponding to the sizes of five femoral components — XS to XL). This guide will be used to make the holes necessary for proper positioning of the posterior femoral section guide and drilling spigot for the distal femoral condyle. It is also used to receive the two fixation contact points of the femoral component, whether cemented or not. This part of the ancillary material makes it possible to control flexion and the components' position in varus/valgus, ideally placing the femoral component in neutral rotation at 10° flexion and 7° valgus. The femoral component is best positioned at 10° flexion to

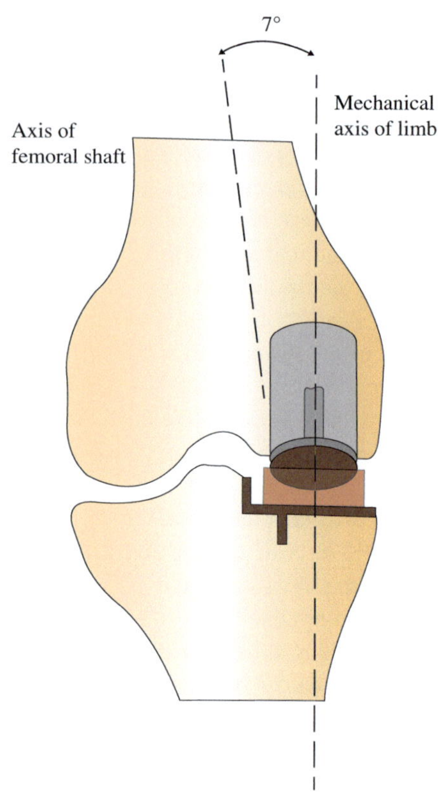

Fig. 7.9 The femoral component is placed parallel to the femoral mechanical axis thanks to the intramedullary rod links to a 7° instrumentation spider-link

increase the area of contact between the femoral component and the mobile insert and allow hyperflexion. Adjustment to 7° valgus compared to the diaphyseal axis will position the component along an axis parallel to the mechanical axis of the femur (Fig. 7.9).

The mediolateral position of the femoral positioning guide is not controlled automatically by instrumentation and must be adjusted manually. The objective should be to position it at the centre of the femoral condyle, avoiding putting it in the medial half of the medial femoral condyle. The two borders of the guide match the width of the corresponding femoral component, such that any medial or lateral overlap can be identified and avoided.

Once this guide has been positioned, first the 4- and then the 6-mm holes are drilled. They will be used for positioning the posterior femoral resection guide, which is the first femoral resec-

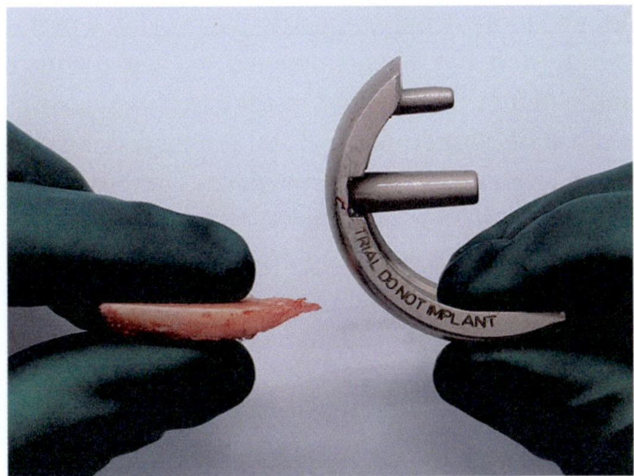

Fig. 7.10 Sagittal view of the posterior cut. The amount of bone and cartilage (+ saw blade thickness) is equal to the thickness of the femoral component

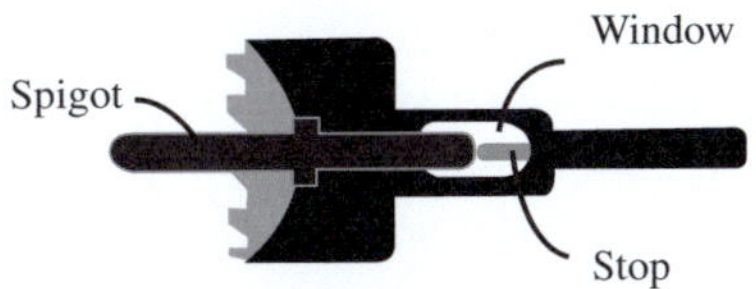

Fig. 7.11 Milling of the distal femoral condyle and spigot. The different spigot sizes allow a 1 mm incremental milling

tion to be performed. This resection, generally in a healthy bone and cartilage area, should remove a quantity of bone equal to the thickness of the femoral component minus the thickness of the saw blade, thereby recreating a physiological posterior offset condyle (Fig. 7.10).

The distal femoral condyle is then resurfaced by milling. In order to do this, spigots with collars of variable thickness will make it possible to adjust the depth of drilling. They are inserted into the 6-mm hole and referenced in two points: the bottom of the 6-mm drill hole and the worn surface of the distal femur. The spigots are available with collars of incremental 1-mm sizes ranging from 0 to 7 mm. Length of the spigot is identical on both sides of the collar, meaning that it can be inserted in both directions. The first milling should be with a spigot of 0 because it will remove the least amount of bone, enabling clean milling. The drill fitting into the spigot has a window through which the spigot can be seen, preventing milling of the distal condyle going further than required (Fig. 7.11). Usually a first milling with spigot 0 will not create a spherical surface of the distal femur yet.

After this first milling, a zero point is established. This will be the reference for the following measurements. The next stage is the *first measurement of the difference between the reference space in flexion and the space in extension*. When the spaces in flexion and extension

are determined, the intramedullary rod and all retractors should be removed because they exert traction on the ligaments and other soft tissue, affecting the ligament balance and opening the internal compartment. Therefore, it is also important to check thoroughly for the absence of osteophytes that can place the MCL under tension at the level of the femoral condyle, particularly under the femoral insertion of the MCL, and if applicable excise them. The osteophytes on the tibial side should not be removed since removal poses a high risk of damaging the MCL.

To evaluate the difference between the physiological space in flexion and the space in extension, a trial tibia and trial femur are inserted. The space in extension is evaluated in 20° flexion, relaxing the posterior capsule. Measuring the joint space in complete extension exerts tension on the capsule, limiting opening of the internal compartment, and may also be misleading in cases of permanent flexion. In anteromedial knee OA, fixed flexion deformity normally does not exceed 15° and measurement of the space in extension in 20° of flexion is therefore considered more reliable. The space in flexion is evaluated at 90° of the previous position, i.e. 110° flexion. 110° flexion also corresponds to a position that is perpendicular overall between the femoral and tibial components: with the femoral component placed at 10° flexion and the metal-back tibial implant with 7° posterior slope. After drilling with spigot 0, the flexion space evaluated at 110° must be larger than the extension space evaluated at 20° because in the flexion space is final (the posterior cut will not be altered), but the extension space has not been finalised to match the flexion space (more bone has to be removed from the distal femur).

Tests are performed using trial spacers that measure the residual space between the femoral and tibial components. At this stage, the single-pegged femoral trial and tibial trial without keel are used. These trial spacers place the MCL under tension and thus correct the joint space. In flexion, the medial compartment is generally the same size as the G-clamp used at the start of the procedure. If a 4 G-clamp was used, usually the flexion space should be 4 mm with the femoral and tibial trial in place.

Key is to determine the difference between the space in flexion and the space in extension. The space in extension should be subtracted from the space in flexion. If the flexion space is 4 (a number 4 spacer is the most appropriate) and the extension is 1 (a spacer of 1 is the most appropriate), there is a difference of 3. The spigots determine the depth of milling and so the quantity of bone that will be removed from the distal femur. Therefore, if the difference between flexion and extension is 3, it is necessary to choose a spigot of 3 for the *second milling*. This one will remove 3 mm of extra bone from the distal femur. It is crucial to gently insert this spigot to prevent damaging the 6 mm hole, since the basis of the 6 mm hole is the reference for distal femoral bone removal.

After this second milling, the sharp edges of bone on the side and the bone cuff around the 6 mm hole are removed, creating a spherical distal femoral condyle. It is important not to exert force on the spigots in order not to distort this reference point, particularly from the time when the cuff of bone has been removed.

Next the flexion and extension spaces must be measured again. If the spaces are balanced, the procedure can be finished by completing the femoral and tibial preparation. If the space in extension is less than the space in flexion, a third milling should be performed. If the difference is equal to 1 (e.g. flexion space of 4, extension space of 3), it is necessary to choose a larger size spigot. If the last milling has been performed with a spigot of 3, with the residual difference equal to 1 the spigot to use is 4 (3 + 1) (Fig. 7.12). Nevertheless, it is necessary to remember that during successive millings, the spigot may be lodged more deeply, in particular, as stated previously, if it has been impacted by force with a large mallet. This would result in excessive withdrawal of bone from the distal femur, risking creating a too much extension space. Therefore, it is important to perform successive millings step-by-step without skipping steps so as not to risk over-milling the distal condyle.

Precautions should also be taken when treating avascular necrosis of the distal femoral condyle because a major bone defect may exist in the distal femur. In this case, it is recommended to perform the first milling with a 0 spigot without milling up to the stop, leaving about 2 mm of margin. If the first test shows a difference in flexion/extension space greater than 2 mm, a second milling with the same 0 spigot can be performed advancing the drill up to the stop.

In rare cases of excessive milling, the space in extension can again be distalised by inserting a 3.5-mm cortical screw, parallel and next to the 6-mm hole. By using piling and adjusting its depth, good balance of the spaces can be reached, particularly by retesting with the trial components (Fig. 7.13). In this specific case, the final implant always has to be cemented.

Moreover, it is important to note that the sphero-spherical shape of the femoral component enables a certain tolerance in its positioning and a difference in varus/valgus, flexion/extension and rotation ranging up to 10° is considered acceptable (Fig. 7.14).

Once a proper balance of the spaces has been obtained, it is very important, using the appropriate ancillary material, to excise posterior osteophytes and remove a possible anterior conflict between the mobile insert and femur with an appropriate drill. Indeed, posterior conflicts on osteophytes and anterior bone are the main causes of dislocation or wear of mobile inserts. For this, the anti-impingement guide should be used. Therefore, this step should not be neglected under any circumstances.

Finalisation of the tibia preparation comes last. With the aid of specific instrumentation for preparation of the tibia, it can be verified that the chosen size is fully suitable before the tibial

Fig. 7.12 How to choose the spigot to mill the distal femoral condyle and to balance space in flexion and extension. (**a**) Flexion space: 4 mm and extension space: 1 mm. To balance the space you have to increase the space in extension by 4–1 = 3 mm. Thus, you have to mill 3 more mm on the femoral distal condyle; (**b**) If a 0 spigot was used in **a**, then we have to choose a spigot that will allowed us to mill 3 more mm. Then we will use a 3–0 = 3 spigot!; (**c**) Perfect milling; (**d**) Perfectly balanced flexion and extension spaces

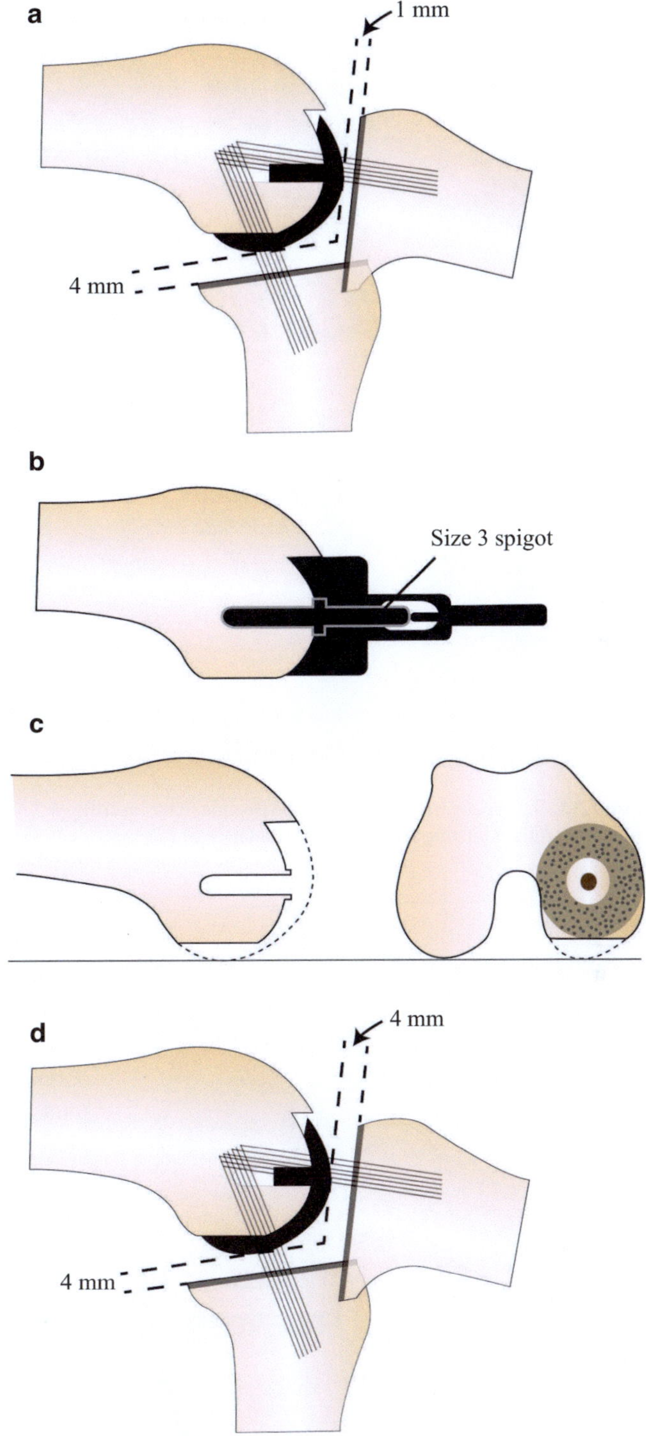

insertion pin is made. This stage is important and should be performed preferably with a reciprocating "toothbrush" saw blade to avoid making a slot that is too deep or too posterior, with resulting damage to the posterior cortex, two errors that risk to fracture the tibial plateau.

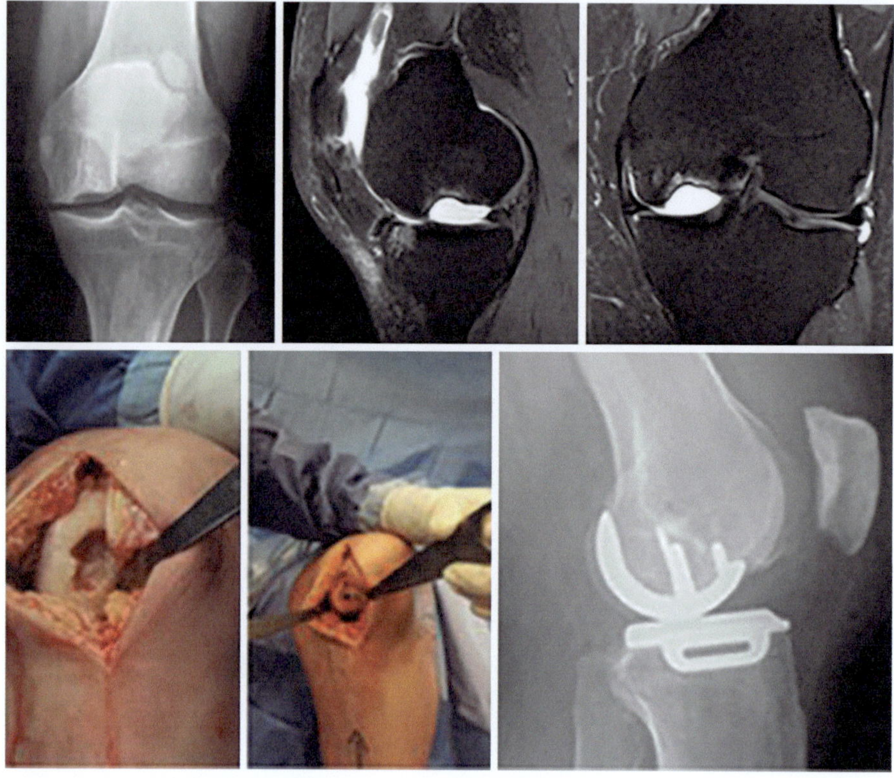

Fig. 7.13 The space in extension can be distalised by inserting a 3.5-mm cortical screw, parallel and next to the 6-mm hole. By using adjusting its depth, good balance of the spaces can be reached

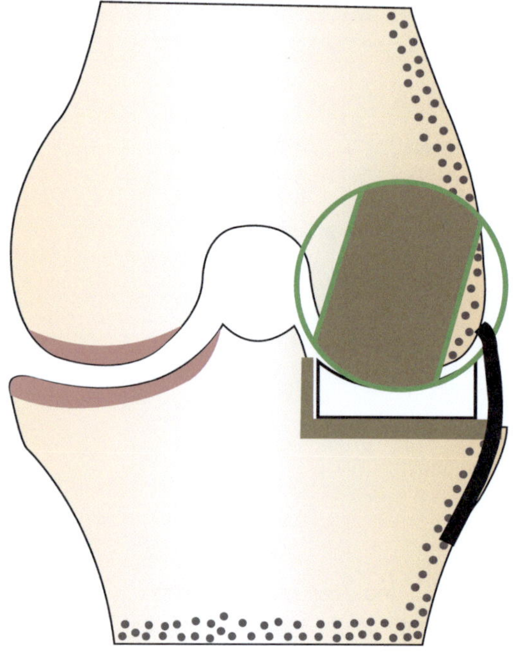

Fig. 7.14 A femoral malposition up to 10° in any direction is considered acceptable

Once the final implants have been placed, it is possible to perform a final test with trial mobile inserts to define the right thickness/height and verify the absence of conflict (anterior, posterior or against the lateral wall of the metal back) or dislocation. If doubt persists between two thicknesses/sizes, in our view, it is preferable to prefer a smaller thickness PE to limit the risk of excess MCL tension and overloading of the external compartment, promoting the occurrence of pain, PE dislocation, and OA progression. The most commonly used PE thicknesses are 3, 4, and 5 mm. Use of PE of more than 6 mm is suspect and should raise questions and, in particular, suspicions of damage to the MCL.

7.6 Take-Home Message

Due to the specific characteristics of anteromedial knee osteoarthritis (including a functionally intact ACL), the main indication for internal

UKA, cartilage is conserved in the posterior part of the tibia and posterior femoral condyle. The MCL and joint capsule are retightened in flexion, preserving their physiological characteristics.

The Oxford knee replacement is a mobile polyethylene insert whose femoral joint surface is fully congruent with the sphero-spherical femoral component. Consequently, it reproduces similar knee kinematics to physiological condition with almost no wear.

Its principle is to copy the physiological space existing in flexion to the space in extension (where wear occurs). By using the isometric characteristics of a healthy MCL and placing it under physiological tension, we are able to measure the difference in space and perform progressive and controlled drilling of the distal femoral condyle, giving a good ligament balance and recreating a joint space and physiological joint biomechanics.

References

1. Victor J, Wong P, Witvrouw E, Sloten JV, Bellemans J. Quelle est l'isométrie de la sphère fémoro-patellaire, de la sphère collatérale superficielle et des ligaments collatéraux latéraux du genou ? Am J Sports Med. 2009;37(10):2028–36. https://doi.org/10.1177/0363546509337407.
2. Price AJ, Svard U. Une deuxième décennie d'analyse de survie sur l'arthroplastie unicompartimentale du genou à Oxford. Clin Orthop Relat Res. 2011;469(1):174–9. https://doi.org/10.1007/s11999-010-1506-2.
3. Gulati A, Chau R, Simpson DJ, Dodd CA, Gill HS, Murray DW. Influence de l'alignement des composants sur les résultats pour le remplacement du genou unicompartimental. Knee. 2009;16(3):196–9. https://doi.org/10.1016/j.knee.2008.11.001.
4. Chau R, Gulati A, Pandit H, Beard DJ, Price AJ, Dodd CA, Gill HS, Murray DW. Porte-à-faux du composant tibial après un remplacement du genou unicompartimental - est-ce important ? Genou. 2009;16(5):310–3. https://doi.org/10.1016/j.knee.2008.12.017.

Lateral Unicompartmental Knee Arthroplasty

8

Axel Schmidt, Matthieu Ollivier,
and Jean-Noël Argenson

8.1 Introduction

Lateral unicompartmental knee arthroplasty (UKA) accounts for a minority of all UKA performed for osteoarthritis [1], about 10% [2]. Its rarity is related to the low incidence of genu valgum deformity [3, 4] and better long-term tolerance of lateral osteoarthritis (OA) compared to medial osteoarthritis [3, 4]. The specificity of the indications and the anatomical and kinematic characteristics of the external knee compartment make lateral UKA surgery more challenging to perform than medial UKA.

Alternatives to external UKA for the treatment of symptomatic, early-stage (Ahlbäck grades 1 and 2) isolated external unicompartmental OA in young and active patients are distal femoral and/or proximal tibial varus derotation osteotomies, which can correct a valgus deformity and therefore decrease the load exerted in the lateral compartment [5]. However, the results and survival rates for varus osteotomies are generally less predictable, the surgical technique is more difficult to perform than valgus osteotomy and postoperative follow-up is longer than for UKA [6]. Total knee replacement is the other surgical option for external tibiofemoral osteoarthritis treatment but is a more complicated procedure with longer postoperative follow-up [7–9].

8.2 Anatomy

The asymmetry between the lateral and medial tibiofemoral space is explained by the anatomical characteristics specific to each compartment [10].

Concerning the lateral tibial plateau, the anatomical specificities are convexity of the cartilage surface, a lower anteroposterior and mediolateral size than the medial plateau, a long axis of 10–15° of internal rotation, and a lower external tibial slope than in the internal compartment [11]. The lateral femoral condyle, often hypoplastic in valgus deformity of the knee, is divergent with a longer anteromedial axis oriented in a posterolateral direction.

Congruence between the femoral condyle and tibial plateau closely depends on the presence, shape, and mobility of the lateral meniscus. In cases of meniscectomy, stability is altered, quickly resulting in the osteoarthritic degenerative alterations that explain the high number of young subjects who develop lateral osteoarthritis after meniscectomy [12].

All these anatomical specificities in the lateral tibiofemoral compartment will affect the surgical technique, implants' positioning, and even the choice of implant used [13, 14].

A. Schmidt (✉) · M. Ollivier · J.-N. Argenson
Institut du Mouvement et de l'Appareil Locomoteur (Institute of Movement and the Musculoskeletal System), CHU (University Hospital Centre) Sud, Marseille, France

© The Author(s), under exclusive license to Springer Nature Switzerland AG 2024
A. Clavé, F. Dubrana (eds.), *Unicompartmental Knee Arthroplasty*,
https://doi.org/10.1007/978-3-031-48332-5_8

Although cartilage wear develops primarily in the anterior part of the medial compartment, osteoarthritis often starts in the posterior part of the lateral compartment [15]. This particularity is important to orient the paraclinical preoperative diagnosis, with Rosenberg X-ray views making it possible to assess the severity of wear correctly.

8.3 Kinematics of a Native Knee and with UKA

The biomechanics and kinematics differ between the medial and lateral tibiofemoral compartment. These variations will explain the technical particularities during lateral UKA placement.

Kinematics of a native knee consists of progressive external rotation of the femur on the tibia during flexion in combination with posterior recession of the femoral condyles, which is greater for the lateral femoral condyle (10 mm) than for the medial condyle (2 mm). This involves the concept of "medial pivoting of the knee": the medial compartment is the area of knee stability while the lateral compartment is the area of mobility [16].

The femur is in neutral position at $0°$ rotation during extension and will turn progressively during flexion up to $7°$ external rotation in the middle of flexion. Translation of the medial femoral condyle seems to be correlated with the integrity of the ACL (anterior cruciate ligament) [17] while mobility of the lateral femoral condyle in the tibial plateau seems to be independent of osteoarthritic degenerative changes and ACL status.

At the end of extension, between $0°$ and $20°$ flexion, external rotation of the tibia occurs after tension is exerted by the two cruciate ligaments, making it possible to block the knee. Therefore, the tibia is in a position of maximum stability with the femur. This process, called "the screw-home mechanism", is key to knee stability in normal gait [18]. External rotation of the tibia during extension should be understood by the operator, who must position the femoral implant as laterally as possible. Excess internal translation of the femoral component may result in conflict with the mass of spinous processes in extension.

8.4 Indications and Preoperative Assessment

The indications for lateral UKA are based on anatomical and radiological criteria grouped in Table 8.1 [19].

Age is no longer an absolute contraindication for UKA [20–22]. In particular, good results have been reported in cases of post-traumatic osteoarthritis in patients under 60 years of age [23, 24].

Table 8.1 Indications and contraindications of lateral UKA

Indications	Contraindications
– Primitive lateral osteoarthritis (secondary to constitutional valgus knee).	– OA in other compartments: Internal tibiofemoral, patellofemoral (particularly at the expense of the lateral facet).
– Avascular osteonecrosis (femoral condyle or tibial plateau).	– Chronic anterior laxity.
	– Frontal laxity.
– Post-traumatic secondary OA (fracture mainly of the lateral tibial plateau).	– Valgus deformity >15° or nonreducible [25].
	– Preoperative knee flexion deformity >15°.
	– Knee stiffness (flexion <100°).
	– History of femoral or tibial osteotomies.
– Lateral post-meniscectomy OA.	– Inflammatory disorders.

8.5 Clinical Examination

The preoperative clinical examination should be especially attentive to detail and look for several points considered as contraindications to perforoint amplitudes will be assessed as well as the origin of pain, which should be localised precisely in the lateral tibiofemoral compartment ("finger sign") with no sign of associated patellofemoral or internal tibiofemoral damage.

Alignment of the lower limb should be assessed to look for a valgus knee deformity, which will be quantified (absolute value and reducibility) and compared to the opposite limb. The assessment of sagittal and frontal ligament laxities will make it possible to evaluate the integrity of the central pivoting and collateral ligaments. Special attention should be paid during examination of the ACL because clinical signs can be a little difficult to interpret in light of pain associated with OA and intra-articular effusion.

8.6 Imaging

The standard preoperative radiological assessment should include anteroposterior and profile views of the knee with weightbearing on one foot, an axial view of the patella in 45° flexion, an anteroposterior schuss view, pan-goniometry of the lower limbs and weightbearing views in varus and valgus. This preoperative assessment makes it possible to evidence an isolated characteristic of external tibiofemoral OA, with no internal tibiofemoral or patellofemoral damage, and to quantify the severity of OA according to the Ahlbäck classification. X-ray views with weightbearing will make it possible to assess reducibility of the deformity in the frontal plane and thickness of the cartilage in the internal compartment in X-ray views in varus position. Pangoniometry will assess the overall deformity of the lower limbs and look for the origin of a valgus deformity by calculating the femoral and tibial mechanical angles (Figs. 8.1 and 8.2).

Specificity of preoperative planning for lateral UKA:

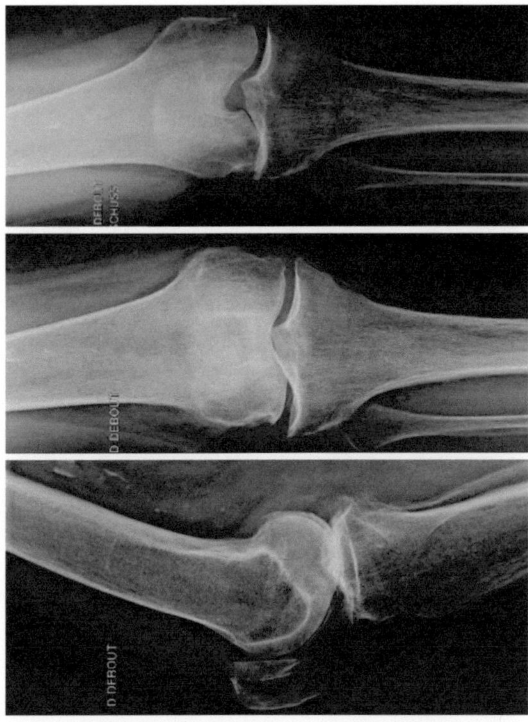

Fig. 8.1 X-ray of the right knee (anteroposterior, profile and anteroposterior schuss views) revealing isolated lateral tibiofemoral OA

Preoperative, clinical, and X-ray assessment should seek to determine the origin of the valgus deformity in order to differentiate six situations:

- Lateral femoral condyle dysplasia [26].
- Post-traumatic valgus secondary to a fracture of the tibial plateau or lateral condyle [23].
- Lateral post-meniscectomy pain syndrome [27].
- Avascular osteonecrosis of the femoral condyle or lateral tibial plateau.
- Valgus secondary to coxofemoral disorder in a native or prosthetic hip [28].
- Valgus secondary to congenital tibial deformity [29].

Femoral condyle hypoplasia is the most common cause [4]. In specific cases, the position of the femoral component should be adapted to the severity of the dysplasia. In cases of severe hypoplasia, the femoral implant should be positioned more distally and more posteriorly to correct dys-

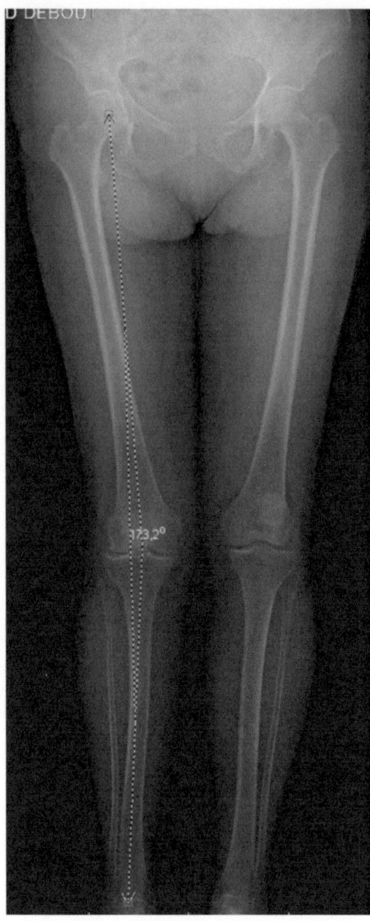

Fig. 8.2 Pan-goniometry of the lower limbs evidencing valgus disorder (HKA angle = 187°)

plasia at its origin in both the sagittal plane and frontal plane, in order to restore an intra-articular space that is closer to the knee's normal anatomy.

In cases of post-traumatic [23] or post-meniscectomy OA and osteonecrosis, there is no bone dysplasia to be compensated. However, poor quality of subchondral bone as well as an architectural anomaly (of the tibial plateau or femoral condyle) secondary to comminution and depression should be anticipated. A precise pre-operative assessment by CT scan will make it possible to plan potential bone graft procedures or insertions of screws for reinforcement in order to obtain a satisfactory bone support for placement of the implant. Cases of post-traumatic OA affect patients who are often younger than the population normally concerned. Placement of a UKA makes it possible to correct the intra-articular deformity secondary to a fracture. Lustig et al. [23] have reported improvement in pain and function with post-traumatic lateral UKA, as well as excellent survival at 5 and 10 years with 80% good results at 15 years. Even though the number of indications is very limited and it involves a rigorous procedure, lateral UKA can be an effective option for treatment of post-traumatic OA. Survival of implants in this context seems comparable to survival of lateral UKA for primary OA.

The last two situations are less common and are more often indications for treatment with TKR or tibial osteotomies [29].

## 8.7	Surgical Technique

### 8.7.1	Approach

A lateral parapatellar approach is traditionally used for this procedure even though some authors have reported the possibility of performing it with a medial parapatellar approach [30].

The skin incision extends from the lateral upper pole of the patella and ends distally 2 cm below the joint space on the lateral border of the ATT. Lateral arthrotomy is then performed, and the patella will be pushed back medially.

To improve intra-articular exposure, the lateral facet (external vertical patellectomy) and lateral patellar osteophytes can be resected in combination with excision of the lateral portion of Hoffa's fat pad tissue.

The entire joint is then explored, making it possible to confirm the isolated characteristic of OA and the absence of anterior laxity (integrity of the ACL).

During exposure of the external tibiofemoral joint, it is important that release of the peripheral capsule around the tibial plateau and osteophytes be as minimal as possible to leave the peripheral ligament structures intact. This is an essential point during UKA placement, ensuring final undercorrection that is favourable to good ligament tension [31]. In fact, similarly to medial

UKA, the principles of ligament balance on both the lateral collateral ligament and fascia lata are not applicable in external unicompartmental surgery.

In a first phase, osteophytes in the intercondylar notch are resected to prevent conflict with the ACL, responsible for secondary rupture. Regarding osteophytes in the lateral femoral condyles, it is important to conserve them initially because they will aid subsequent positioning of the femoral implant [32]. In fact, the latter should be positioned as laterally as possible when the knee is in flexion, which implies that in some cases it will be partially pressing on the condylar osteophytes.

Before any bone resection, it is useful to note the contact point between the anterior part of the femoral condyle and the anterior part of the tibial plateau when the knee is in extension. This point will serve as a marker subsequently for the positioning of implants (size and direction).

8.7.2 First Stage: Tibial Resection

Horizontal tibial resection is performed with an extramedullary guide. The objective is to perform bone resection that is the most economical and conservative possible, orthogonal to the mechanical tibial axis, in order to avoid having to increase the thickness of the tibial insert to restore alignment and stability [2].

In fact, in valgus knee deformity, where OA generally affects the femoral condyle more [31], minimal bone resection will ensure a larger area of resection, enabling better weightbearing on the tibial cortex for the future implant. If the surgeon wants to conserve the patient's valgus deformity partially, this should not be done during tibial resection but preferably during femoral resection, where generally the origin of valgus knee deformity lies. There is very little metaphysis tibial deformity in valgus knee deformity.

The tibial slope of the lateral compartment, which is lower than that of the medial compartment [11], should be reproduced to prevent insta-

bility in flexion in cases of excessive slope, or stiffness in cases of an insufficient slope generating a tight lateral compartment [33, 34]. An excessive slope will also have the effect of increasing anterior tibial translation, which is the source of secondary lesions of the ACL [35].

To conclude, sagittal tibial resection should be performed as close as possible to the tibial spine mass while conserving them. It is performed with the knee in flexion and should follow a line connecting two markers for identification:

- With the knee in flexion, it involves the most medial point of the middle of the anteroposterior axis of the external tibial plateau, behind the ACL insertion.
- With the knee in extension, the most medial point of the anterior part of the external tibial plateau, in front of the ACL insertion.

Because of the natural orientation of the external tibial plateau in external rotation ("screw-home mechanism" [18]), this line will cross the patellar ligament, which must be carefully retracted to avoid injuring it during bone resection.

8.7.3 Second Stage: Femoral Resections

Distal femoral resection should be as minimal as possible to "distalise" the femoral implant, compensating on the one hand for possible hypoplasia of the femoral condyle and on the other hand for wear, essentially femoral in valgus knee deformity. Since wear develops mainly in the posterior part of the lateral compartment, cartilage often persists in the distal femoral condyle, even in cases of post-traumatic OA after a tibial plateau fracture. This cartilaginous remainder should be removed to resect the distal condyle [2].

Each implant has specific characteristics, but the major principles and stages are similar. The distal femoral resection can be performed using two different techniques:

- Independent resections: performed with the aid of an intramedullary resection guide.
- The opening of an intramedullary femoral guide is centred above the apex of the intercondylar notch. Distal femoral resection is performed depending on the HKS angle (angle between the mechanical femoral axis and the anatomical femoral axis, generally between 4° and 6°).
- Dependent sections: the knee is placed in extension after resection of the tibia. The distal femoral resection guide is placed in the tibiofemoral space as done with a spacer.

The posterior femoral resection and bevelling will then be performed using guides for appropriate resection size.

Posterior femoral resection should be as minimal as possible to compensate for posterior condylar offset and therefore obtain a tibiofemoral space in flexion similar to the tibiofemoral space in extension. With this technique, the femoral implant will not reproduce the patient's initial anatomy but will be used to compensate for hypoplasia of the femoral condyle.

Rotation of the resection guide is essential because it will determine the rotation of the future implant. Considering the natural divergent aspect of the lateral femoral condyle compared to the medial condyle, it will be necessary to position the resection guide in order to avoid having excess internal rotation of the implant in flexion, which would result in a conflict with the anterior tibial spines during a shift to extension.

Size of the resection guide is a compromise between an anatomical position centred on the femoral condyle and the long axis of impact perpendicular to the tibial plateau. Special attention should be paid so as not to "overdimension" the femoral implant. There should instead be a tendency to "underdimension" the femoral component. The anterior limit of impact should be located at the level of the mark previously made before bone resection, at the anterior contact point between the femur and tibia on the knee in extension. This marker lies about 1–2 mm below the border between bone and cartilage created by distal femoral resection and will make it possible

to avoid subsequent conflict between the implant and patella due to excess anterior coverage.

Once the posterior section and the bevel have been performed, it is essential to look for and resect any possible posterior osteophytes in order to obtain the best joint amplitude and prevent conflict between the polyethylene insert during major flexion.

8.7.4 Third Stage: Positioning the Implants

The size of the tibial implant is chosen once all bone resections have been performed. It involves the best compromise between maximum tibial coverage without over dimensioning or overlapping the implant in the frontal and sagittal planes. The tibial implant should be as close as possible to the tibial spine mass and have 15–20° internal rotation.

The femoral implant should be placed, with the knee in flexion, in external rotation and as laterally as possible, sometimes meaning that it lies partially on osteophytes [32]. This technique makes it possible to obtain ideal contact with the tibia without entering into conflict with the tibial spines during a shift in position of the knee in extension related to the divergent anatomical shape of the lateral femoral condyle during flexion.

The knee is then placed in maximum flexion and in internal rotation to facilitate final preparation of the tibia, consisting of creating anchoring contact points for the keel pin of the final implant in the subchondral bone.

The knee's stability is then tested with the test implants and a test insert. During movements of flexion/extension, the medial part of the femoral implant should remain opposite to the middle of the tibial implant. It is important to look for a conflict between the femur and the tibial spine mass in extension, which would be secondary to lack of external rotation in flexion of the femoral implant. Testing the spaces in flexion and extension will assess residual frontal laxity, patellar travel, and the absence of conflict between the patella and femoral implant, leaving the surgeon to choose the correct thickness of the PE insert, often thicker in lateral UKA than for medial UKA because of femoral dysplasia.

At the end of the surgical procedure, it is necessary to make certain that slight residual lateral laxity is still present when the knee is tested by blocking it in varus with 15° flexion (unlocked knee). In fact, it is essentially to undercorrect the deformity in lateral UKA in order to avoid any overconstraint of the medial compartment, which is essential for long-term survival [24] (development of OA in the medial compartment).

The strategy of lateral UKA corresponds to a resurfacing procedure whose goal is to correct only intra-articular wear while leaving the extra-articular deformity intact. In any event, it does not involve a procedure whose purpose is correction of the lower limb deformity.

The final tibial implant is cemented and placed first in the knee in complete flexion and in internal rotation to increase exposure of the lateral compartment. The femoral implant is then cemented, and the PE insert is placed after careful cleaning of the metal-backed tibia (Fig. 8.3).

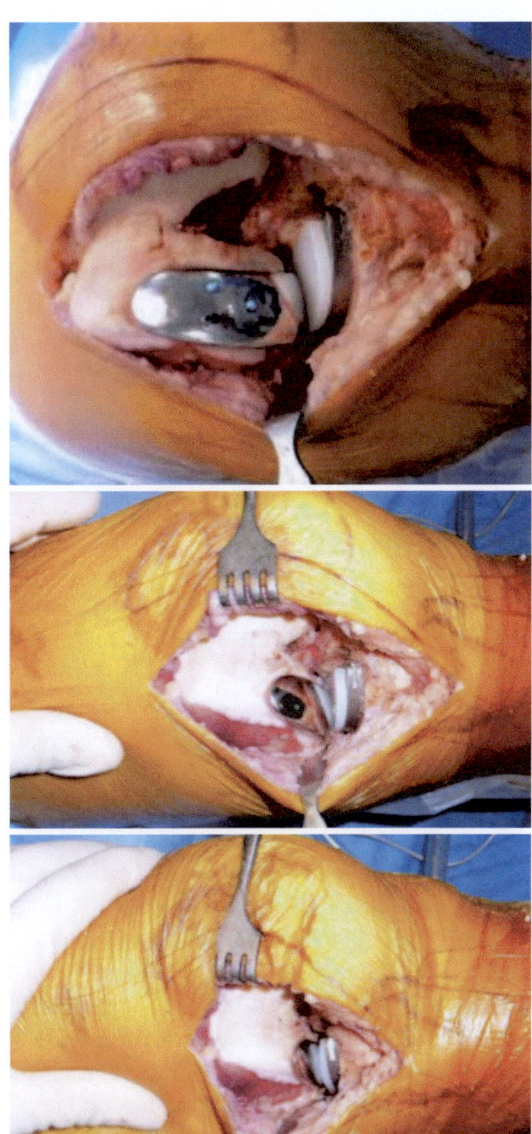

Fig. 8.3 Perioperative views of a Zimmer/Lima ZUK metal-backed implant for lateral UKA (left panel: knee in complete extension, middle panel: knee in mid-flexion, right panel: knee in 90° flexion)

8.8 Traditional Technical Errors and Perioperative Difficulties

Overcorrection of a valgus deformity towards an axis in varus will result in excess constraint in the medial tibiofemoral compartment and early development of medial OA.

The divergent anatomical shape of the lateral femoral condyle during flexion should be considered to avoid conflict between the implant and tibial spines during extension. Special attention should be paid during tibial resection to avoid an excess slope that would affect ligament alignment.

The tibial implant should be positioned with internal rotation of 15–20° and aligned with a natural tibial slope.

8.9 Results and Survival of Lateral UKA

Concerning modern UKA, the literature reveals very good results with mean and long-term survival greater than 90% [19, 36, 37]. In cases of failure, surgical revision is easier with better results and more satisfied patients with UKA revision by TKR than TKR revision by TKR [38].

Long-term clinical and radiological results of lateral UKA are good with functional scores, patient satisfaction, and survival at 10, 16, and 22 years comparable to the results of medial UKA [32]. Recent studies report lower rates of revision than those recorded in the first studies on lateral UKA. In a 2002 series with 21-year follow-up, Ashraf et al. [39] found 10-year survival of 83% and 74% for 15 years. Currently, studies report survival greater than 90% in the medium term and 80% in the long term [40, 41].

This improvement in results is related to better preoperative selection of patients, surgical techniques, and prosthetic implants.

8.10 Failure and Revision

The main reason for failure of lateral UKA is OA progression in other compartments, particularly the medial compartment. In a retrospective series

on tibial "all-polyethylene" cemented fixed implants and on resurfacing on the femoral component, Lustig et al. [24] reported excellent long-term survival with rates of 94.4% at 10 years and 91.4% at 15 years, as well as very satisfactory clinical scores (Fig. 8.4). The main factor in failure resulting in repeat surgery in this study was OA progression in the medial tibiofemoral compartment. No case of patellofemoral OA was reported. These results were confirmed by Deroche et al. [40], who found OA progression in the medial compartment as the main cause of failure (87.5%) in a series of identical implants, followed by aseptic loosening of the tibial implant (12.5%). With mean follow-up of 17.9 years, the revision surgery rate was 20.5%, and for patients who did not undergo revision, the satisfaction rate was excellent at 90.5% with good clinical results. Survival was 82.1% at 15 years and 79.4% at 20 years.

Excellent results have also been reported with cemented implants consisting of a metal-backed tibial implant (Fig. 8.5) and using a so-called resection technique in the short [42] and long terms [32]. Argenson et al. [32] found excellent survival with these implants of 92% at 10 years and 84% at 16 years for isolated involvement of the lateral compartment (essential OA, post-traumatic OA, osteonecrosis).

Concerning mobile-bearing plateau implants, Fornell et al. [41] found excellent survival of 97.5% at 5 years with a 2.4% revision rate at 49 months' follow-up. The main reason for failure in series with the mobile-bearing plateau in the lateral compartment was dislocation of the insert [43]. Long-term survival of the implant will also depend on postoperative alignment. In fact, a defect in alignment with postoperative varus will have the consequence of worsening the development of OA in the medial compartment. A defect in postoperative alignment in the upper frontal plane with 7° residual valgus deformity has been reported as a risk factor for early failure with a risk 7 times higher for re-revision [44].

External OA can also affect young and active patients who wish to resume physical activity similar to their preoperative level quickly. Canetti

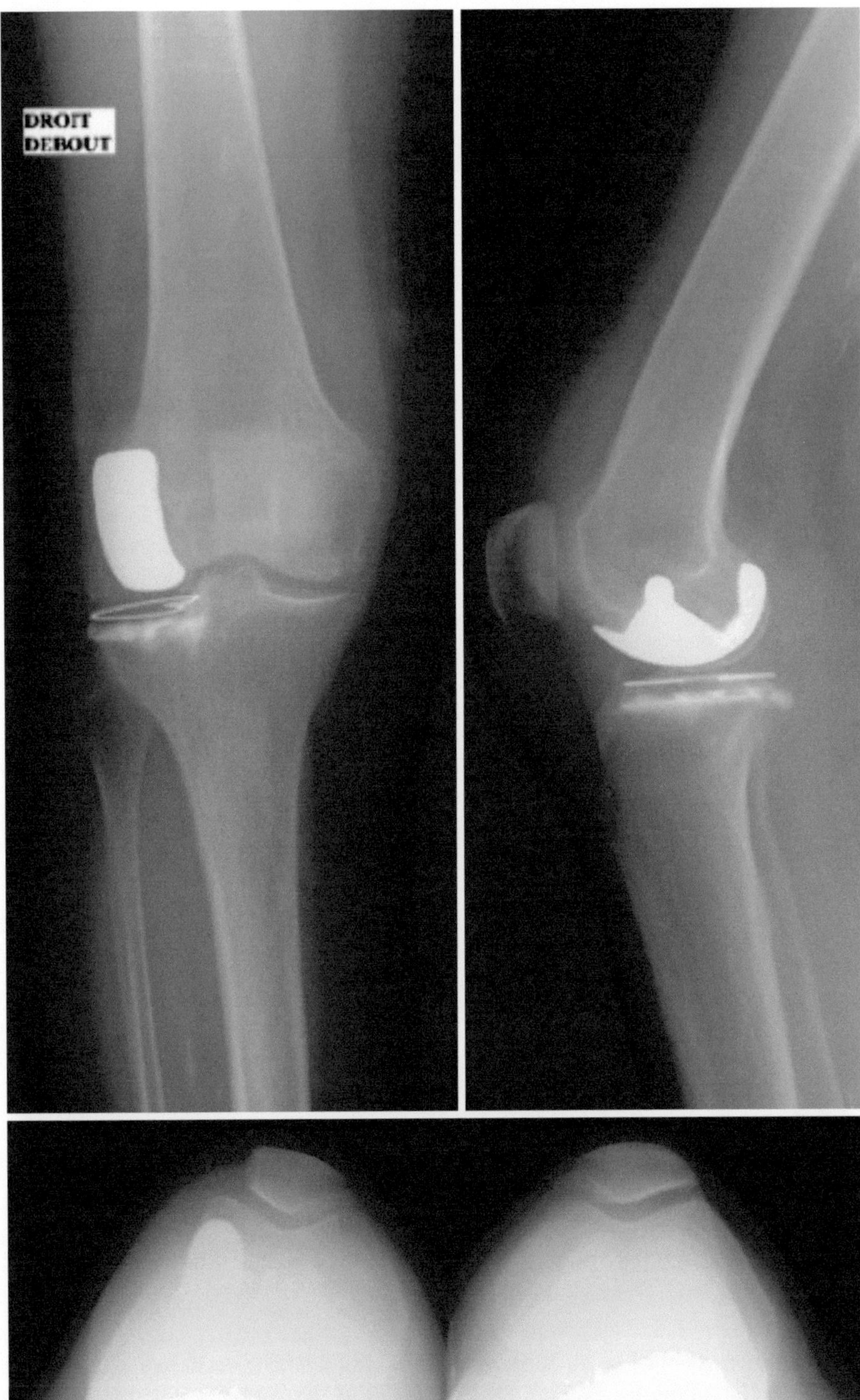

Fig. 8.4 Postoperative repeat X-ray control for lateral UKA with a full-PE tibial implant from the company Corin (image used with the permission of Dr. Guillaume Demey)

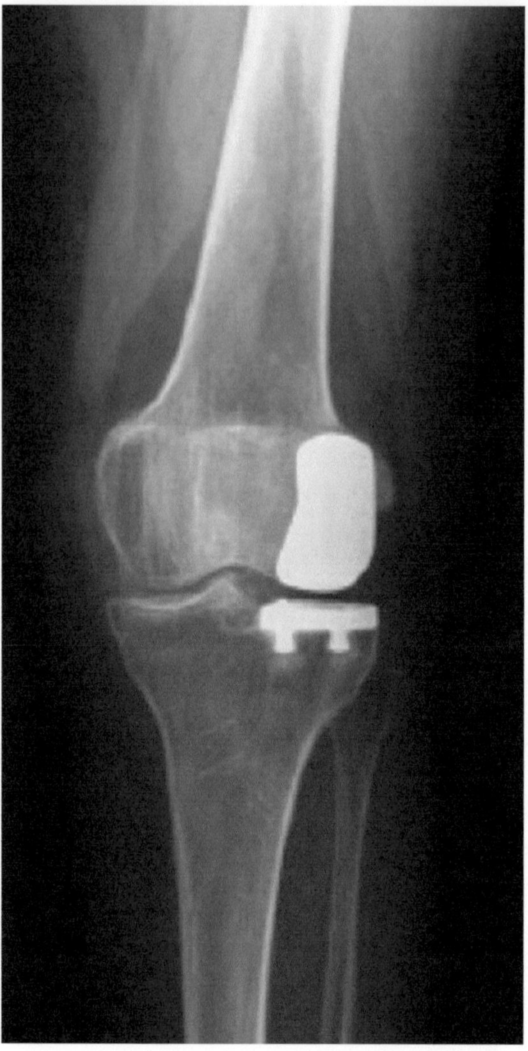

Fig. 8.5 Postoperative repeat X-ray control of lateral UKA with a Zimmer/Lima ZUK metal-backed tibial implant

et al. [45] found a rate of return to contact sports with low or moderate impact of between 94% and 100% after 4.2–10.5 months in a series of athletic patients who underwent surgery either by conventional or robot-assisted technique. In a review of the literature, Witjes et al. [46], who combined 7 studies (including 2 on lateral UKA), found a rate of return to high-impact sports in 8%, 22% for intermediate impact, and 70% for low-impact activities.

8.11 Conclusion

With appropriate surgical technique (positioning, implant size) and selected patients, lateral unicompartmental knee arthroplasty is an effective procedure for isolated damage in the lateral compartment with good long-term results similar to those with medial UKA [31, 32].

Given the anatomical and biomechanical differences between the medial compartment and lateral compartment, the technical specificities should be known and mastered when performing lateral UKA. Lateral UKA should be considered as a resurfacing procedure without correction of the deformity to prevent early failure related to development of medial tibiofemoral OA. Implants with a fixed plateau may be preferable considering the important mobility of the lateral tibiofemoral compartment.

References

1. Parratte S, Ollivier M, Lunebourg A, Abdel MP, Argenson J-N. Long-term results of compartmental arthroplasties of the knee: long term results of partial knee arthroplasty. Bone Joint J. 2015;97-B(10 Suppl A):9–15. https://doi.org/10.1302/0301-620X.97B10.36426.
2. Scott RD. Lateral unicompartmental replacement: a road less traveled. Orthopedics. 2005;28(9):983–4.
3. Ranawat AS, Ranawat CS, Elkus M, Rasquinha VJ, Rossi R, Babhulkar S. Total knee arthroplasty for severe valgus deformity. J Bone Joint Surg Am. 2005;87(Suppl 1(Pt 2)):271–84. https://doi.org/10.2106/JBJS.E.00308.
4. Rossi R, Rosso F, Cottino U, Dettoni F, Bonasia DE, Bruzzone M. Total knee arthroplasty in the valgus knee. Int Orthop. 2014;38(2):273–83. https://doi.org/10.1007/s00264-013-2227-4.
5. Madelaine A, Lording T, Villa V, Lustig S, Servien E, Neyret P. The effect of lateral opening wedge distal femoral osteotomy on leg length. Knee Surg Sports Traumatol Arthrosc. 2016;24(3):847–54. https://doi.org/10.1007/s00167-014-3387-5.
6. de Andrade MAP, Gomes DCFF, Portugal AL, de A e. Silva GM. Distal femoral varusing for osteoarthritis of valgus knee: a long-term follow-up. Rev Bras Ortop. 2015;44(4):346–50. https://doi.org/10.1016/S2255-4971(15)30165-8.
7. Arirachakaran A, Choowit P, Putananon C, Muangsiri S, Kongtharvonskul J. Is unicompartmental knee

arthroplasty (UKA) superior to total knee arthroplasty (TKA)? A systematic review and meta-analysis of randomized controlled trial. Eur J Orthop Surg Traumatol. 2015;25(5):799–806. https://doi.org/10.1007/s00590-015-1610-9.

8. Drager J, Hart A, Khalil JA, Zukor DJ, Bergeron SG, Antoniou J. Shorter hospital stay and lower 30-day readmission after unicondylar knee arthroplasty compared to total knee arthroplasty. J Arthroplast. 2016;31(2):356–61. https://doi.org/10.1016/j.arth.2015.09.014.

9. Zuiderbaan HA, van der List JP, Chawla H, Khamaisy S, Thein R, Pearle AD. Predictors of subjective outcome after medial unicompartmental knee arthroplasty. J Arthroplast. 2016;31(7):1453–8. https://doi.org/10.1016/j.arth.2015.12.038.

10. Miyatake N, Sugita T, Aizawa T, et al. Comparison of intraoperative anthropometric measurements of the proximal tibia and tibial component in total knee arthroplasty. J Orthop Sci. 2016;21(5):635–9. https://doi.org/10.1016/j.jos.2016.06.003.

11. Weinberg DS, Williamson DFK, Gebhart JJ, Knapik DM, Voos JE. Differences in medial and lateral posterior tibial slope: an osteological review of 1090 tibiae comparing age, sex, and race. Am J Sports Med. 2017;45(1):106–13. https://doi.org/10.1177/0363546516662449.

12. Longo UG, Ciuffreda M, Candela V, et al. Knee osteoarthritis after arthroscopic partial meniscectomy: prevalence and progression of radiographic changes after 5 to 12 years compared with contralateral knee. J Knee Surg. 2019;32(5):407–13. https://doi.org/10.1055/s-0038-1646926.

13. Demange MK, Von Keudell A, Probst C, Yoshioka H, Gomoll AH. Patient-specific implants for lateral unicompartmental knee arthroplasty. Int Orthop. 2015;39(8):1519–26. https://doi.org/10.1007/s00264-015-2678-x.

14. Greco NJ, Cook GJE, Lombardi AV, Adams JB, Berend KR. Lateral unicompartmental knee arthroplasty utilizing a modified surgical technique and specifically adapted fixed-bearing implant. Surg Technol Int. 2019;34:371–8.

15. Gulati A, Chau R, Beard DJ, Price AJ, Gill HS, Murray DW. Localization of the full- thickness cartilage lesions in medial and lateral unicompartmental knee osteoarthritis. J Orthop Res. 2009;27(10):1339–46. https://doi.org/10.1002/jor.20880.

16. Argenson J-NA, Komistek RD, Aubaniac J-M, et al. In vivo determination of knee kinematics for subjects implanted with a unicompartmental arthroplasty. J Arthroplasty. 2002;17(8):1049–54. https://doi.org/10.1054/arth.2002.34527.

17. Du PZ, Markolf KL, Boguszewski DV, McAllister DR. Femoral contact forces in the anterior cruciate ligament deficient knee: a robotic study. Arthroscopy. 2018;34(12):3226–33. https://doi.org/10.1016/j.arthro.2018.06.051.

18. Kim HY, Kim KJ, Yang DS, Jeung SW, Choi HG, Choy WS. Screw-home movement of the tibiofemoral joint during normal gait: three-dimensional analysis. Clin Orthop Surg. 2015;7(3):303–9. https://doi.org/10.4055/cios.2015.7.3.303.

19. Walker T, Aldinger PR, Streit MR, Gotterbarm T. Lateral unicompartmental knee arthroplasty – a challenge. Oper Orthop Traumatol. 2017;29(1):17–30. https://doi.org/10.1007/s00064-016-0476-2.

20. Fabre-Aubrespy M, Ollivier M, Pesenti S, Parratte S, Argenson J-N. Unicompartmental knee arthroplasty in patients older than 75 results in better clinical outcomes and similar survivorship compared to Total knee Arthroplasty. A matched controlled study. J Arthroplasty. 2016;31(12):2668–71. https://doi.org/10.1016/j.arth.2016.06.034.

21. Price AJ, Dodd C, Svard UGC, Murray DW. Oxford medial unicompartmental knee arthroplasty in patients younger and older than 60 years of age. J Bone Joint Surg Br. 2005;87(11):1488–92. https://doi.org/10.1302/0301-620X.87B11.16324.

22. Parratte S, Argenson J-NA, Pearce O, Pauly V, Auquier P, Aubaniac J-M. Medial unicompartmental knee replacement in the under-50s. J Bone Joint Surg Br. 2009;91(3):351–6. https://doi.org/10.1302/0301-620X.91B3.21588.

23. Lustig S, Parratte S, Magnussen RA, Argenson J-N, Neyret P. Lateral unicompartmental knee arthroplasty relieves pain and improves function in posttraumatic osteoarthritis. Clin Orthop Relat Res. 2012;470(1):69–76. https://doi.org/10.1007/s11999-011-1963-2.

24. Lustig S, Lording T, Frank F, Debette C, Servien E, Neyret P. Progression of medial osteoarthritis and long term results of lateral unicompartmental arthroplasty: 10 to 18 year follow-up of 54 consecutive implants. Knee. 2014;21(Suppl 1):S26–32. https://doi.org/10.1016/S0968-0160(14)50006-3.

25. Kozinn SC, Scott R. Unicondylar knee arthroplasty. J Bone Joint Surg Am. 1989;71(1):145–50.

26. Feldman DS, Goldstein RY, Kurland AM, Sheikh Taha AM. Intra-articular osteotomy for genu valgum in the knee with a lateral compartment deficiency. J Bone Joint Surg Am. 2016;98(2):100–7. https://doi.org/10.2106/JBJS.O.00308.

27. Pengas IP, Nash W, Khan W, Assiotis A, Banks J, McNicholas MJ. Coronal knee alignment 40 years after total meniscectomy in adolescents: a prospective cohort study. Open Orthop J. 2017;11:424–31. https://doi.org/10.2174/1874325001711010424.

28. Barrios JA, Heitkamp CA, Smith BP, Sturgeon MM, Suckow DW, Sutton CR. Three- dimensional hip and knee kinematics during walking, running, and single-limb drop landing in females with and without genu valgum. Clin Biomech (Bristol, Avon). 2016;31:7–11. https://doi.org/10.1016/j.clinbiomech.2015.10.008.

29. van Lieshout WAM, van Ginneken BJT, Kerkhoffs GMMJ, van Heerwaarden RJ. Medial closing wedge high tibial osteotomy for valgus tibial deformities: good clinical results and survival with a mean 4.5 years of follow-up in 113 patients. Knee Surg Sports Traumatol Arthrosc. 2019. https://doi.org/10.1007/s00167-019-05480-9.

30. Sah AP, Scott RD. Lateral unicompartmental knee arthroplasty through a medial approach. Surgical technique. J Bone Joint Surg Am. 2008;90(Suppl 2 Pt 2):195–205. https://doi.org/10.2106/JBJS.H.00257.

31. Ollivier M, Abdel MP, Parratte S, Argenson J-N. Lateral unicondylar knee arthroplasty (UKA): contemporary indications, surgical technique, and results. Int Orthop. 2014;38(2):449–55. https://doi.org/10.1007/s00264-013-2222-9.

32. Argenson J-NA, Parratte S, Bertani A, Flecher X, Aubaniac J-M. Long-term results with a lateral unicondylar replacement. Clin Orthop Relat Res. 2008;466(11):2686–93. https://doi.org/10.1007/s11999-008-0351-z.

33. Karimi E, Norouzian M, Birjandinejad A, Zandi R, Makhmalbaf H. Measurement of posterior tibial slope using magnetic resonance imaging. Arch Bone Jt Surg. 2017;5(6):435–9.

34. Moreland JR, Bassett LW, Hanker GJ. Radiographic analysis of the axial alignment of the lower extremity. J Bone Joint Surg Am. 1987;69(5):745–9.

35. Dejour H, Bonnin M. Tibial translation after anterior cruciate ligament rupture. Two radiological tests compared. J Bone Joint Surg Br. 1994;76(5):745–9.

36. Vasso M, Del Regno C, Perisano C, D'Amelio A, Corona K, Schiavone Panni A. Unicompartmental knee arthroplasty is effective: ten year results. Int Orthop. 2015. https://doi.org/10.1007/s00264-015-2809-4.

37. Pandit H, Jenkins C, Gill HS, Barker K, Dodd C, Murray DW. Minimally invasive Oxford phase 3 unicompartmental knee replacement: results of 1000 cases. J Bone Joint Surg Br. 2011;93(2):198–204. https://doi.org/10.1302/0301-620X.93B2.25767.

38. Lunebourg A, Parratte S, Ollivier M, Abdel MP, Argenson J-NA. Are revisions of unicompartmental knee arthroplasties more like a primary or revision TKA? J Arthroplasty. 2015;30(11):1985–9. https://doi.org/10.1016/j.arth.2015.05.042.

39. Ashraf T, Newman JH, Evans RL, Ackroyd CE. Lateral unicompartmental knee replacement survivorship and clinical experience over 21 years. J Bone Joint Surg Br. 2002;84(8):1126–30.

40. Deroche E, Batailler C, Lording T, Neyret P, Servien E, Lustig S. High survival rate and very low wear of lateral unicompartmental arthroplasty at long term: a case series of 54 cases at a mean follow-up of 17 years. J Arthroplasty. 2019;34(6):1097–104. https://doi.org/10.1016/j.arth.2019.01.053.

41. Fornell S, Prada E, Barrena P, García-Mendoza A, Borrego E, Domecq G. Mid-term outcomes of mobile-bearing lateral unicompartmental knee arthroplasty. Knee. 2018;25(6):1206–13. https://doi.org/10.1016/j.knee.2018.05.016.

42. Kim KT, Lee S, Kim J, Kim JW, Kang MS. Clinical results of lateral unicompartmental knee arthroplasty: minimum 2-year follow-up. Clin Orthop Surg. 2016;8(4):386–92. https://doi.org/10.4055/cios.2016.8.4.386.

43. Pandit H, Jenkins C, Beard DJ, et al. Mobile bearing dislocation in lateral unicompartmental knee replacement. Knee. 2010;17(6):392–7. https://doi.org/10.1016/j.knee.2009.10.007.

44. Perkins TR, Gunckle W. Unicompartmental knee arthroplasty: 3- to 10-year results in a community hospital setting. J Arthroplast. 2002;17(3):293–7.

45. Canetti R, Batailler C, Bankhead C, Neyret P, Servien E, Lustig S. Faster return to sport after robotic-assisted lateral unicompartmental knee arthroplasty: a comparative study. Arch Orthop Trauma Surg. 2018;138(12):1765–71. https://doi.org/10.1007/s00402-018-3042-6.

46. Witjes S, Van Geenen RCI, Koenraadt KLM. Expectations of younger patients concerning activities after knee arthroplasty: are we asking the right questions? Qual Life Res. 2017;26(2):403–17. https://doi.org/10.1007/s11136-016-1380-9.

Kinematic Alignment Technique for Medial Unicompartmental Knee Arthroplasty

Charles C. J. Rivière, Philippe Cartier, and Cédric Maillot

9.1 Summary

The kinematic alignment (KA) technique for unicompartmental knee arthroplasty (UKA) has been performed successfully for decades, even though the terminology "kinematic" is of more recent introduction. This chapter helps the surgeon understand the theoretical bases and surgical principles of the technique. The objective is to encourage surgeons to use the KA technique because it is a simple, safe, more anatomical, more physiological and probably clinically advantageous method compared to traditional mechanical alignment for UKA. More investigations are necessary to better define its clinical impact and if there are limits to follow for the alignment of prosthetic components.

C. C. J. Rivière (✉)
Clinique du Sport Bordeaux-Mérignac, Mérignac, France

The Lister Hospital, London, UK

P. Cartier
Clinique Hartmann, Neuilly-sur-Seine, France

C. Maillot
Hôpitaux Universitaire Beaujon – Bichat, APHP, Paris, France

9.2 Definition

The traditional technique for partial or total knee arthroplasty (TKA) consists of reproducing the systematised positioning of prosthetic components, neglecting anatomical variations of the knee between each subject. Therefore, the standard for decades has been to align the prosthetic components perpendicularly on the femoral and tibial mechanical axes in the frontal plane, and to produce an identical tibial slope for all patients; this is called the mechanical alignment (MA) technique for TKA [1] and UKA [2]. At the cost of altering the knee anatomy and physiological ligament balance, the MA technique was supposed to ensure surgical reproducibility and clinical results. Nevertheless, functional performance and patient perception of MA knee replacements were sometimes disappointing [3, 4], despite the precise implantation of sophisticated implants [5, 6]. This has led to the development of more personalised and physiological implantation techniques that better reflect the individual anatomy of the knee and balance of soft tissue, known under the term kinematic alignment (KA) (Fig. 9.1) [1, 7].

Based on the same principle as KA-TKA, the aim is to co-align the UKA components with the kinematic axes that dictate native movement of the tibia around the femur [8, 9], and to resect an equivalent bone and cartilage thickness to that of the implant. Therefore, the components are

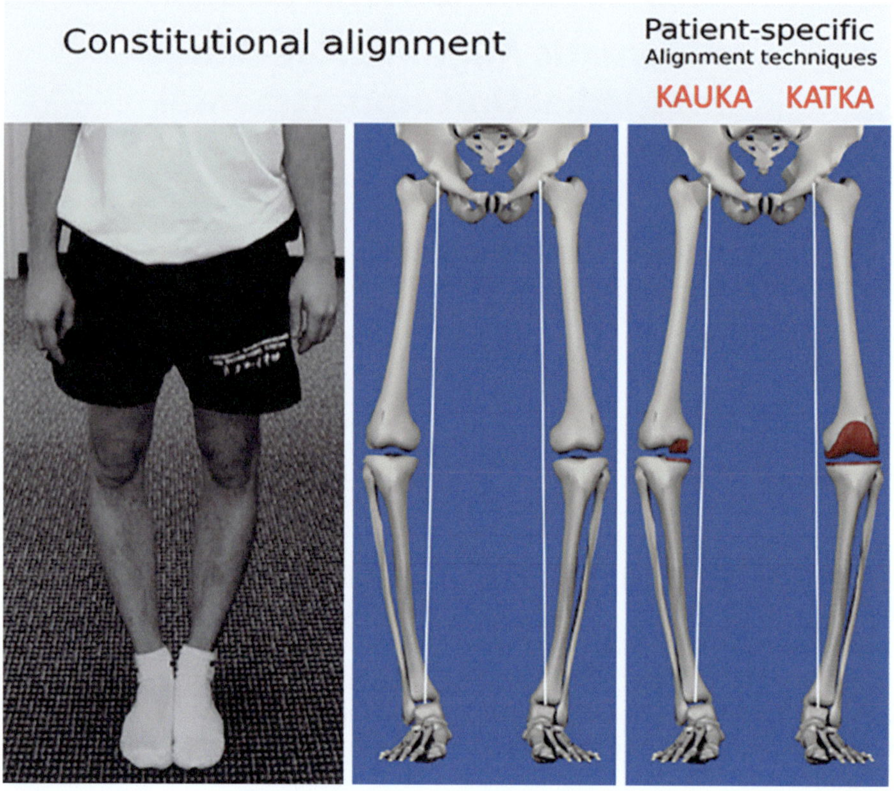

Fig. 9.1 This figure illustrates the kinematic alignment (KA) technique for unicompartmental knee arthroplasty (UKA) and total knee arthroplasty (TKA). The KA technique aims to restore the anatomy and ligament balance of the pre-arthritic knee; these are de facto personalised and physiological methods of implanting prosthetic knee components

aligned in parallel to the cylindrical axis and perpendicular to the tibial longitudinal axis, respectively (Fig. 9.2). In simplified terms, the KA technique for UKA aims to produce "true'" joint surfacing by restoring the level and three-dimensional orientation of the native joint space in the implanted knee compartment (Fig. 9.3). In cases of medial KA-UKA, the native medial and posterior slopes of the medial tibial plateau, as well as the frontal and axial constitutional orientation of the medial femoral condyle, are restored (Fig. 9.3). The KA technique for UKA was popularised decades ago under the name "Cartier's Angle" [10, 11]. Philippe Cartier developed it in the 1970s under the influence of studies by Christophe Lévigne and Michel Bonnin (Lyon

School, France) on the metaphyseal–epiphyseal axis of the proximal tibia [12].

The terminology describing the alignment technique is derived from the reference marker used to align UKA components: the KA and MA techniques align the UKA components on the kinematic axes of the knees and on the mechanical axis of the long bones, respectively (Figs. 9.4 and 9.5). Because of the different objective of alignment, the KA and MA techniques differ in almost each stage of the implantation procedure (see the following section on surgical technique) [8]. In clinical assessment of UKA, therefore, it is important to consider the alignment technique by differentiating between KA and MA positioning of the components [8] (Fig. 9.4).

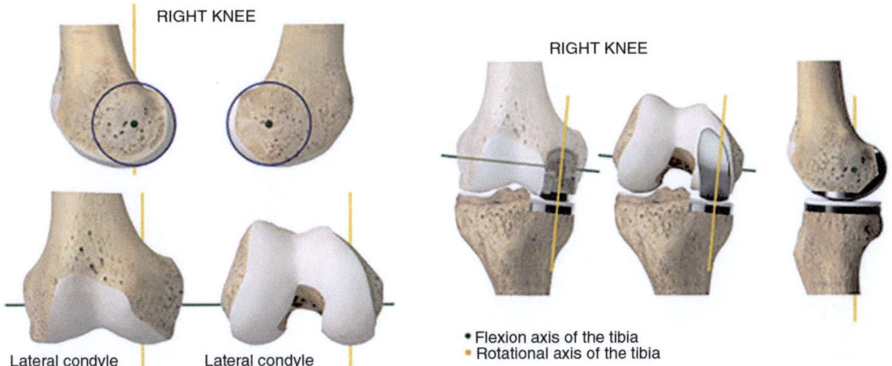

Fig. 9.2 This figure illustrates the "academic" definition of the kinematic alignment (KA) technique for medial UKA. Implants are parallel to the cylindrical axis (green line) and perpendicular to the tibial longitudinal axis (yellow line). These kinematic axes dictate movement of the tibia around the femur during flexion–extension movement of the knee. (courtesy of Medacta)

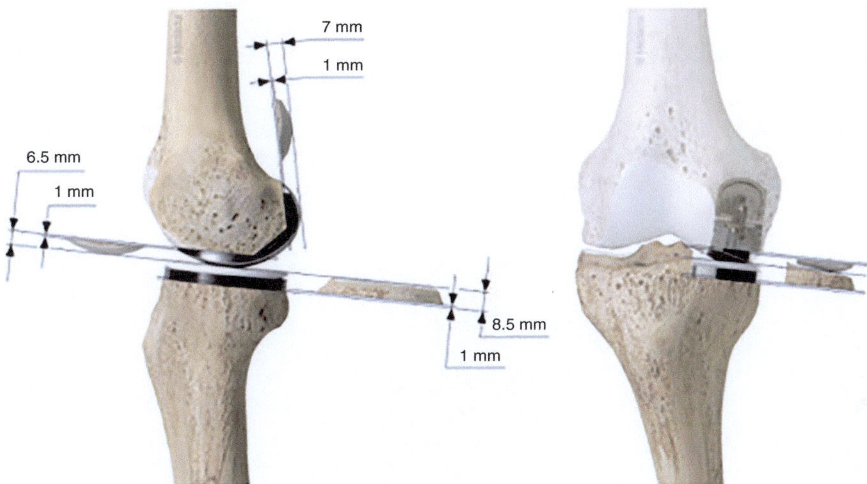

Fig. 9.3 This figure illustrates the "simplified" definition of the kinematic alignment (KA) technique for medial UKA. Positioning of the implants results in "true resurfacing" of the medial compartment of the knee. The thickness of the implant is equal to the total thickness of the bone section, the sawblade line of 1 mm and 2 mm of cartilage loss. Therefore, the physiological soft tissue balance and kinematics of the knee are restored, probably facilitating optimal clinical results. (courtesy of Medacta)

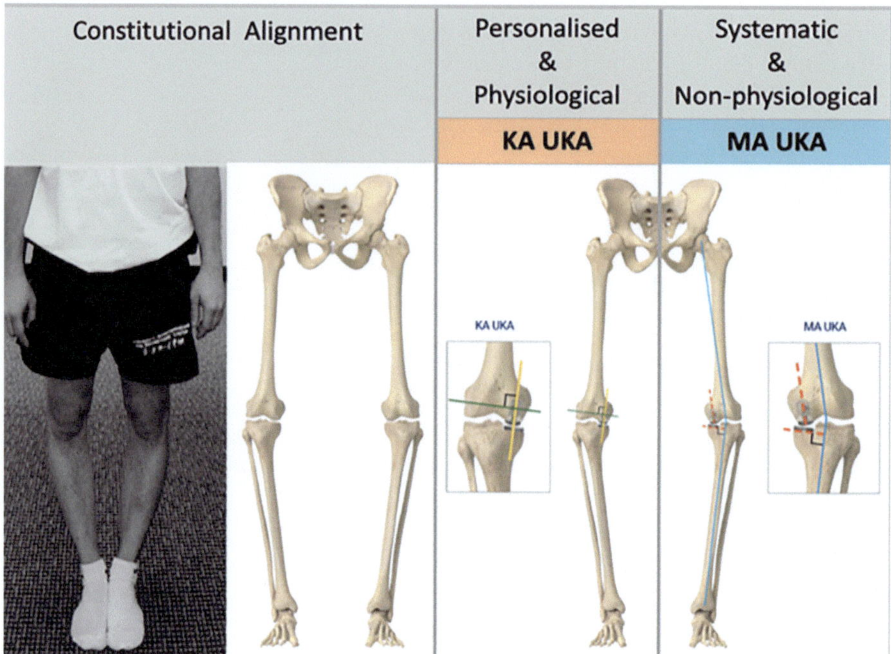

Fig. 9.4 This figure illustrates the two principal techniques for medial UKA alignment. The kinematic alignment (KA) technique positions the prosthetic components on the kinematic axis of the knee, which dictates movement of the tibia around the femur. The mechanical alignment (MA) technique positions the components by taking as reference the mechanical axis of the long bones

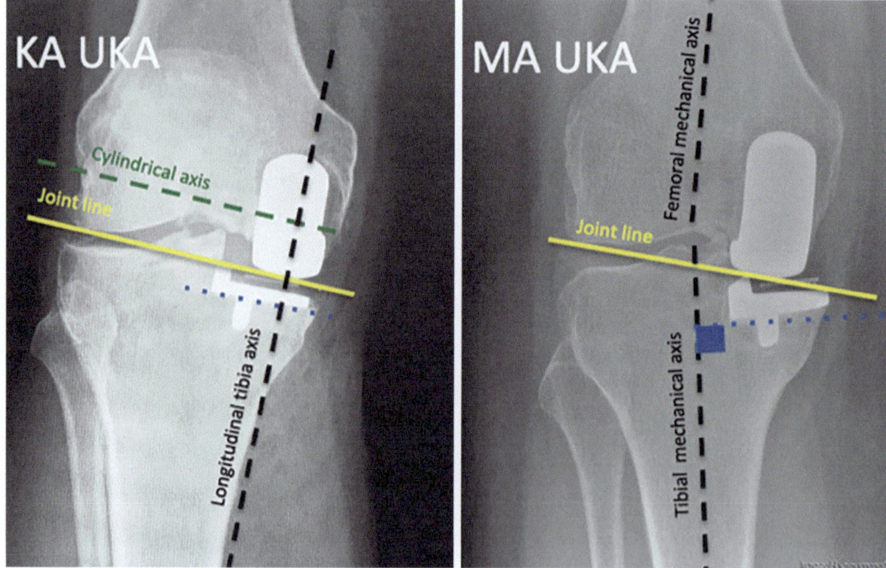

Fig. 9.5 This X-ray composite image illustrates the radiographic aspect of medial KA-UKA (left image) and MA-UKA (right image). During the KA technique, the UKA components are positioned along the mechanical axis of the tibia and femur. Note alteration of the anatomy during MA-UKA, resulting in a tibial implant concentrating stress on the medial cortex during weightbearing of the limb. The bony section is represented by a blue dotted line

9.3 Utility of the KA Technique

The KA technique enables personalised and relatively physiological implantation as a result of conservation of the ligament balance, knee kinematics and transmission of stresses to the metaphyseal bone. The KA technique also optimises dynamic interaction (i.e., throughout the knee movement arc) between the components, thereby reducing the risk of edge loading between the femoral component and the polyethylene insert (Figs. 9.4 and 9.5).

By leaving the medial compartment anatomy of the knee intact, i.e. height and orientation of the joint surfaces, the KA technique is biomechanically healthy:

- The components are aligned on the native kinematic axes of the knee, which dictate physiological movement of the tibia around the femur.
- The natural tension of the medial collateral ligament (MCL) and physiological kinematics of the knee are promoted.
- The tibial component is perpendicular to the subchondral trabecula whose orientation is dictated by Wolff's law, adapted to mechanical stress [13], and is oriented parallel to the ground during walking [14]. This relatively physiological weightbearing of the tibial bone, which seems able to reduce shearing stress at the implant–bone fixation interface, may be beneficial to the implants' lifespan.

While the KA and MA techniques for medial UKA are designed to restore constitutional alignment of the lower limb and knee in erect posture, the KA technique is likely to better reproduce natural frontal alignment of the limb when the knee is flexed. This is the result of conservation of the posterior tibial slope solely with the KA technique. Consequently, KA enables more physiological biomechanics of the knee by reduced alteration of the anatomy and soft tissue balance.

Similar to KA-TKA, compliance with the anatomy of the knee during implantation of the UKA components may make it possible to obtain optimal clinical results [1, 8, 15]. This approach is repeated by many studies which have reported the harmful effect of a change in the anatomy of the medial tibial plateau during medial UKA implantation [16–19].

9.4 Scientific Evidence

The KA technique for UKA has many theoretical advantages compared to the MA technique, most of which remain to be scientifically demonstrated. This paucity of scientific evidence is explained by the fact that UKA alignment techniques to date have been seldom or poorly discussed and that no study has been designed to compare the value of KA and MA techniques [8].

The KA technique conserves tibial bone stock and exerts stress on the metaphyseal tibial bone in a more physiological manner [20–22] than the MA technique. By reducing stress on the tibial metaphyseal cortex, the KA technique may reduce the risk of fracture of the tibial plateau and of secondary residual pain in remodelling metaphyseal bone [20–22].

By restoring the posterior slope of the native tibial plateau, the KA technique makes it possible to conserve the physiological tension of the medial collateral ligament when the knee is flexed. This can potentially reduce the frequency of complications such as pain and residual stiffness in UKA [23].

The KA technique enables the prosthetic components to interact optimally throughout the knee's arc of motion. This optimal dynamic interaction of the components can reduce complications related to the "edge-loading effect", i.e. dislocation of the mobile polyethylene insert or accelerated wear on a fixed polyethylene insert.

It has been demonstrated that kinematically aligned Oxford® UKA components adapt better to supporting bone with significant reduction in the risks of overlap or prosthetic underdimensioning in comparison to MA positioning [9]. This may be clinically beneficial by reducing the risk of residual pain and optimising the implants' lifespan.

Lastly, it is biomechanically healthy to perform KA-UKA that places the tibial component perpendicular to the subchondral trabeculae [13] and parallel to the ground during walking [14]. By reducing the shearing stress at the tibial implant fixation interface and constraining the metaphyseal bone in a relatively physiological manner, the KA technique could benefit the long-term results of UKA.

Many studies have reported good long-term results of KA-UKA: acceptable lifespan of implants, high functional performance, often natural perception of the prosthetic joint and high patient satisfaction after KA-UKA [10, 12, 24–27].

By simulating the Oxford® medial KA-UKA in 40 models of an OA knee, Rivière et al. [9] observed that frontal, sagittal and axial orientations of Oxford® KA components were always within the alignment range recommended by the Oxford group.

Three radiostereometric studies have demonstrated that fixation of KA components is reliable given their low migration during the first 2 years after implantation and that the limit of 6° varus orientation for the tibial component could be recommended [28–30].

Many studies have reported the harmful effect of a change to the anatomy of the medial tibial plateau during implantation of a UKA [16–19].

A systematic review concluded in the good safety and efficacy of KA-UKA in the medium and long terms [8]. No fracture of the tibial plateau and low rates of unexplained proximal tibial pain (0.8%), tibial implant loosening (2%) and aseptic failure of the implant (5.6%) were reported in an assessment of 593 KA-UKA with 3.2 and 12 years' follow-up [8]. Alignment of the lower limb and tibial component was slightly in the varus position (mean values of 3° to 5°), and the tibial component remained parallel to the ground with the patient in the erect position.

The author has manually performed 150 Oxford® medial KA in the last 2 years. Among these, one patient was suffering from residual anterior knee pain and underwent revision surgery (TKA); no other complications or revisions were evidenced (data from the National Joint Registry). The Oxford Knee Scores (OKS) and patient satisfaction at 1-year follow-up were 44 (median value) and 98% (unpublished data), respectively.

9.5 Surgical Technique

KA for UKA is a technique with independent sectioning that can be performed simply and reliably with manual instrumentation. Measuring the thickness of bone resection with vernier callipers makes it possible to control the quality of bone resection, and potentially decide on bone resection in case of an imperfect first cut. Sophisticated technological assistance with three-dimensional planning (e.g. personalised surgical [31] and robotic instrumentation) can also be useful.

It is likely that most UKA implants currently available on the market (fixed or mobile insert, metal-backed or full-polyethylene, implants with resurfacing or not) are suitable for the KA technique, provided that the instrumentation so permits.

As previously mentioned, KA and MA surgical techniques differ at this stage of the implantation procedure except for axial and sagittal rotation of the tibial and femoral components, respectively (Table 9.1). The first author implanted the Oxford® UKA (Zimmer Biomet) following the KA technique and using so-called Phase 3® manual instrumentation. This rudimentary instrumentation was preferable to more recent Microplasty® instrumentation because the latter requires the operator to perform MA-UKA. Please refer to video 1 illustrating the KA technique for implantation of an Oxford® medial UKA. In video 1, you will see the "tibia first" technique, followed by measured resection of the posterior condyle, and then distal femoral reaming to balance the space in subextension (more precisely at 10° knee flexion).

Tibial resection for medial Oxford® UKA (Fig. 9.6): The posterior slope is guided by a pin inserted in the joint space and resting on the anterior and posterior borders of the medial tibial plateau. The medial slope is guided by the anteroposterior axis of the flexion facet of the

Table 9.1 Different recommendations for positioning medial UKA implants between mechanical alignment (MA) and kinematic alignment (KA) techniques. The two surgical techniques differ significantly because only flexion of the femoral component and axial rotation of the tibial component follow the same recommendations

		MA technique	KA technique
Femoral component	**Flexion**	Identical	
	Frontal section	Perpendicular to the mechanical axis	Parallel to the tibial section
	Posterior section	Parallel to the MA tibial section	Parallel to the KA tibial section
Tibial component	**Axial rotation**	Identical (parallel to the lateral wall of the medial femoral condyle)	
	Frontal orientation	Perpendicular to the mechanical axis of the tibia	Perpendicular to the anteroposterior axis of the flexion facet of the medial condyle
	Posterior slope	Systematic slope whose value ranges between 2° and 7° depending on the implant used	Parallel to the slope of the medial tibial plateau

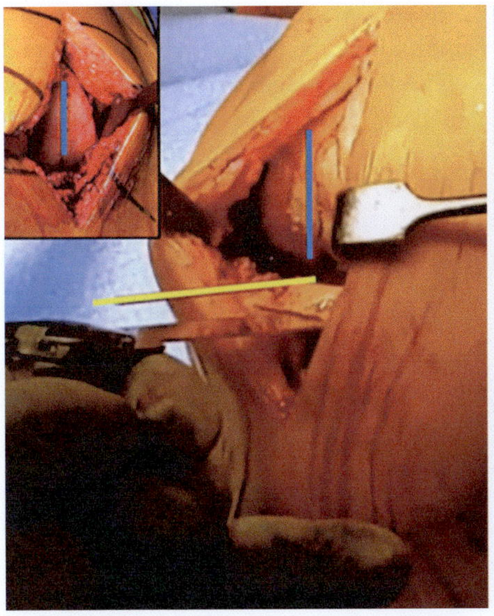
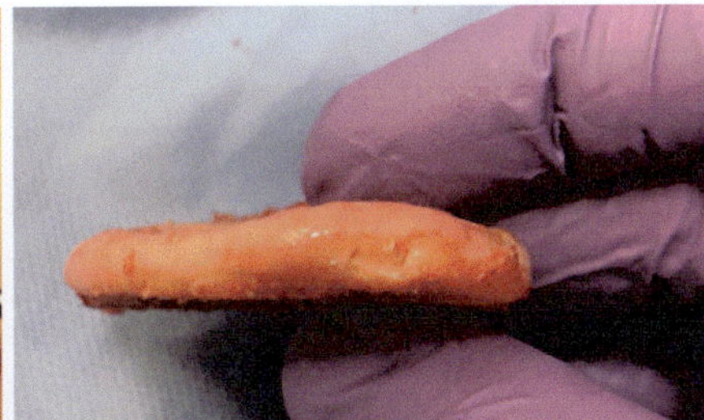
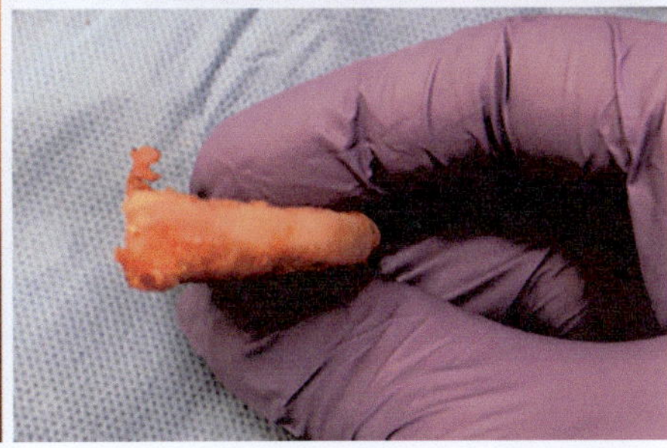

Fig. 9.6 This composite image shows the anatomical markers used to align the tibial component during medial KA-UKA. Images on the left show the anteroposterior axis of the flexion facet of the condyle (blue lines) and a pin inserted in the joint space in the anterior and posterior borders of the medial plateau. They will be used to adjust frontal rotation (varus–valgus) and the posterior slope of the tibial component, respectively. The images on the right show the resultant tibial resection, which aims to restore the medial (upper image) and posterior (lower image) tibial slopes

medial condyle [32]; the tibial section has to be perpendicular to this axis. Once performed, tibial resection is verified visually to assess the posterior slope (it should follow the native slope) and the anteroposterior and mediolateral dimensions, which should not exceed those of the tibial trial base. The thickness of the tibial cut is measured with vernier callipers; the objective is to equalise the thickness of the Oxford® tibial implant (minimum 6.5 mm) after considering cartilage loss (2 mm), possible bone loss (rare during isolated anteromedial wear) and thickness of the saw-blade (1 mm). The tibial section is generally oriented in slight varus during medial UKA, but this varies by subject. Following these recommendations, the tibial component will be aligned parallel to the femoral cylindrical axis and perpendicular to the tibial longitudinal axis, respectively. Considering the thickness of the resected bone measured with vernier callipers, the surgeon can determine the thickness of the polyethylene insert necessary to restore the pre-arthritis height of the medial tibial plateau joint surface.

Femoral resection for medial Oxford® UKA (Fig. 9.7): Axial and frontal rotations of the femoral component are determined by following the anteroposterior axis of the flexion facet and the medial wall (after removing medial osteophytes) from the medial femoral condyle, respectively (Fig. 9.7). Frontal alignment can be guided by a pin inserted along the medial wall of the condyle (after resectioning osteophytes) between the medial collateral ligament and the condylar bone,

which provides information on the frontal orientation of the medial femoral condyle. The femoral component is generally oriented in slight valgus position during medial UKA, with valgus varying among patients depending on the original knee anatomy (Fig. 9.7). The thickness of the posterior femoral section is then verified with vernier callipers; its thickness has to be equal to that of the prosthetic posterior condyle after considering the thickness of the sawblade (1 mm) and possible cartilage loss (rare in isolated anteromedial wear). The last stage, which is very simple, consists of balancing the spaces at 90° and 10° flexion with slight distal femoral reaming. Considering that the Oxford® femoral component is an implant with resurfacing of approximately 3 mm in thickness and that the condylar cartilage measures about 2 mm in thick-

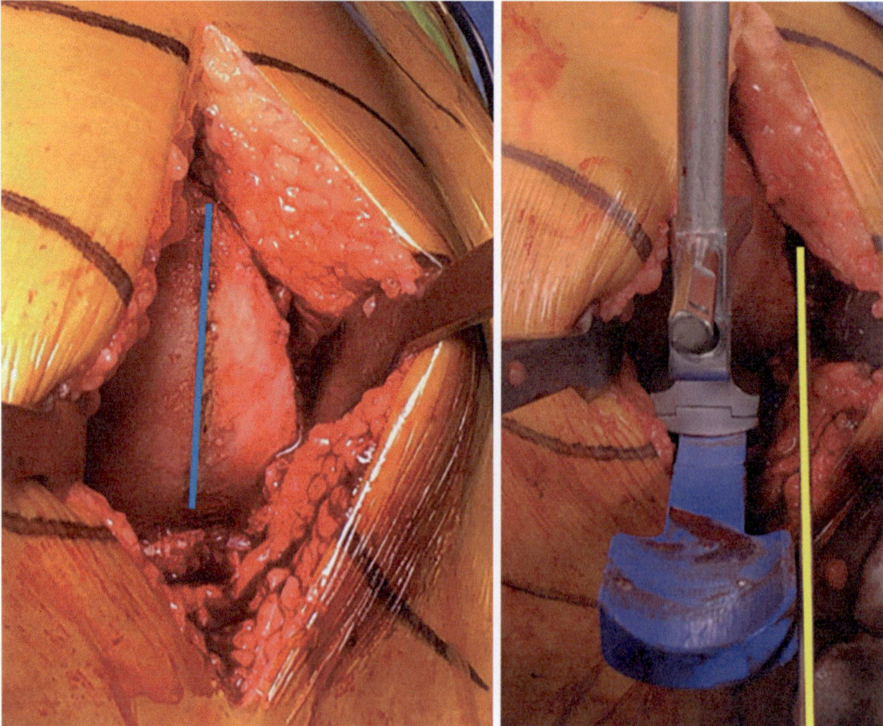

Fig. 9.7 These composite images show the anatomical markers used to align the femoral component during execution of medial KA-UKA. The image on the left shows the anteroposterior axis of the flexion facet of the condyle which can be marked by electrocauterisation; this line is used to adjust the axial rotation and mediolateral transla-tion of the femoral component. The image on the right shows the femoral height aligned on the anteroposterior axis of the flexion facet of the condyle, and a pin positioned along the medial wall of the condyle and indicating the frontal orientation of the condyle

ness, reaming of the distal femur should not remove more than 1–2 mm of subchondral bone. By following these stages, the femoral component will be aligned perpendicular to the femoral cylindrical axis.

Thanks to quality control of bone sections, which is performed at each stage of surgery with the aid of vernier callipers, the decision on the polyethylene insert's thickness can be deduced. It is essential to ensure that residual laxity of 1–2 mm remains when stress is exerted on the flexed knee in the valgus position. It is possible to underdimension the insert by 1– 2 mm if desired to protect the lateral compartment of the knee by undercorrecting alignment of the limb.

9.6 Conclusion

The kinematic alignment (KA) technique for unicompartmental knee arthroplasty (UKA) has been performed successfully for decades. This chapter helps the surgeon understand the theoretical bases and surgical principles of the technique. The objective is to encourage surgeons to use the KA technique because it is a simple, safe, more anatomical, more physiological and probably clinically advantageous method compared to traditional mechanical alignment for UKA. Other investigations are necessary to better define its clinical impact and the limits of prosthetic component alignment.

Acknowledgements We wish to thank Medacta for providing the images illustrating kinematic alignment of the MOTO® implant.

References

1. Rivière C, Iranpour F, Auvinet E, et al. Alignment options for total knee arthroplasty: a systematic review. Orthop Traumatol Surg Res. 2017;103(7):1047–56.
2. Whiteside LA. Making your next unicompartmental knee arthroplasty last. J Arthroplast. 2005;20:2–3.
3. Baker PN, Petheram T, Avery PJ, Gregg PJ, Deehan DJ. Revision for unexplained pain following unicompartmental and total knee replacement. J Bone Joint Surg Am. 2012;94(17):e126.
4. NJR 15th Annual report 2018.
5. Ollivier M, Parratte S, Lunebourg A, Viehweger E, Argenson J-N. The John Insall award: no functional benefit after unicompartmental knee arthroplasty performed with patient-specific instrumentation: a randomized trial. Clin Orthop Relat Res. 2016;474(1):60–8.
6. Fu J, Wang Y, Li X, et al. Robot-assisted vs. conventional unicompartmental knee arthroplasty: systematic review and meta-analysis. Orthopade. 2018;47(12):1009–17.
7. Rivière C, Vigdorchik JM, Vendittoli P-A. Mechanical alignment: the end of an era! Orthop Traumatol Surg Res. 2019;105(7):1223–6.
8. Rivière C, Sivaloganathan S, Cartier P, Villet L, Vendittoli PA, Cobb J. Kinematic Alignment Is A Reliable Technique For Implanting medial UKA: a systematic review. KSSTA. 2020;30(3):1082–94.
9. Rivière C, Harman C, Leong A, Cobb J, Maillot C. Kinematic alignment technique for medial OXFORD UKA: an in-silico study. Orthop Traumatol Surg Res. 2019;105(1):63–70.
10. Deschamps G, Chol C. Fixed-bearing unicompartmental knee arthroplasty. Patients' selection and operative technique. Orthop Traumatol Surg Res. 2011;97(6):648–61.
11. Cartier P. Story of my passion. Knee. 2014;21(1):349–50.
12. Cartier P, Sanouiller JL, Grelsamer RP. Unicompartmental knee arthroplasty surgery: 10-year minimum follow-up period. J Arthroplast. 1996;11(7):782–8.
13. Sampath SA, Lewis S, Fosco M, Tigani D. Trabecular orientation in the human femur and tibia and the relationship with lower-limb alignment for patients with osteoarthritis of the knee. J Biomech. 2015;48(6):1214–8.
14. Asada S, Inoue S, Tsukamoto I, Mori S, Akagi M. Obliquity of tibial component after unicompartmental knee arthroplasty. Knee. 2019;26(2):410–5.
15. Rivière C, Iranpour F, Auvinet E, et al. Mechanical alignment technique for TKA: are there intrinsic technical limitations? Orthop Traumatol Surg Res. 2017;103(7):1057–67.
16. Chatellard R, Sauleau V, Colmar M, Robert H, Raynaud G, Brilhault J. Medial unicompartmental knee arthroplasty: does tibial component position influence clinical outcomes and arthroplasty survival? Orthop Traumatol Surg Res. 2013;99(4):S219–25.
17. Lee SY, Bae JH, Kim JG, et al. The influence of surgical factors on dislocation of the meniscal bearing after Oxford medial unicompartmental knee replacement: a case–control study. Bone Joint J. 2014;96-B(7):914–22.
18. Lo Presti M, Raspugli GF, Reale D, et al. Early failure in medial unicondylar arthroplasty: radiographic analysis on the importance of joint line restoration. J Knee Surg. 2019;32(09):860–5.
19. Zambianchi F, Digennaro V, Giorgini A, et al. Surgeon's experience influences UKA survivorship: a comparative study between all-poly and metal

back designs. Knee Surg Sports Traumatol Arthrosc. 2015;23(7):2074–80.

20. Dai X, Fang J, Jiang L, Xiong Y, Zhang M, Zhu S. How does the inclination of the tibial component matter? A three-dimensional finite element analysis of medial mobile-bearing unicompartmental arthroplasty. Knee. 2018;25(3):434–44.

21. Inoue S, Akagi M, Asada S, Mori S, Zaima H, Hashida M. The valgus inclination of the Tibial component increases the risk of medial tibial condylar fractures in unicompartmental knee arthroplasty. J Arthroplast. 2016;31(9):2025–30.

22. Zhu G-D, Guo W-S, Zhang Q-D, Liu Z-H, Cheng L-M. Finite element analysis of mobile-bearing unicompartmental knee arthroplasty: the influence of Tibial component coronal alignment. Chin Med J. 2015;128(21):2873–8.

23. Wahal N, Gaba S, Malhotra R, Kumar V, Pegg EC, Pandit H. Reduced bearing excursion after Mobile-bearing unicompartmental knee arthroplasty is associated with poor functional outcomes. J Arthroplast. 2018;33(2):366–71.

24. Heyse TJ, Khefacha A, Fuchs-Winkelmann S, Cartier P. UKA after spontaneous osteonecrosis of the knee: a retrospective analysis. Arc Orthop Trauma Surg. 2011;131(5):613–7.

25. Heyse TJ, Khefacha A, Peersman G, Cartier P. Survivorship of UKA in the middle-aged. Knee. 2012;19(5):585–91.

26. Franz A, Boese C, Matthies A, Leffler J, Ries C. Mid-term clinical outcome and reconstruction of posterior Tibial slope after UKA. J Knee Surg. 2019;32(05):468–74.

27. Bruni D, Akkawi I, Iacono F, et al. Minimum thickness of all-poly tibial component unicompartmental knee arthroplasty in patients younger than 60 years does not increase revision rate for aseptic loosening. Knee Surg Sports Traumatol Arthrosc. 2013;21(11):2462–7.

28. Soavi R, Loreti I, Bragonzoni L, La Palombara PF, Visani A, Marcacci M. A roentgen stereophotogrammetric analysis of unicompartmental knee arthroplasty. J Arthroplast. 2002;17(5):556–61.

29. Ensini A, Barbadoro P, Leardini A, Catani F, Giannini S. Early migration of the cemented tibial component of unicompartmental knee arthroplasty: a radiostereometry study. Knee Surg Sports Traumatol Arthrosc. 2013;21(11):2474–9.

30. Barbadoro P, Ensini A, Leardini A, et al. Tibial component alignment and risk of loosening in unicompartmental knee arthroplasty: a radiographic and radiostereometric study. Knee Surg Sports Traumatol Arthrosc. 2014;22(12):3157–62.

31. Jones GG, Clarke S, Harris S, et al. A novel patient-specific instrument design can deliver robotic level accuracy in unicompartmental knee arthroplasty. Knee. 2019;26(6):1421–8.

32. Freeman MA, Pinskerova V. The movement of the normal tibio-femoral joint. J Biomech. 2005;38(2):197–208.

10

Computer-Assisted and Robotic Unicompartmental Knee Arthroplasties

Constant Foissey, Cécile Batailler, Elvire Servien, and Sébastien Lustig

10.1 Introduction

The development of ancillary instruments (instrumentation) for the unicompartmental knee arthroplasties (UKA) has made it possible to improve positioning of the implant and its reproducibility. Each stage in this progression has increased the reliability of UKA:

- In the early 1970s, Marmor [1] developed a rudimentary instrumentation device allowing near-'freehand' placement of the implant.
- In the 1980s, Cartier [2] introduced a tibial cutting guide and a test condyle with contact points.
- In the 1990s, an intra-medullary rod was considered for a femoral implant, but that undermined the mini-invasive aspect of the procedure.
- Computer-assisted navigation was developed towards the end of the 1990s and quickly presented encouraging results [3–6].
- Lastly, robotic-assisted surgery developed progressively with the introduction of Acrobot® in 2003, MAKO® in 2015 and Navio®.

UKA is a rare surgical procedure in France. In 2011, 9500 UKA were performed versus 70,200 TKR [7]. The surgical technique is demanding and the operator must follow strict rules to obtain optimal function and survival. The different parameters to be considered are as follows:

- The tibiofemoral mechanical axis [8]
- Ligament tension
- Tibial slope [9]
- Positioning in the sagittal plane of the femur [10]
- Rotation of the implants [11]
- Size of the implants [12]
- Contact point: centring the femoral implant on the tibia across all degrees of mobility
- Restoration of the joint space [13]

The latest technological advances make it possible to control these parameters to different degrees. Navigation can be performed in two different ways: by navigating tibial resection alone or by navigating tibial and femoral resection [14]. The first procedure makes it possible to control the first three parameters whilst the second controls the first four. Robotic assistance makes it possible to control all these parameters.

C. Foissey · C. Batailler (✉) · E. Servien · S. Lustig
Service de chirurgie orthopédique, Hôpital de la
Croix Rousse, Hospices civils de Lyon, Lyon, France

10.2 Navigation and Medial UKA

10.2.1 Installation of UKA with Isolated Navigation on the Tibial Plateau

The system described uses OrthoPilot® (B. Braun–Aesculap), which does not require preoperative imaging and functions with perioperative dynamic image acquisition of the hip, knee, ankle and visible femoral and tibial points.

The femoral and tibial sensors are inserted percutaneously. The approach is standard.

Once the markers are acquired, the axis of the limb appears and reducibility of the deformity can be tested.

The tibial sectioning guide is positioned, and navigation can start by adjusting varus/valgus, the tibial slope and height of the resection by computer-acquired data (Fig. 10.1). Once the correct position has been found, the sectioning guide is attached to the bone and tibial cutting of the bone is performed with the oscillating saw.

The remaining cutting takes place without navigation with a femoral cut dependent on the tibial cut, taking care not to place the condyle in recurvatum in order to avoid conflict with the patella. The navigator is again used when tests are performed to verify the axis (177°±2°) and safety margin. A safety margin >1° contraindicates use of a mobile plateau due to the risk of its dislocation.

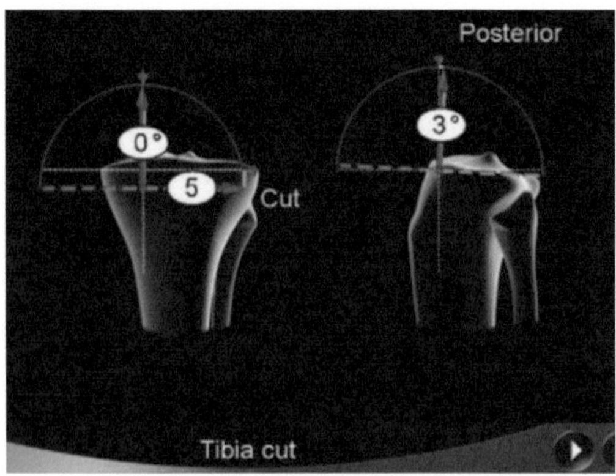

Fig. 10.1 Computer showing the choice of tibial section: 0° varus, 3° slope and 5-mm resection

Once all parameters have been validated, the final implants are sealed. Another control of the tibiofemoral mechanical axis can then be performed with the final implants.

This system is independent of the type of medial UKA installed.

10.2.2 Placement of a UKA with Navigation on the Tibial Plateau and Femoral Condyle

Preoperative preparation requires radiographic measurement of two elements:

- Frontal orientation of the femoral epiphysis: the angle between the femoral mechanical axis and the tangent to the femoral condyles.
- The presumed size of the femoral component (seen in the profile X-ray view).

The acquisition system allows a mini-invasive approach without cutting into the tendon insertion of the vastus medialis [15]. The acquisitions are similar to the technique previously described. The same applies to the tibial cut.

The tibiofemoral space is then measured in flexion and in extension. Depending on the gap in flexion and extension, femoral cuts are planned: frontal and sagittal orientation, height of distal and posterior resection, thickness of the tibial component, residual laxity in flexion and extension.

Once the data are validated, a semicircular frame is fixed under navigation control directly to the femoral reference screw (Fig. 10.2).

All cuts are made by adjusting the different section guides on this frame: with a saw for the posterior tibial cut and the bevel and milling of the femur for the distal section (Fig. 10.3).

The procedure ends as in the previous technique. The navigator is again used at the time testing is conducted to verify the axis (177°±2°) and safety margin. Once all parameters have been validated, the final implants are sealed. Another control of the tibiofemoral mechanical axis can then be performed with the final implants.

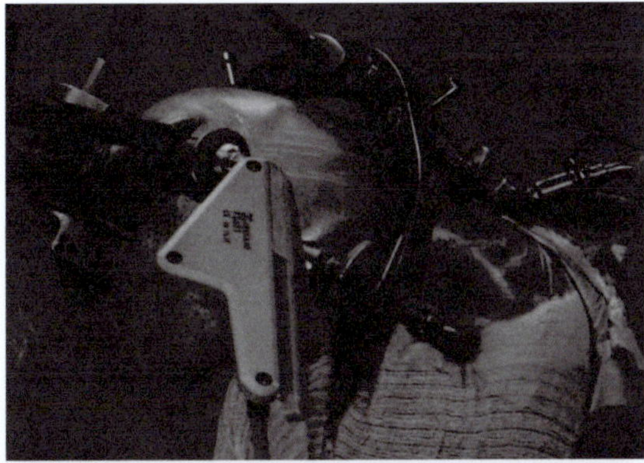

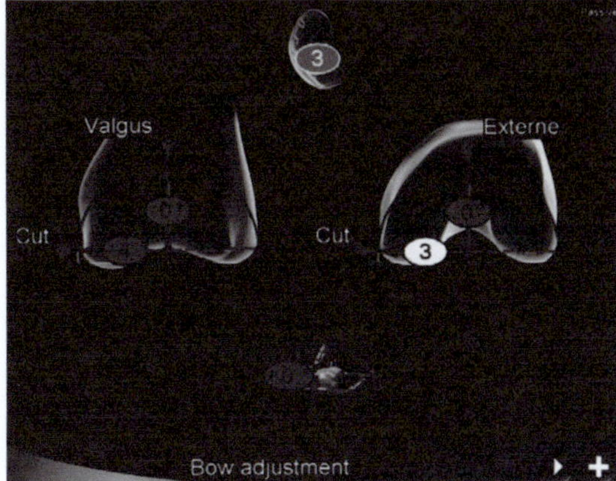

Fig. 10.2 Mini-invasive implantation of a UKA: preoperative and control views under navigation of the femoral section guide

Various navigation systems can be used with different systems to make the cuts. However, the acquisition of preoperative parameters and planning are similar between each one.

10.2.3 Results of Medial UKA Implanted with Navigation

In the context of medial UKA with isolated navigation on the tibial plateau, a 2009 study [3] comparing 20 navigated UKA versus 20 standard UKA on the accuracy of the postoperative HKA (hip–knee–ankle) angle compared to the target objective (178°) found 85% accuracy with navigation vs. 60% without navigation ($p < 0.05$).

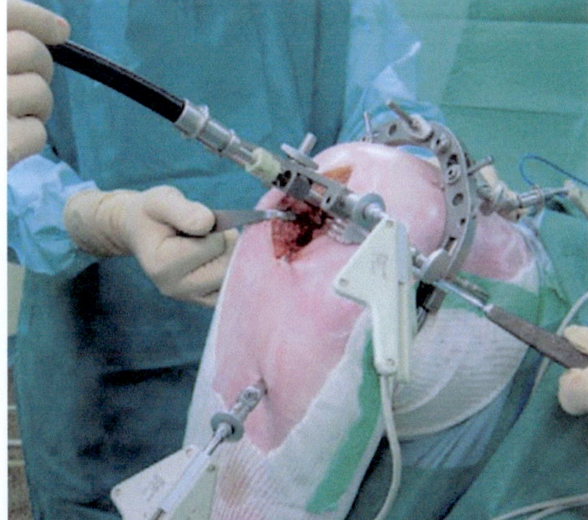

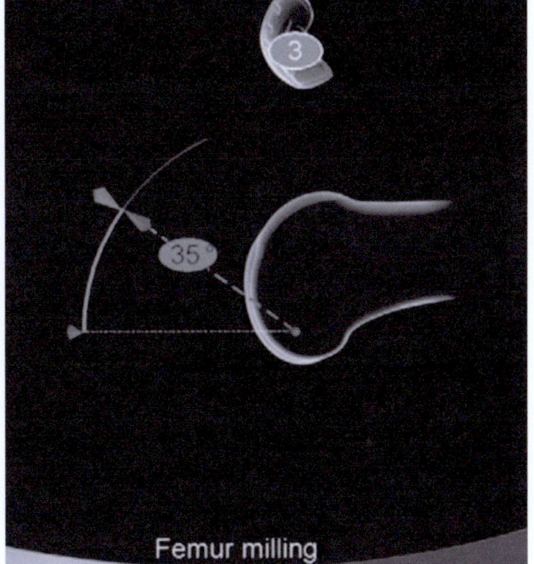

Fig. 10.3 Femoral cuts

These results were confirmed in 2012 [16] with 93.9% accuracy for HKA, 84.8% for the mechanical tibial axis, and 100% for the posterior tibial slope in 33 medial UKA surgically implanted with assistance from the OrthoPilot® system.

In 2011 [17], a review of 81 medial UKA with tibial and femoral navigation found 94% accuracy regarding HKA, with implantation considered as radiologically perfect in 77% of cases and 97% 2-year survival.

10.3 Robotic-Assisted Medial UKA

Various robotic systems can be used for implanting a medial UKA. This involves mainly the NAVIO® system from Smith & Nephew and the MAKO® system from Stryker. The essential difference between the two lies in the need to perform a preoperative CT scan or not.

10.3.1 Surgical Technique—Navio® System (Smith & Nephew)

The NAVIO® system (Smith & Nephew) does not require preoperative imaging. It is based on kinematic preoperative image acquisitions of the hip, knee and ankle via bone morphing and on acquisition of points of interest.

10.3.1.1 Positioning of the Patient

The patient is placed in the supine position, with a side block and distal block to maintain the knee at 90°.

The NAVIO® PFS console consists of three components (Fig. 10.4):

- An infrared camera placed 1 m from the area of interest.
- A touchscreen.
- A console that controls the robotic-assisted drill connected to it by a cable.

No cutting ancillary instrument is necessary.

The only preoperative imaging is a standard radiographic assessment.

The first stage is positioning the femoral and tibial sensors on the skin (Fig. 10.5). These sensors should be visible throughout the procedure and for extreme amplitudes of the knee.

A medial parapatellar incision is made conventionally from the upper pole of the patella to about 1 cm below the joint space over a length of about 10 cm. Arthrotomy is performed at the mid-vastus medialis. It is important that osteophytes be removed before any image acquisition in order to have an appropriate ligament balance.

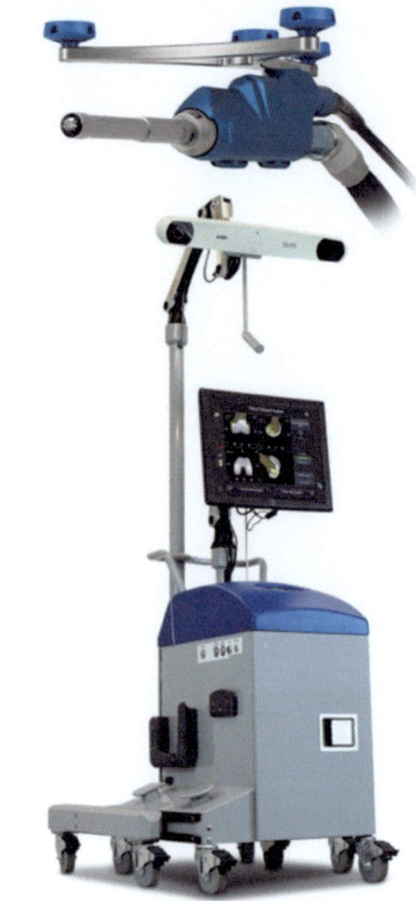

Fig. 10.4 The Navio® system

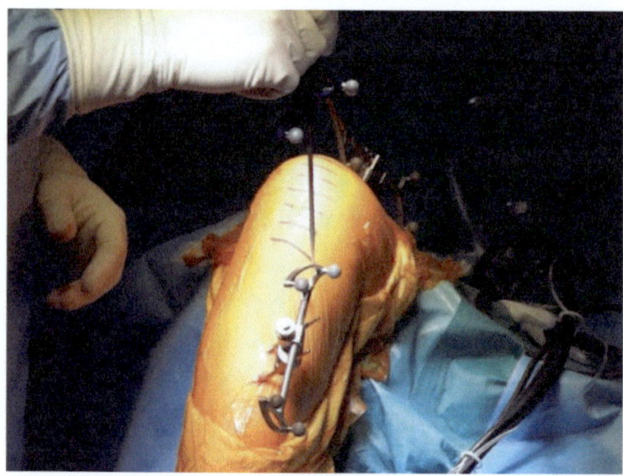

Fig. 10.5 Positioning of the patient and sensors

10.3.1.2 Acquisition of Points of Interest

In order to ensure that the sensors are stable throughout the procedure, a reference point is identified in the tibia and femur, making it possible to verify at any time with a probe that the sensors have not moved.

The centre of the hip, ankle and knee axis of flexion are acquired by complete flexion–extension movement without stress in the varus/valgus position. The same flexion–extension movement is then performed with stress in valgus to record the reducibility of the deformity. This dynamic acquisition is essential because it enables the system to consider ligament laxity during the planning stage. It is also essential that the deformity be reduced with moderation.

The points of interest are then acquired on the femur: the centre of the knee, the most distal point of the medial condyle, the most posterior point and the most anterior point of the medial condyle. Femoral acquisition continues with a phase of bone morphing from the area of interest using the probe (Fig. 10.6).

The same sequence is then repeated in the tibia: the centre of the tibia, the most distal point of the tibial cup, the most posterior point, the most medial point and the most anterior point. The anteroposterior axis of the tibia is also recorded to finish tibial acquisition with a bone morphing phase.

10.3.1.3 Planning

This enables effective dynamic planning, reflecting the reducibility of the deformity.

The first stage consists of choosing the femoral implant's size, which can be modified at any time during planning (Fig. 10.7).

Key Points

– *Obtain ideal bone coverage without overdimensioning to avoid having an implant that overlaps, entering into conflict with the patella, tibial spine mass or soft tissue, or on the contrary an underdimensioned implant that risks sinking in a secondary phase.*
– *Moderately increasing flexion of the femoral implant can make it possible to obtain an appropriate size with optimal bone coverage.*

The desired position for the femoral component is then determined in the three spatial planes. Exact positioning of the implant compared to the shape of the femoral condyle is depicted with the angular values (varus/valgus, flexion, rotation) (Fig. 10.8). Usually, it is necessary to distalise somewhat the femoral implant in order to compensate for distal wear and to follow the bony

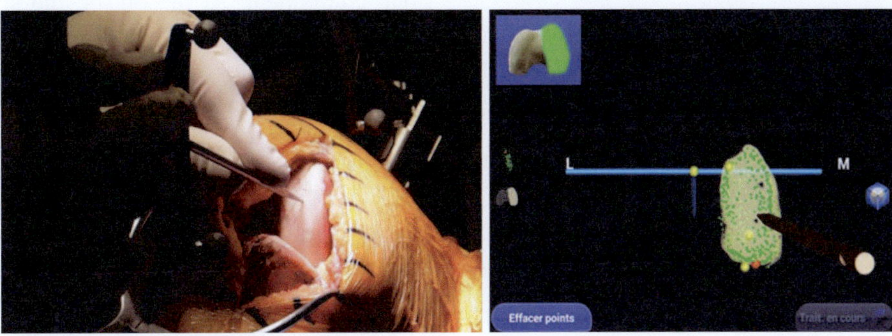

Fig. 10.6 Bone morphing of the femoral condyle

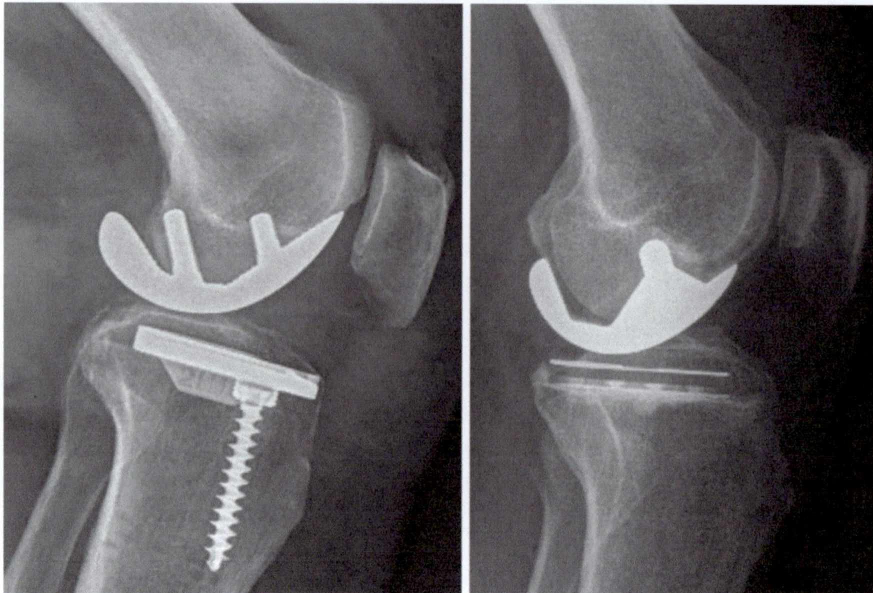

Fig. 10.7 Over- and underdimensioned femoral implants

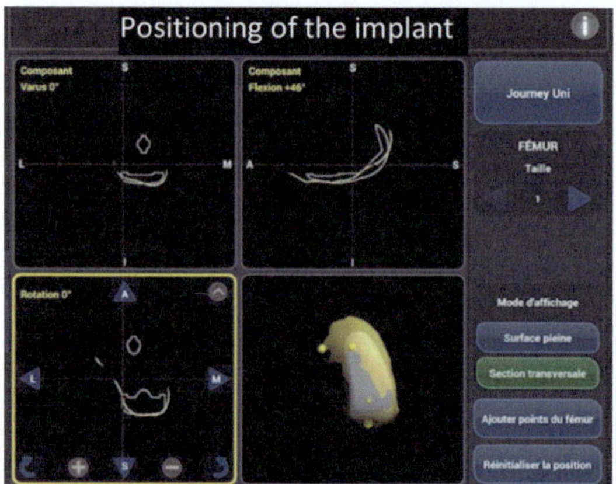

Fig. 10.8 Planning the positioning of the femoral implant: 0° varus, 0° rotation, and 45° flexion

contour posteriorly to avoid increasing posterior femoral offset and to tighten the knee in flexion.

Key Points

The objective is to:

- *Preserve the height of the joint space.*
- *Prevent a conflict anteriorly with the tibial spine mass.*

- *Avoid any conflict with the patella (hence the importance of marking the most anterior point).*

Usually, the femoral component should be as close as possible to the intercondylar notch in order to improve the contact points between the femoral and tibial implants.

The same stages are then performed for the tibial component. At the outset, the size of the implant and thickness of the polyethylene are decided. The positioning in varus/valgus, the tibial slope, rotation and mediolateral positioning of the implant are then chosen in line with the tibial spines.

Key Points

- *Tibial bone cutting should be minimal (usually 4–5 mm).*
- *The tibial slope is adapted to the patient's anatomy; it is higher in the medial positioning (equal to or less than 5°) than in the lateral position and determines flexion, stability and survival.*
- *The tibial cut is usually orthogonal in the tibial mechanical axis. In cases of a major varus*

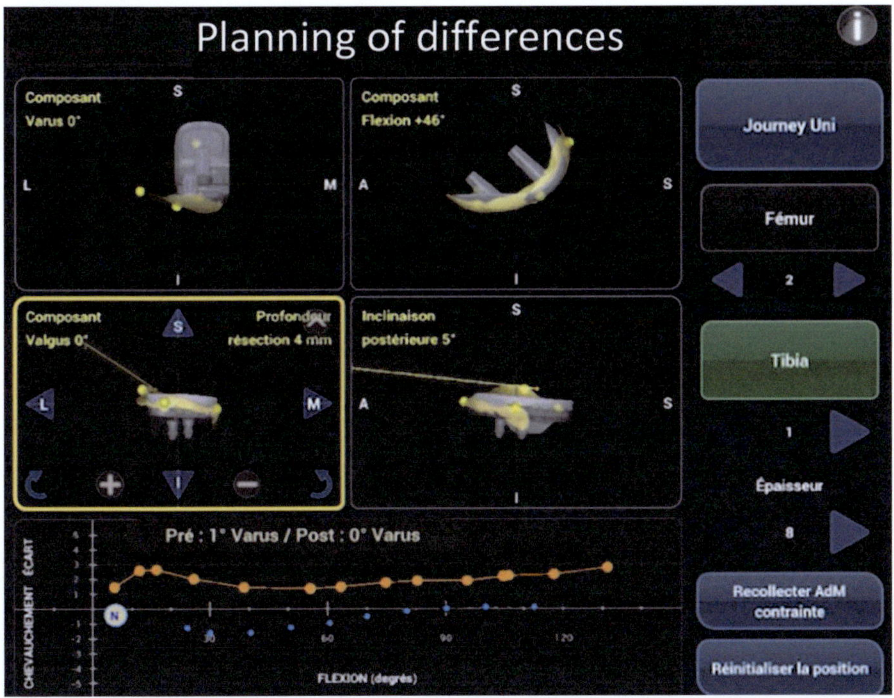

Fig. 10.9 Planning the overall balancing of the knee according to the positioning of the femoral and tibial implants

deformity, it is preferable to maintain a few degrees of varus in the tibial section in order to improve the contact points between the femoral and tibial implants.

The next step makes it possible to visualise the results of planning in terms of angular correction (preoperative versus postoperative) between 0° and 120° of flexion, as well as ligament balance (Fig. 10.9). At this stage, the positioning of the tibial (varus/valgus, slope, rotation, section height) and femoral (varus/valgus, flexion, rotation, cut height) implants can be changed to visualise directly the effects on final angular correction and ligament balance. These parameters consider not only static acquisition but also initial dynamic acquisition and therefore reducibility of the deformity with each degree of flexion.

Key Points
– *Obtain slight undercorrection to avoid contra-lateral decompensation (overcorrection) or*

conversely rapid failure of the implant (undercorrection).
– *Importance of the ligament balance in the frontal plane, for which we strive to maintain a residual safety margin balanced in flexion and in extension.*

The last stage in planning consists of visualising the contact points between the two implants during flexion, which, if necessary, makes it possible to lateralise or medialise one or both of the implants to better centre this contact point (Fig. 10.10).

Key Point
Avoid any risk of impingement responsible for premature wear of the polyethylene.

10.3.1.4   Preparation of Bone Surfaces

Generally, we start with the femur, which is the most readily accessible. An automatic feedback system

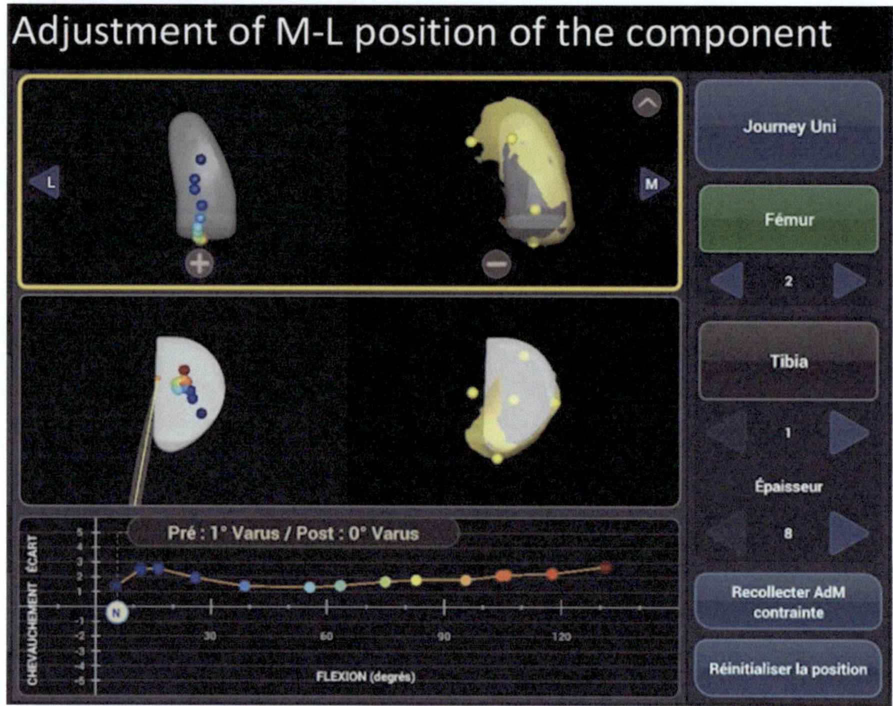

Fig. 10.10 Adjustment of the mediolateral positioning of the implants to centre the tibiofemoral contact point

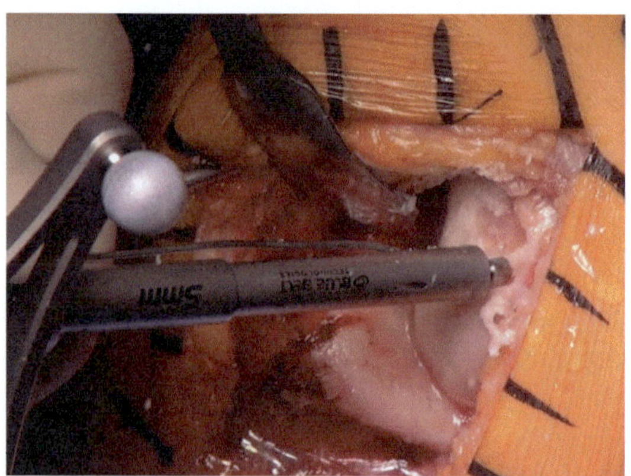

Fig. 10.11 Milling of the femoral condyle. The mill automatically retracts when the operator strays outside the planned area

makes it possible to mill only the planned area. If the operator strays outside this area, the milling cutter retracts, making erroneous bone resection impossible in an unwanted area (Fig. 10.11). The depth of bone to be removed is continuously visualised by changing colour (Fig. 10.12).

Once the femur is prepared, we move onto the tibia, following the same procedure. It is possible to use the most anterior part of the bone cut to press with a saw and saw the most posterior part of the tibia.

A rasp (grater) makes it possible to flatten the bone sections once milling is complete. The meniscus, readily accessible at this stage, is then removed.

The last stage consists of milling the anchoring points of the femoral implant (Fig. 10.13).

10.3.1.5 Tests and Final Implants

It is then possible to insert the test implants and to visualise onscreen the angular correction obtained, as well as the balancing on all amplitudes of flexion (Fig. 10.14). Cementing and fixation of the final implants are done according to the operator's usual practice. It is then possible to recheck the angular correction and balancing of the knee with the final implants.

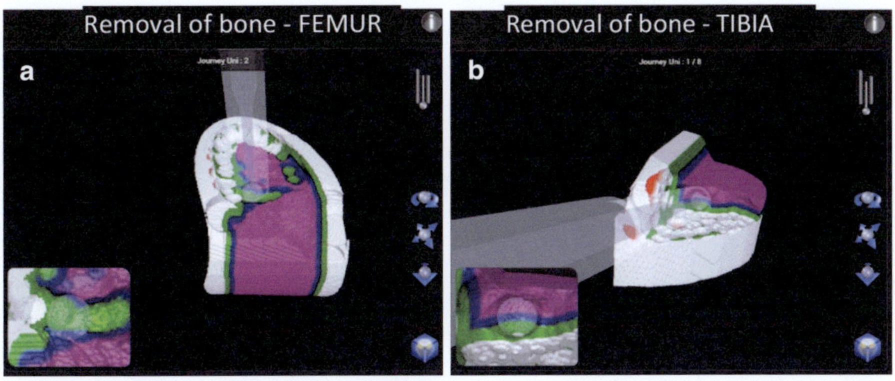

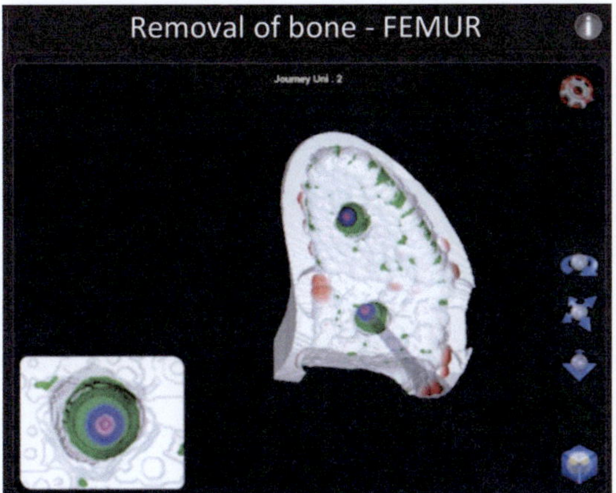

Fig. 10.12 Onscreen visualisation of milled areas of bone yet to be removed (**a**) distal femur, (**b**) tibia

Fig. 10.13 Milling of the femoral points

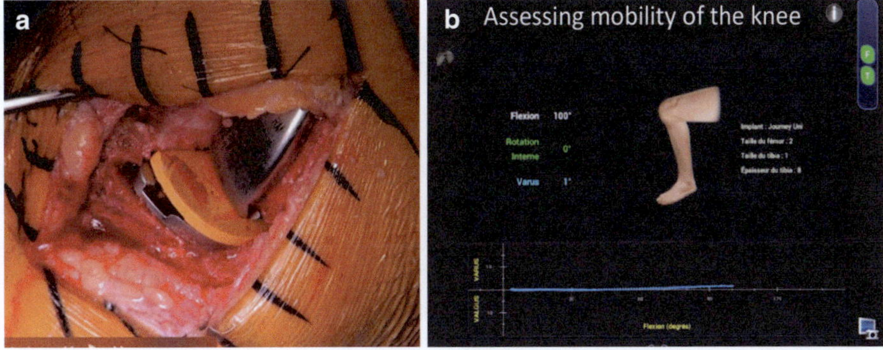

Fig. 10.14 Positioning of the test implants (11a) and control of balancing on all joint amplitudes (11b)

10.3.2 Surgical Technique—MAKO° System (Stryker)

The MAKO® system bases its modelling on a preoperative CT scan. This makes it possible to plan the positioning of the implant, as well as the desired sizes, upstream of the procedure.

10.3.2.1 Positioning of the Patient

The patient is placed in the supine position, with an uncumbersome lateral block (in order not to hinder the robot's progression) and a distal block to maintain the knee at 90°.

The MAKO® system consists of four components:

- An infrared camera placed 1 m from the area of interest.
- A screen for the surgeon.
- A control console for the engineer.
- A robotic arm, which is positioned on the side to be treated with surgery, close to where the surgeon stands.

No cutting ancillary instrument is necessary.

A CT scan is performed preoperatively according to a precise protocol in order to plan the implants' positioning. Planning can be undertaken a few days prior to the procedure or just before. It will be adjusted during the procedure following acquisition of the ligament balance.

Positioning of the femoral and tibial sensors percutaneously is similar to that of the Navio® system. The incision and approach are also unremarkable. Osteophytes must be removed after acquisition of the reference points (osteophytes potentially comprise areas of acquisition) and before the ligament balance.

10.3.2.2 Acquisition of Points of Interest

Acquisition of the centre of the hip and the centre of the knee is approximately identical to that of the NAVIO® system. For modelling the knee, however, the CT scan makes it possible to avoid bone morphing. Therefore, the acquisition points performed on the femur and tibia make it possible to couple the patient's knee with the preoper-

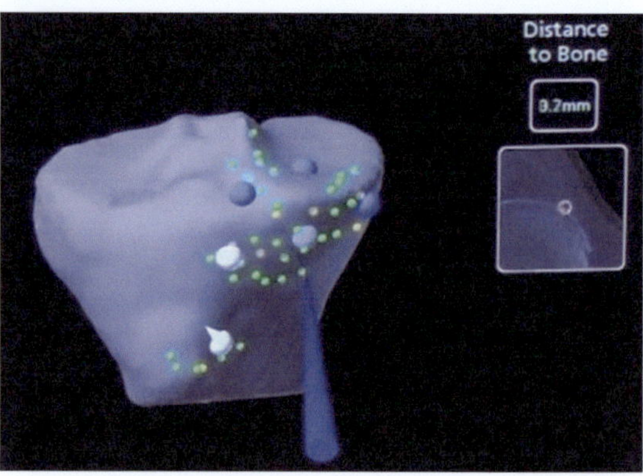

Fig. 10.15 Modelling of the knee by coupling with the preoperative CT scan: acquisition of specific points

ative scan by precise modelling perioperatively the knee that has undergone surgery (Fig. 10.15).

Acquisition of ligament balance is relatively similar to the NAVIO® system. The lower limb deformity is acquired extension, with 90° flexion and maximum flexion, by simulating weightbearing. Reduction of the deformity is acquired in complete extension and then every 20° to obtain the ligament balance throughout amplitude of the joint.

10.3.2.3 Planning

Preoperative planning makes it possible to choose the most appropriate implant size in order to have optimal bone coverage without overlap, and then to position precisely the femoral and tibial implants in the 3D reconstruction obtained with the CT scan (Fig. 10.16). The positioning can be modified in the three spatial planes (coronal, sagittal and axial) for the two implants by also adjusting the heights of the bone cuts.

Perioperatively, planning can be adjusted to reflect the ligament balance acquired at the start of the procedure, as well as contact points between the femur and tibia on the entire joint amplitude.

10.3.2.4 Preparation of Bony Areas

Lastly, the bone cuts will be made with a robotic arm controlled by the surgeon with haptic feedback allowing a certain rapidity (Fig. 10.17). The robotic arm can use either a narrow saw or milling cutter, as chosen by the surgeon. Once the

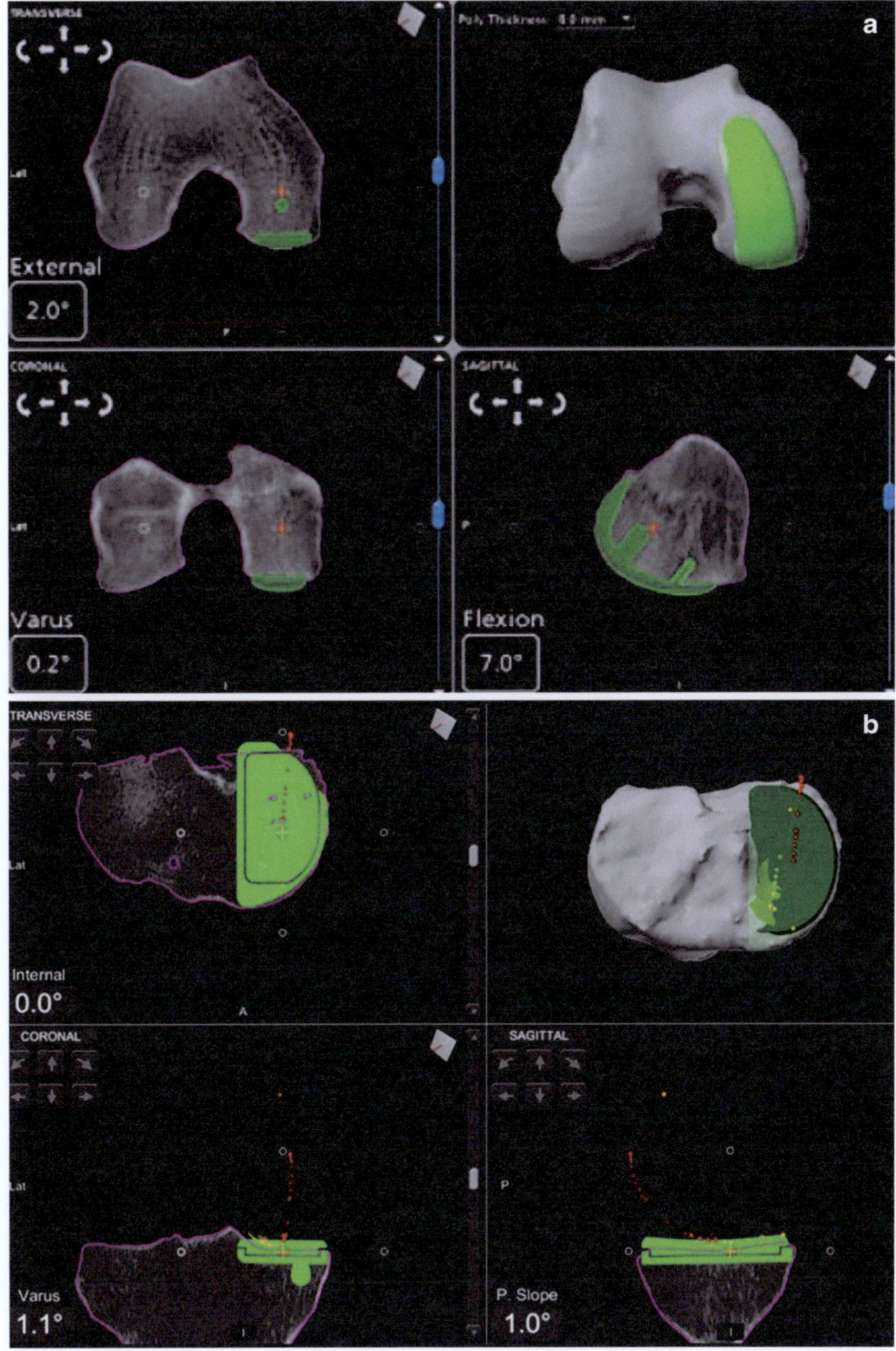

Fig. 10.16 Planning the positioning of the implant with CT scan acquisition (**a**) and control of the femur–tibia contact points perioperatively (**b**)

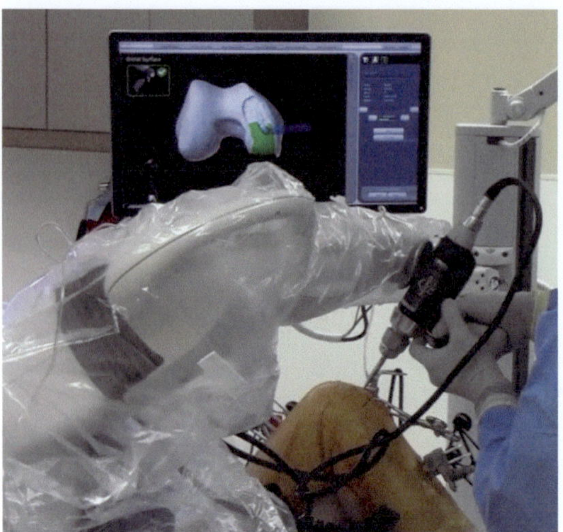

Fig. 10.17 Robotic arm with haptic feedback

bone cuts have been made, tests may be conducted in a conventional manner. The lower limb axis and residual laxity will be determined by the robotic system during the tests.

10.3.3 Results

In a retrospective study, 80 robotic UKA versus 80 standard UKA with 1.5 years' follow-up were analysed in our department [18]. We found a significant decrease in aberrant values regarding the HKA angle, tibial slope and orientation of the tibial section, which falls within the logic of results reproducibility. Analysis of revisions revealed the absence of revision due to malposition of the implants. The last advantage found was the absence of a learning curve; none of the first implants placed by younger surgeons using robotic control presented any aberrant values. Robotic planning readily enables acquisition of precise techniques prior to validation, which is highly valuable in a university department.

Restitution of the joint space in the resurfacing implants was also studied [19] and a significant difference was found in favour of a robotic procedure with a mean decrease of 1.4 mm vs. 4.7 mm. Therefore, the femoral implant was less distalised, with good restitution of the joint space and decreased thickness of the tibial cut. This

reduction in excessive tibial cuts lowers the risk of complications in the tibial implant (postoperative pain, early loosening, secondary displacement).

Other robotic systems requiring a preoperative scan (Acrobot® and Mako®) found similar results [3, 11, 12]. The literature did not report any difference in terms of precision of the cuts, clinical result or survival of implants between the MAKO® and NAVIO® technologies [20, 21]. However, an advantage was reported in favour of the MAKO® system in the dimensioning of the implants. The NAVIO® system is dependent on the acquisition of points of interest, which can prove difficult behind the femur and tibia. Use of the MAKO® system, coupled with CT scans, enables better restitution of the posterior femoral offset and less underdimensioning with the posterior part of the tibia [22]. Lastly, the MAKO® technology has enabled faster procedure times thanks to preoperative planning and the robotic arm [20, 21].

Robotisation significantly decreases improper positioning and alignment errors. Consequently, it is possible to expand certain indications and regularly perform procedures that are known to be demanding and difficult, such as lateral UKA, bicompartmental arthroplasties and reconstruction of the anterior cruciate ligament (ACL) associated with UKA.

References

1. Marmor L. The Marmor knee replacement. Orthop Clin North Am. 1982;13(1):55–64.
2. Cartier P, Cheaib S. Unicondylar knee arthroplasty: 2–10 years of follow-up evaluation. J Arthroplast. 1987;2(2):157–62.
3. Ayach A, Plaweski S, Saragaglia D. Computer-assisted uni knee arthroplasty for genu varum deformity. Results of axial correction in a case-control study of 40 cases. In: 9th annual meeting of CAOS-International proceedings; 2009. p. 4–7.
4. Cossey AJ, Spriggins AJ. The use of computer-assisted surgical navigation to prevent malalignment in unicompartmental knee arthroplasty. J Arthroplast. 2005;20(1):29–34.
5. Jenny J-Y, Boeri C. Unicompartmental knee prosthesis implantation with a non-image-based navigation system: rationale, technique, case-control

comparative study with a conventional instrumented implantation. Knee Surg Sports Traumatol Arthrosc. 2003;11(1):40–5.

6. Jung KA, Kim SJ, Lee SC, Hwang SH, Ahn NK. Accuracy of implantation during computer-assisted minimally invasive Oxford unicompartmental knee arthroplasty: a comparison with a conventional instrumented technique. Knee. 2010;17(6):387–91.

7. Haute Autorité de Santé. Rapport d'évaluation - Implants articulaires du genou. 2012.

8. Lustig S, Lording T, Frank F, Debette C, Servien E, Neyret P. Progression of medial osteoarthritis and long term results of lateral unicompartmental arthroplasty: 10 to 18 year follow-up of 54 consecutive implants. Knee. 2014;21(Suppl 1):S26–32.

9. Nunley RM, Nam D, Johnson SR, Barnes CL. Extreme variability in posterior slope of the proximal tibia: measurements on 2395 CT scans of patients undergoing UKA? J Arthroplast. 2014;29(8):1677–80.

10. Kaya Bicer E, Servien E, Lustig S, Demey G, Ait Si Selmi T, Neyret P. Sagittal flexion angle of the femoral component in unicompartmental knee arthroplasty: is it same for both medial and lateral UKAs? Knee Surg Sports Traumatol Arthrosc. 2010;18(7):928–33.

11. Servien E, Fary C, Lustig S, Demey G, Saffarini M, Chomel S, et al. Tibial component rotation assessment using CT scan in medial and lateral unicompartmental knee arthroplasty. Orthop Traumatol Surg Res. 2011;97(3):272–5; https://www.em-consulte.com/en/article/288184.

12. Servien E, Saffarini M, Lustig S, Chomel S, Neyret P. Lateral versus medial tibial plateau: morphometric analysis and adaptability with current tibial component design. Knee Surg Sports Traumatol Arthrosc. 2008;16(12):1141–5.

13. Weber P, Schröder C, Laubender RP, Baur-Melnyk A, von Schulze PC, Jansson V, et al. Joint line reconstruction in medial unicompartmental knee arthroplasty: development and validation of a measurement method. Knee Surg Sports Traumatol Arthrosc. 2013;21(11):2468–73.

14. Jenny J-Y, Saragaglia D. Navigation informatisée des prothèses unicompartimentales du genou. In: Prothèses partielles de genou. ELSEVIER MASSON. (Cahiers d'enseignement de la SOFCOT); 2012.

15. Jenny J-Y. Navigated unicompartmental knee replacement. Sports Med Arthrosc Rev. 2008;16(2):103–7.

16. Saragaglia D, Picard F, Refaie R. Navigation of the tibial plateau alone appears to be sufficient in computer-assisted unicompartmental knee arthroplasty. Int Orthop. 2012;36(12):2479–83.

17. Jenny J-Y, Saussac F, Louis P. Navigated, minimal invasive, mobile bearing unicompartmental knee prosthesis. A 2-year follow-up study. Orthopaedic Proc. 2012;94-B(SUPP_XXXVII):271.

18. Batailler C, White N, Ranaldi FM, Neyret P, Servien E, Lustig S. Improved implant position and lower revision rate with robotic-assisted unicompartmental knee arthroplasty. Knee Surg Sports Traumatol Arthrosc. 2018;27:1232. https://doi.org/10.1007/s00167-018-5081-5.

19. Herry Y, Batailler C, Lording T, Servien E, Neyret P, Lustig S. Improved joint-line restitution in unicompartmental knee arthroplasty using a robotic-assisted surgical technique. Int Orthop. 2017;41(11):2265–71.

20. Leelasestaporn C, Tarnpichprasert T, Arirachakaran A, Kongtharvonskul J. Comparison of 1-year outcomes between MAKO versus NAVIO robot-assisted medial UKA: nonrandomized, prospective, comparative study. Knee Surg Relat Res. 2020;32(1):13.

21. Porcelli P, Marmotti A, Bellato E, Colombero D, Ferrero G, Agati G, et al. Comparing different approaches in robotic-assisted surgery for unicompartmental knee arthroplasty: outcomes at a short-term follow-up of MAKO versus NAVIO system. J Biol Regul Homeost Agents. 2020;34(4 Suppl. 3):393–404. Congress of the Italian Orthopaedic Research Society

22. Batailler C, Bordes M, Lording T, Nigues A, Servien E, Calliess T, et al. Improved sizing with image-based robotic-assisted system compared to image-free and conventional techniques in medial unicompartmental knee arthroplasty. Bone Joint J. 2021;103-B(4):610–8.

Hubert Lanternier and Arnaud Clavé

11.1 Introduction

Although total knee arthroplasty is still the "gold standard" with medium- and long-term survival rates of 92–100% [1, 2], the good results of unicompartmental knee arthroplasty (UKA), particularly functional, have made them an alternative choice for younger patients with high functional demand who have unicompartmental knee osteoarthritis (OA) [3].

Nevertheless, implant failure on the tibial side remains a major cause of failure [4]. Over time, this has led to the development of different types of tibial components. Currently, we can identify two major groups:

– Full-polyethylene (FPE) implants.
– Metal-back implants for which a polyethylene (PE) insert can be either fixed or mobile.

The progressive introduction of metal-back implants has come to supplement the traditional, older "full-polyethylene" offering, and coexistence of the two concepts is prompting reflection on their mechanical, biological, and surgical specificities and respective indications.

11.2 The Different Types of Tibial Implants

The "full-polyethylene" implant (Fig. 11.1) is a UHMWPE single block, generally with a flat joint surface, which will be cemented directly onto the tibial section. Its minimum thickness to limit complications due to wear and creep was validated by the SOFCOT consensus in 1995 and was set at 9 mm.

Metal back refers to the implantation on the tibial section of a metal baseplate, generally made of Stellite (chromium–cobalt) and more rarely titanium, for which bone anchoring can be achieved with or without cementing. Similarly, there are different manufacturer designs, including stemmed implant and variable number of contact points (or a screw-in type), making it possible to reinforce the metal-back implant's fixation to the tibial bone. This metal-back implant is designed to receive a polyethylene insert, either fixed or mobile. For fixed plateau, the polyethylene is generally flat and noncongruent (Fig. 11.2) with the minimum thickness validated at the 1995 SOFCOT symposium of 6 mm and 9 mm for the screw-in format. This thickness was determined to limit the risk of wear. Using a metal-back

H. Lanternier
Department of Orthopaedic Surgery and
Traumatology, Polyclinique de l'Europe,
Saint-Nazaire, France

A. Clavé (✉)
Department of Orthopaedic Surgery and
Traumatology, Saint George Private Hospital,
Nice, France

LaTIM UMR 1101 INSERM-UBO, Brest, France

© The Author(s), under exclusive license to Springer Nature Switzerland AG 2024
A. Clavé, F. Dubrana (eds.), *Unicompartmental Knee Arthroplasty*,
https://doi.org/10.1007/978-3-031-48332-5_11

131

implant involves the thinnest possible PE to limit the depth/height of tibial cut. To reduce stress and therefore creep and wear on the PE, Goodfellow had the idea in the 1970s of developing a mobile plateau concept. The PE has become concave and congruent with the femoral implant and has two surfaces for sliding, one with the femoral implant and the other with the metal-back tibial implant (Fig. 11.3). As the femoral implant has a spherical shape, the contact surface is optimised, theo-

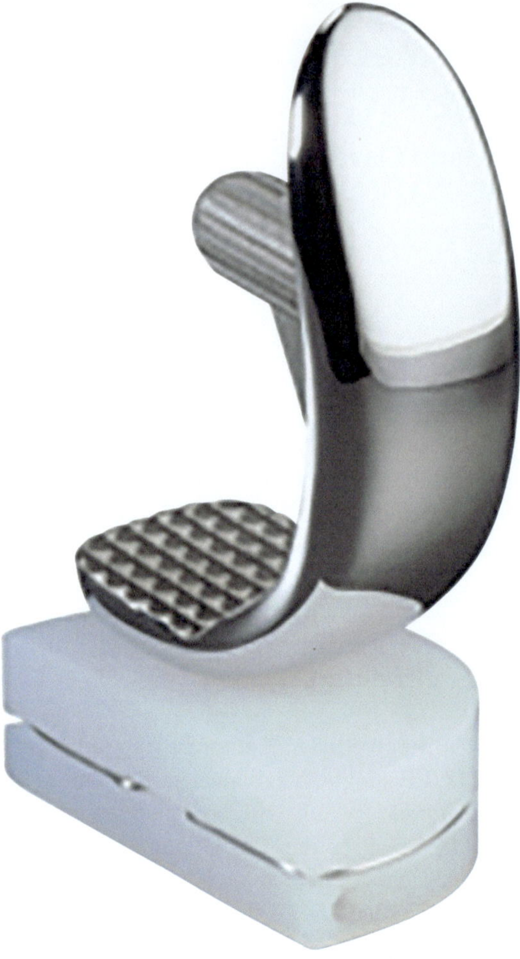

Fig. 11.1 P Uni Full-Polyethylene HLS Univ-evolution™, Tornier (Courtesy of Tornier/Stryker)

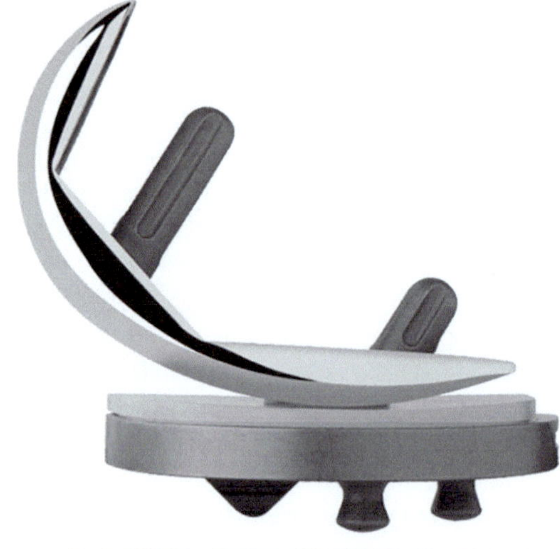

Fig. 11.2 P Uni Fixed Metal-Back Uni-highFlex™, Zimmer (Courtesy of Zimmer-Biomet)

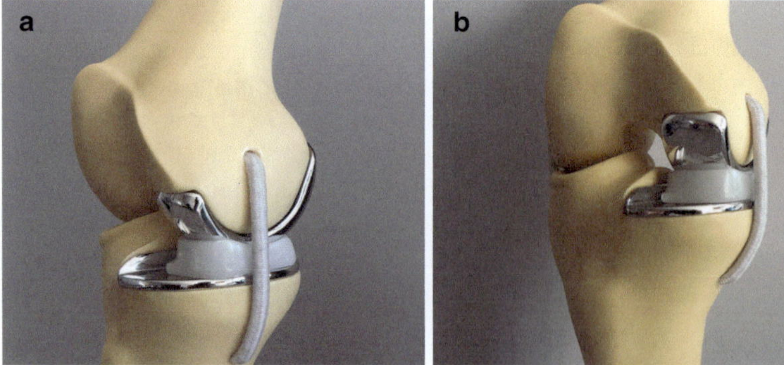

Fig. 11.3 P Uni Mobile Metal-Back Oxford™, Zimmer Biomet (**a**) 3/4 view from the medial side (**b**) Frontal view

retically decreasing and better distributing stresses and shearing forces. The advantage is the possibility of using thinner PE.

11.3   The Problem

Tibial replacement requires a highly specific unicompartmental implant procedure since it is necessary to resect a sufficient thickness of bone to leave room for a suitable thickness of polyethylene (PE). To do that, we have to sacrifice the underlying subchondral bone layer, thereby losing a solid and stable support, as the underlying cancellous bone is less dense. Nothing very different from total knee replacement you might think, if it were not for three major differences.

The first one lies in the surface area of support provided. In the case of UKA, it is much less than half of what is available for TKR since the latter has the entire surface of tibial spine mass shifted from stability to transfer of weightbearing.

The second specificity lies in the lesser quality of the bone segment offered to support the UKA. In fact, a TKR can be supported by dense bone close to cortical bone throughout the periphery, while UKA is deprived of this benefit near to the tibial spine mass since the resection here exposes low-density cancellous bone that does not have the primary purpose of stress transfer during compression. In summary, two thirds of the peripheral bone are dense and much more suitable for weightbearing than in the central third. The bony base of a UKA, therefore, is much less homogeneous.

The third difference lies in the level of ligament balance needed to maintain residual varus: this point can only be acquired by sufficient bone resection, often deeper than in a TKR. And the problem worsens because we know that the deeper we descend into bone, the more the surface area decreases and bone density diminishes.

Therefore, tibial implantation is demanding: a small surface area, little homogeneity and low-density bone. The surgeon, aware of these delicate parameters, will strive to perform a precise,

economical resection while gaining in surface area by going as close as possible to the central pivotal point.

It is then important to choose the most appropriate implant and fixation for this specific context. The design of the tibial implant, which is available in several sizes, should cover maximum surface area without entering into conflict with the capsular ligaments.

The type of implant (full PE or metal back) in contact with bone will govern the transfer of weightbearing, which we will describe.

11.4   Biomechanical: Stress, Wear and Creep

11.4.1   Finite Element Model Parts/ Transition of Rigidity/ Elasticity/Young's Modulus

It is important to know the finite element model parts and their mechanical characteristics [5–7].

Young's modulus (elasticity modulus) is the constant that connects the compression or traction stress and start of deformation before the limit of elasticity.

- PE, a constant element in UKA, has a Young's modulus evaluated between 0.4 and 0.7 GPa; it is homogeneous [7].
- The alloy (Cr–Co) used for metal-back implants is also homogenous with a much higher Young's modulus of 193 GPa [5] to 225 GPa [7].
- The polymethylmethacrylate cement is around 4 GPa [7].
- Lastly, the mechanical characteristics of the tibial bone chosen to receive the implant are extremely variable according to its cortical or cancellous structure and depending on the subjects. Furthermore, resistance in compression, the one that interests us, is more important than in distraction. The literature reports very different figures with maximum values of 30 GPa for cortical bone and minimum 0.3 GPa for cancellous bone [6, 7].

Therefore, the metal alloy has a very high modulus while the PE, cement and cancellous bone have much lower and "relatively" similar moduli. Implant fixation must incorporate these elements because much demand is placed on the sealing interface between a rigid and less rigid body (Table 11.1).

11.4.2 Stress and Strain

In 2010, Small et al. [8] studied in vitro in a validated biomechanical model the effect of metal backing (mobile metal-back vs. full PE study) on the stress transmitted and found on the tibia and its subchondral bone depending on flexion of the knee (extension, 45° and 90° flexion). For full-PE implants, they found statistically higher stresses in the four weightbearing positions with, depending on the area, significant differences ranging from +57% to +223%. They concluded, therefore, that mobile metal-back implants enable better distribution of stresses on the surface area of the tibia and up to 3 cm below the tibial implant (Fig. 11.4). The areas of excess stress were more common and more pronounced in the absence of metal-back implants, which induced both higher testing of the bone–implant interface (cemented or not) which transmits the stresses and greater risk of collapse of the underlying bone structure. These localised excess stresses and their less good distribution to the underlying tibia, moreover, were responsible for the poor results obtained by full PE in a clinical study by Aleto [4]. In fact, 87% of the revised full-PE internal UKA versus 53%

Table 11.1 Material properties assigned lo finite element model part.20, 21 Cortical and cancellous bone properties apply to loading in compression

Model	Part	Elastic modulus (GPa)	Poisson's ratio	Elements
AP	Cortical bone	16.7	0.3	105,375
	Cancellous bone	0.155	0.3	93,880
	PMMA cement	2.4	0.3	19,691
	AP tibia	0.69	0.46	23,950
MB	Cortical bone	16.7	0.3	105,375
	Cancellous bone	0.155	0.3	96,340
	PMMA cement	2.4	0.3	6,371
	MB tibial tray (CoCr)	210	0.3	16,594
	Polyethylene insert	0.69	0.46	22,313

AP all-polyethyne, *MB* metal-backed, *GPa* gigapascal, *PMMA* polyethylmethacrylate, *CoCr* cobalt chrome
Mechanical properties assigned to finite element model parts (Scott CEH et al.) [7].

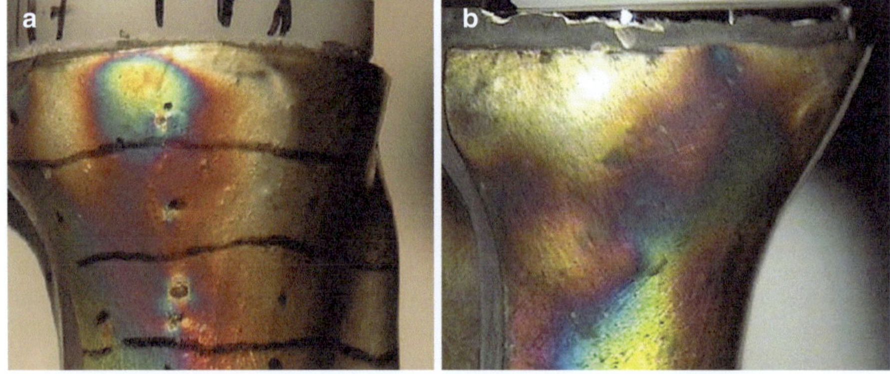

Fig. 11.4 Distribution and intensity of stress on the tibia depending on the type of tibial implant: (**a**) Full PE: stress hotspot in posteromedial view, (**b**) mobile metal back: gradual distribution of intensity and distribution of stress [8]

for MB ($p = 0.04$) were due to collapse of the fixed tibial plateau [4].

Several teams have studied the stress exerted on PE and its distribution based on the type of tibial plateau. Simpson et al. [9] developed an experimental model enabling analysis of the peaks of stress and strain exerted on the four types of tibial plateaus: mobile metal back, partially congruent fixed metal back, flat fixed metal back and full PE. Their results showed that the intensity of the contact stress, identical for the fixed metal back and full PE (44.3, 48.6 and 45.9 MPa), was much lower on the mobile metal-back implants (2.7 MPa). This was due to more uniform stress distribution over a wider surface area of the PE with mobile metal-back implants (Fig. 11.5). Therefore, only these PE had peaks of contact forces below the PE level of resistance (17 MPa); the other models were subject to stresses three times higher (Fig. 11.6). Similarly, in a study of stresses by von Mises, the peaks of stress were lower than the limit of PE fatigue only for mobile metal-back implants (Fig. 11.7). Moreover, these peaks of stresses varied inversely with the thickness of the PE, and the authors observed that for fixed metal-back

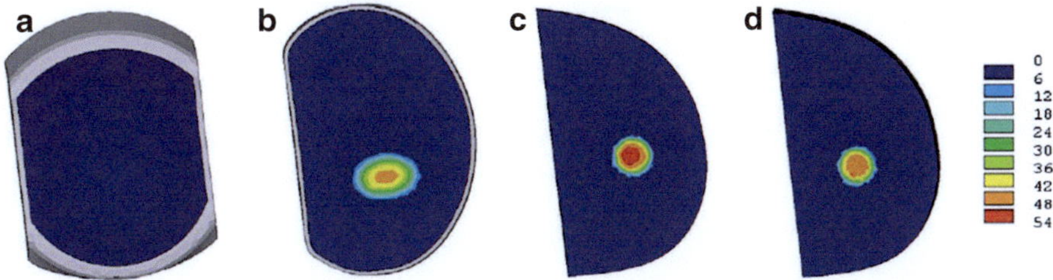

Fig. 11.5 Peak of intensity of contact stress (in MPa) depending on the type of plateau: (**a**) mobile metal back, (**b**) semi-congruent fixed metal back, (**c**) fixed metal back, (**d**) full PE [9]

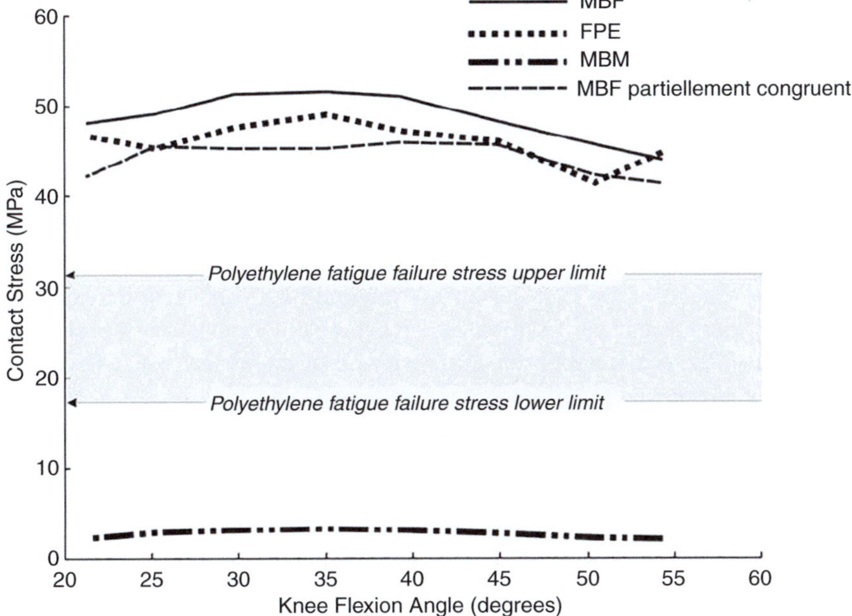

Fig. 11.6 Comparison of contact stress peaks depending on the type of plateau (on y-axis flexion of the knee in degrees, on x-axis pressure in MPa) [9]

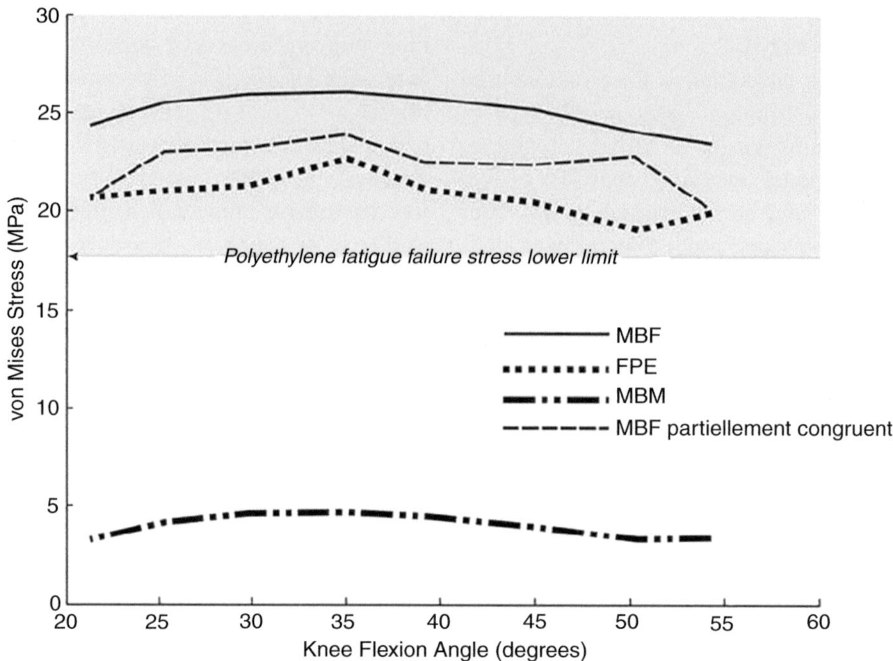

Fig. 11.7 Comparison of stress peaks from von Misses depending on the type of plateau (on y-axis flexion of the knee in degrees, on x-axis pressure in MPa) [9]

implants with PE of 8.5 mm, those in the von Mises study were greater than the limit of PE fatigue, an observation that was identical with full PE of 15 mm. These results, therefore, call into question the minimum thickness of 6 mm and 9 mm for fixed metal-back and full-PE implants. On the contrary, peaks of PE stresses of mobile metal-back implants of 3.5 mm and 2.5 mm were less than the limit of fatigue.

11.4.3 Volume and Reasons for Wear

The main industrial and mechanical factors that affect wear are type of PE, its method of sterilisation and thickness, congruence of parts and contact surface area [10, 11].

Several studies have examined PE wear and creep in vivo on specimens explanted to replace an implant. Ashraf et al. [12] reported a mean linear wear rate of 0.15 mm/year for fixed plateau implants (full PE and fixed metal back) in 2004. The total mean wear rate was highly related to the duration of implantation. Argenson and

O'Connor [13], as well as Psychoyiosis et al. [14] or Price et al. [15], reported much lower linear wear rates ranging from 0.01 to 0.08 mm/year for mobile inserts (Oxford™, Biomet Warsaw, USA).

It is interesting to note that in these two studies, the difference in wear was observed less in terms of volumetric wear: 17.3 mm³/year for full-PE and fixed metal-back implants [12] and 6 to 47 mm³/year for mobile metal-back implants [13, 14]. A possible explanation is that in congruent fixed plateaus, wear is distributed mainly in the "femoral-meniscal" area of excess stress while for mobile plateaus, wear occurred over a larger section of the plateau and in both the "femoral-meniscal" and "tibial-meniscal" areas.

We note that these values are not very different to what Wroblewski found in 1985 for Charnley total hip replacements (16 mm³/year) [16].

In vitro studies that examine PE wear in UKA are rare in the literature and find more wear for mobile metal-back implants than for fixed plateaus (fixed metal back or full PE) [17]. Kretzer et al. found a mean wear rate in vitro of 10.7 mg and 5.38 mg/10^6 cycles for medial and lateral mobile metal-back implants (Univation Mobile™, Aesculap, Germany) versus 7.51 mg and 3.04 mg/10^6 cycles for the fixed metal back. Moreover, higher generation of PE debris occurred with mobile inserts. These statistically significant differences led the author to conclude in the existence of a greater risk of aseptic loosening of the implant with mobile inserts [17].

Other studies have examined the characteristics of PE degradation: Manson et al. in 2010 analysed the degree (subjective score) and type of wear for three types of uni replacements, Oxford™ (mobile metal back), Miller-Galante™ (fixed metal back) and Repicci™ (full PE), removed during revision surgery [18]. Seven types of wear were identified: scratching (Fig. 11.8), pitting, burnishing (Fig. 11.9), embedded debris, abrasion (Fig. 11.10), delamination and creep. They found wear scores that were statistically higher (and similar) for the full-PE (33.6) and fixed metal-back implants (33.7) than for mobile metal-back implants (22.6). The latter, however, presented wear on the metal-back side of the PE with a mean score of 16.3 reinforcing the notion of wear on both sides of the mobile plateaus. Concerning the type of wear, the same quantity of pitting and embedded debris lesion types was found for the three groups. The full-PE and fixed metal-back implants showed evidence of wear induced by shearing forces (creep, delamination and burnishing). The mobile metal-

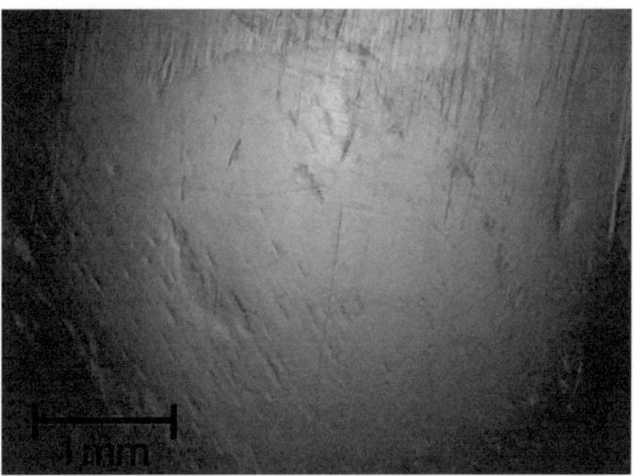

Fig. 11.9 Burnishing-type lesions on the upper aspect of PE in full PE, which are dominant in full-PE and fixed metal-back implants [17]

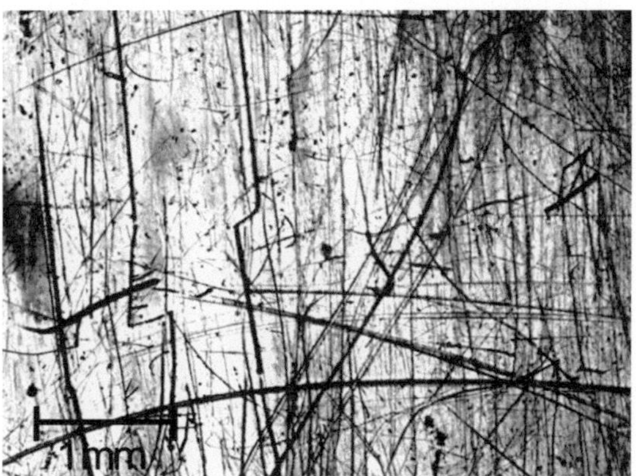

Fig. 11.10 Abrasion-type lesions on the lower aspect of the PE of mobile metal-back implants [17]

back implants mainly presented lesions such as abrasion and scratching. The authors concluded that the mobile metal-back implants showed evidence of wear similar to that found in PE inserts of THR (total hip replacement) and related to abrasion and adhesion forces, while the reasons for the wear of fixed metal-back and full PE are similar to those of TKR in relation to forces and stress of shearing and in fatigue.

In their in vitro study, Kretzer et al. systematically found on the upper sides of the mobile metal-back and fixed metal-back implants, the burnishing processes considered as the least harmful wear [17]. The lower sides of the fixed meta-back implant in contact with the metal back presented evidence of wear manifesting as abra-

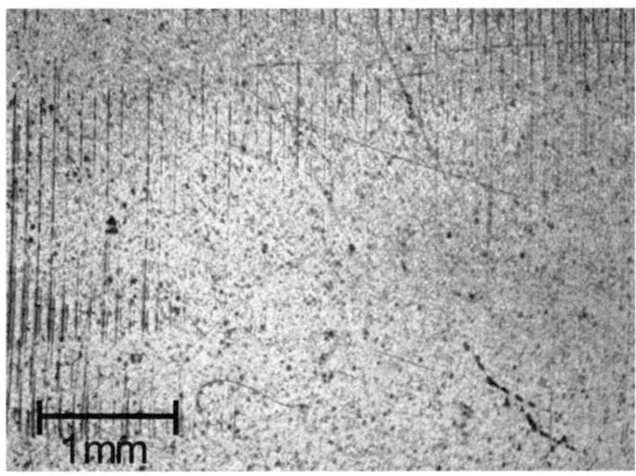

Fig. 11.8 Scratching and creep-type lesions [17]

sion and creep/scratching; these lesions were probably due to micromovements in the PE–metal back interface (backside wear lesion). Significant lesions such as abrasion, on the contrary, were systematically found on the lower side of the mobile metal-back PE inserts [17, 19].

The results of these studies, nevertheless, are to be interpreted with caution due to:

- The low number of cases studied each time.
- PE of unequal manufacture, some old and sterilised with processes that are now implicated in their degradation.
- Performances specific to each implant and probably different, irrespective of the model.
- Studies conducted on specimens explanted for revision surgery and therefore in a "pathological" context.
- Or in vitro studies that cannot perfectly reproduce the complexity of the knee joint kinematics.

11.5 The Strategy, the Options

The type of implant (full PE or metal back) in contact with bone, therefore, will govern the transfer of stresses. The bone implantation surface is irregular in its mechanical characteristics, has a relatively low elasticity modulus and needs to be made weightbearing. The issue is delicate, and the complexity of the situation is confirmed by the frequency of bone–cement borders; two strategies can contradict each other.

If the harmonious transition of elasticity is preferred, the full-PE implant is attractive: bone, cement and PE elasticity moduli are relatively similar. However, PE, if thin [7, 17–19], is susceptible to creep deformation or creep and will struggle to transfer the load equally to the entire bone section.

If homogenous transfer of stress to all considered surfaces is a priority, then very thick and less deformable PE or a metal-back implant should be prioritised. That solution is reassuring but comes at the expense of a brutal transition of elasticity.

11.5.1 Full PE

The full-PE tibial implant is cemented and fixed, and there are two interfaces, bone to cement and cement to PE.

An experimental study by Scott [7] examined the theoretical causes of mechanical disappointment with full PE to reiterate that 40% of revision surgeries may be performed because of unexplained pain, a figure that can appear disconcerting for a surgeon. The study's author, in particular, examined transfer of stresses to the tibial epiphysis to observe that a full-PE implant generates more abnormal stress (possibly causing pain) than metal-back implants, the increase in PE thickness from 6 to 10 mm decreasing but not cancelling out anomalies. These stresses are located in the anteromedial area and descend distally while the metal base that logically ensures their more harmonious distribution is more extensive in surface and less deep.

Hernigou [20] studied a series of removed full-PE implants to confirm that although wear was relatively constant, creep was more pronounced on parts with a lower thickness and particularly in heavy patients, suggesting the relative incompetence of thin and unrigid PE to transfer load harmoniously.

This biomechanical reflection is echoed in clinical studies that report lower survival over time, particularly in heavy and active patients. In a series of 1746 implants, Stefano Bini [21] found a significantly higher risk of revision surgery for full PE in comparison to metal-back implants. KR Berend [22] also found more cases of implant loosening with full PE in heavy patients.

11.5.2 Metal Back

The metal-back implant is attractive in principle: it provides a rigid base that can distribute load over a bone surface inhomogeneously. Moreover, it offers the possibility of uncemented fixation and opens the option of meniscal replacement. Nevertheless, it should be remembered that this strategy will multiply the interfaces and insert a metal part that is very rigid between two elements (bone and PE) which are less so.

The study by Scott [7] showed us that the transmission of stresses was optimised by the metal plate. Michael Berend [23], who conducted a photoelasticity study on the transmission of stresses, found pronounced internal stresses (particularly posterointernal) for a full-PE implant, but he also demonstrated relatively significant internal stresses that are more anterior with metal backs [23]. The stresses were not cancelled out, they were shifted: rearwards, more homogeneous and less deep. He suggested that these stresses could explain internal pain during the first 6 months after the implantation of a metal-back implant, as if it was necessary to allow a stress fracture to heal [23].

The metal-back implant with fixed plateau introduced a new interface, that of industrial fixation of PE on the base. A number of studies in the 1990s [24–26] mentioned the responsibility of micromovements that are likely to release particles that can promote the occurrence of backside wear [17–19, 27]. These reasons for wear are not the same as those resulting from contact of the upper aspect of the PE with the femoral component and may be more hazardous, particularly because the trapped concentration of PE residue near to or in contact with bone is higher. The methods of metal/PE assembly have since improved but the quality of this fixation should be analysed when selecting an implant.

Mobile implants fall within a different logic; they are marked by PE solidity with the aim of decreasing wear: translation movements are shifted to the flat lower aspect while sliding in flexion is allocated to the concave upper aspect, which can be completely congruent with the femoral component. There are two technical specificities to this type of implant. The first, the more difficult, is the need for perfect ligament balance to ensure good implant kinematics and stability, which will obviously contribute to a good clinical result. This is a demanding type of implant. The second, easier one is the quality of exposure during tibial sealing: introduction of a single, relatively thin metal plateau offers better visibility

rearwards and makes it possible to ensure good adaption before adding the PE. The introduction of a full implant with integrated or full PE immediately encumbers the surgical field and hinders good visibility. And it is all the more difficult when the tibial element is installed with procedures directed "below and rearwards", encouraging the implant to slide rearwards during its final impaction. With cumbersome full PE, it is difficult to perform unhindered vertical implantation, a procedure that is somewhat easier with a metal back fin. This subtlety does not pose a problem with TKR because implantation on a dislocated or subluxated tibia occurs mainly from the upper to lower aspect.

11.5.3 Clinical Results

There are clinical studies comparing full-PE implants to metal-back implants, and they present discrepant results. Gleeson et al. compared 47 metal-back mobile implants (Oxford™) and 57 full-PE implants (St Georg™ Sled) at 2 years' follow-up and found a better functional result and lower number of complications (particularly pain) [3]. Bhattacharya et al. in 2012 with slightly longer follow-up (5.6 and 3.7 years on average, respectively) found the opposite results after analysing 49 metal-back mobile (Oxford™) and 91 full-PE implants (Preservation™, DePuy, USA) [28].

A meta-analysis by Smith T.O. in 2009 [29] compared mobile plateaus with fixed plateaus (MBF and full PE) and did not find any difference in clinical results, patient satisfaction or complications, simply reporting a lower frequency of tibial radiological borders with mobile metal-back implants [29]. In a series of 144 full-PE cases (HLS Uni-Evolution™, Tornier, France), however, Lustig found 26.5% of such borders starting with year one, not progressive, with only a 3.5% revision rate because of loosening of the implant [30].

The conclusion of the lower number of clinical studies that have compared full-PE to metal-back implants (and to a greater extent fixed plateaus to mobile plateaus) is that, currently, there is no definitive clinical evidence supporting one type of plateau over another [31], although one randomised study in 2015 favoured metal-back implants [32]. A large number of recent studies report retrospective clinical studies.

The vast majority of them evaluated results by establishing an implant survival curve and clinical score (KSS, HSS, GIUM, Oxford Score, etc.). Few studies detail the different components of the clinical and functional evaluation, particularly the joint amplitudes. The survival rates ranged from 82% to 98% at 10 years for different types of plateaus, and no specific type seems to provide better results, although over the very long-term mobile metal-back implants appear superior with 91% survival at 20 years [33] versus 85% for full-PE implants [34, 35] and 86% at 15 years for fixed metal-back [36] implants. The functional results given by clinical scores do not show any differences between the families. Restoration of more anatomical kinematics of the knee for mobile metal-back implants does not translate into a marked improvement in clinical performance.

As in comparative studies, analysis of retrospective series shows very similar results in terms of functional score or survival, even though they can vary within a given family.

However, although these survival rates appear similar irrespective of the type of plateau, it should be underlined that the authors did not all use the same causes of failure in their calculations, making a strict comparison impossible.

Traditional UKA complications include complications that are more pathognomonic, such as type of tibial plateau, and can be correlated with biomechanical processes.

OA progression in the opposite compartment and infection are not affected by the type of tibial implant [29], although this first point is sometimes debated [19].

On the contrary, PE wear and creep are found mainly in fixed plateau implants and tended initially to involve the old-generation full-PE implants. This trend is declining with new full-PE models for which less revision surgery due to wear has been found.

Full PE are the type of implants most affected by aseptic loosening, which points in the direction of studies by Simpson, Small and Aleto among others on the existence of excess stresses with this type of plateau [4, 8, 24, 25].

This may also account for the higher number of cases of unexplained pain and tibial collapse found in the tibia with full PE [4, 8, 28, 37].

PE dislocations are an almost-exclusive complication of mobile metal-back implants [3, 38].

No consensus is found in the literature on the earlier occurrence of failure depending on the type of plateau. For some authors such as Bhattacharya, full PE is subject to earlier failure [28], but Gleeson found the opposite results in his study with a higher early failure rate for mobile metal-back implants [3].

The complexity of UKA revision UKA for totalisation is assessed differently by the authors [4, 18, 37, 39]. The technical difficulty, correlated with the cause of failure, nevertheless remains more often in the tibial component [4, 39]. Yet one of the advantages of the full-PE implant lies in conservation of tibial bone stock [40]. For some authors, the higher number of tibial plateau collapses with this type of implant requires more frequent bone grafts and reconstitutions, ultimately making revision surgery more complicated [4, 37].

Several authors have shown a correlation between the rate of revision surgery and number of UKA performed each year, suggesting that experience tallies with results, which is especially true for mobile metal-back implants [41, 42]. Mobile metal-back UKA is commonly considered as more technically demanding and requires a steeper learning curve.

11.6 Conclusion

After clarification of these factors, how can we choose?

The literature remains difficult to use: many very large series analyse numerous criteria but overlook the model used [43]; others simply compare uncemented implants (and therefore metal-back implants) to cemented implants that probably combine full PE and metal back but with no precise details [21]. Moreover, full-PE implants are the oldest and series on them may be tainted by implant design, PE quality or manufacturing issues, which can penalise results.

Most clinical series that can be used support metal-back implants with a lower rate of revision surgery due to loosening of the implant, particularly in heavy and active patients [44]. Yet transient upper metaphyseal pain has been reported with both full-PE [7] and metal-back implants [23], perhaps because of conflicts in elasticity or bone stress. This point, which is sometimes observed in clinical practice, is considered temporary and should not lead to hasty revision surgery for unexplained pain during year one postoperatively [23, 41].

The metal-back implant has a good reputation, the survival rate seems better, it opens the door to cementless fixation and enables the use of a mobile insert without cement. It should certainly be preferred in heavy and active subjects.

The full-PE implant also does not lack merit: its favourable elasticity modulus makes it possible to offer appropriate surgery to older, less active patients in the hope of minimising the painful events related to possible conflict in elasticity.

It emerges from the literature that UKA is a good procedure whose conduct should be meticulous and will yield good, lasting results provided that the right indication based on a clinical, radiographic and psychological analysis has been made. The implant model chosen is clearly important, but ranks behind quality of the indication and surgical procedure.

Take-Home Messages
Biomechanical level:

- Metal-back implants enable better distribution of loads and stresses in the implant/bone interface and underlying tibial bone tissue.
- The stresses and strains exerted on PE in mobile metal-back implants remain below the level of its mechanical resistance.

- Mobile metal-back implants enable better restoration of the knee joint's kinematic presentation.

In terms of wear:

- Mobile metal-back implants are less subject to creep and wear than full-PE and fixed metal-back implants, even though volumetric wear in studies seems to question that notion.
- The reasons for wear of full-PE and fixed metal-back implants correspond to stresses and strains in shearing forces and fatigue which are similar to those of TKR, contrary to mobile metal-back implants, where the abrasion events found are similar to those of THR (total hip replacement).

Clinically:

- No difference was found in the functional results and patients' satisfaction rate. The mid- to long-term survival rates are similar to recent series.
- More complications manifesting as aseptic loosening of the implant and collapse of the tibial plateau were found for full PE.
- Dislocation of a PE insert represents an exclusive complication of mobile-insert metal-back implants.
- Difficulties in revision surgery for totalisation are correlated with the reason for failure. Among these, tibial plateau collapses are a cause of complexity.

References

1. McCalden RW, Robert CE, Howard JL, Naudie DD, McAuley JP, MacDonald SJ. Comparison of outcomes and survivorship between patients of different age groups following TKA. J Arthroplast. 2013;28:83–6. https://doi.org/10.1016/j.arth.2013.03.034.
2. Gioe TJ, Killeen KK, Hoeffel DP, Bert JM, Comfort TK, Scheltema K, et al. Analysis of unicompartmental knee arthroplasty in a community-based implant registry. Clin Orthop Relat Res. 2003;416:111–9. https://doi.org/10.1097/01.blo.0000093004.90435.d1.

3. Gleeson RE, EVANS R, Ackroyd CE, WEBB J, Newman JH. Fixed or mobile bearing unicompartmental knee replacement? A comparative cohort study. Knee. 2004;11:379–84. https://doi.org/10.1016/j.knee.2004.06.006.

4. Aleto TJ, Berend ME, Ritter MA, Faris PM, Meneghini RM. Early failure of Unicompartmental knee arthroplasty leading to revision. J Arthroplast. 2008;23:159–63. https://doi.org/10.1016/j.arth.2007.03.020.

5. Silver FH. Biomaterials medical devices & tissue engineering: an integrated approach. New York: Chapmann & Hall; 1993.

6. Baïetto S. Modèles visco-élastiques de remodelage osseux. Approche théorique, numérique et expérimentale. 2004.

7. Scott CEH, Eaton MJ, Nutton RW, Wade FA, Evans SL, Pankaj P. Metal-backed versus all-polyethylene unicompartmental knee arthroplasty: proximal tibial strain in an experimentally validated finite element model. Bone Joint Res. 2017;6:22–30. https://doi.org/10.1302/2046-3758.61.BJR-2016-0142.R1.

8. Small SR, Berend ME, Ritter MA, Buckley CA, Rogge RD. Metal backing significantly decreases Tibial strains in a medial Unicompartmental knee arthroplasty model. J Arthroplast. 2010;26:1–6. https://doi.org/10.1016/j.arth.2010.07.021.

9. Simpson DJ, Gray H, Lima DD, Murray DW, Gill HS. The effect of bearing congruency, thickness and alignment on the stresses in unicompartmental knee replacements. Clin Biomech. 2008;23:1148–57. https://doi.org/10.1016/j.clinbiomech.2008.06.001.

10. Engh GA, Dwyer KA, Hanes CK. Polyethylene wear of metal-backed tibial components in total and unicompartmental knee prostheses. J Bone Joint Surg (Br). 1992;74:9–17.

11. Kendrick BJL, Simpson DJ, Kaptein BL, Valstar ER, Gill HS, Murray DW, et al. Polyethylene wear of mobile-bearing unicompartmental knee replacement at 20 years. J Bone Joint Surg (Br). 2011;93:470–5. https://doi.org/10.1302/0301-620X.93B4.25605.

12. Ashraf T, Newman JH, Desai VV, Beard D, Nevelos JE. Polyethylene wear in a non-congruous unicompartmental knee replacement: a retrieval analysis. Knee. 2004;11:177–81. https://doi.org/10.1016/j.knee.2004.03.004.

13. Argenson J-N, O'Connor JJ. Polyethylene wear in meniscal knee replacement. A one to nine-year retrieval analysis of the Oxford knee. J Bone Joint Surg (Br). 1992;74:228–32.

14. Psychoyios V, Crawford RW, O'Connor JJ, Murray DW. Wear of congruent meniscal bearings in unicompartmental knee arthroplasty: a retrieval study of 16 specimens. J Bone Joint Surg (Br). 1998;80:976–82.

15. Price AJ, Short A, Kellett C, Beard D, Gill H, Pandit H, et al. Ten-year in vivo wear measurement of a fully congruent mobile bearing unicompartmental knee arthroplasty. J Bone Joint Surg (Br). 2005;87:1493–7. https://doi.org/10.1302/0301-620X.87B11.16325.

16. Wroblewski BM. Direction and rate of socket wear in Charnley low-friction arthroplasty. J Bone Joint Surg (Br). 1985;67:757–61.

17. Kretzer JP, Jakubowitz E, Reinders J, Lietz E, Moradi B, Hofmann K, et al. Wear analysis of unicondylar mobile bearing and fixed bearing knee systems: a knee simulator study. Acta Biomater. 2011;7:710–5. https://doi.org/10.1016/j.actbio.2010.09.031.

18. Manson TT, Kelly NH, Lipman JD, Wright TM, Westrich GH. Unicondylar knee retrieval analysis. J Arthroplast. 2010;25:108–11. https://doi.org/10.1016/j.arth.2010.05.004.

19. Kwon O-R, Kang K-T, Son J, Kwon S-K, Jo S-B, Suh D-S, et al. Biomechanical comparison of fixed- and mobile-bearing for unicomparmental knee arthroplasty using finite element analysis. J Orthop Res. 2014;32:338–45. https://doi.org/10.1002/jor.22499.

20. Hernigou P, Poignard A, Filippini P, Zilber S. Retrieved Unicompartmental implants with full PE Tibial components: the effects of knee alignment and polyethylene thickness on creep and Wear. Open Orthop J. 2008;2:51–6. https://doi.org/10.2174/1874325000802010051.

21. Bini S, Khatod M, Cafri G, Chen Y, Paxton EW. Surgeon, implant, and patient variables may explain variability in early revision rates reported for unicompartmental arthroplasty. J Bone Joint Surg. 2013;95:2195–202. https://doi.org/10.2106/JBJS.L.01006.

22. Berend KR, Lombardi AV, Mallory TH, Adams JB, Groseth KL. Early failure of minimally invasive unicompartmental knee arthroplasty is associated with obesity. Clin Orthop Relat Res. 2005;440:60–6. https://doi.org/10.1097/01.blo.0000187062.65691.e3.

23. Berend ME. State of the art in partial knee arthroplasty Mobile bearing. San Francisoc: AAOS; 2012.

24. Parks NL, Engh GA, Topoleski LD, Emperado J. The Coventry Award. Modular tibial insert micromotion. A concern with contemporary knee implants. Clin Orthop Relat Res. 1998;356:10–5.

25. Conditt MA, Thompson MT, Usrey MM, Ismaily SK, Noble PC. Backside wear of polyethylene tibial inserts: mechanism and magnitude of material loss. J Bone Joint Surg Am. 2005;87:326–31. https://doi.org/10.2106/JBJS.C.01308.

26. Steklov N, Chao N, Srivastav S. Patient-specific unicompartmental knee resurfacing arthroplasty: use of a novel interference lock to reduce tibial insert micromotion and backside wear. Open Biomed Eng J. 2010;4:156–61. https://doi.org/10.2174/1874120701004010156.

27. Wasielewski RC, Parks N, Williams I, Suprenant H, Collier JP, Engh G. Tibial insert undersurface as a contributing source of polyethylene wear debris. Clin Orthop Relat Res. 1997;345:53–9.

28. Bhattacharya R, Scott CEH, Morris HE, Wade F, Nutton RW. Survivorship and patient satisfaction of a fixed bearing unicompartmental knee arthroplasty

incorporating an all-polyethylene tibial component. Knee. 2012;19:348–51. https://doi.org/10.1016/j.knee.2011.04.009.

29. Smith TO, Hing CB, Davies L, Donell ST. Fixed versus mobile bearing unicompartmental knee replacement: a meta-analysis. Orthop Traumatol Surg Res. 2009;95:599–605. https://doi.org/10.1016/j.otsr.2009.10.006.

30. Lustig S, Paillot J-L, Servien E, Henry J, Ait Si Selmi T, Neyret P. Cemented all polyethylene tibial insert unicompartimental knee arthroplasty: a long term follow-up study. Orthop Traumatol Surg Res. 2009;95:12–21. https://doi.org/10.1016/j.otsr.2008.04.001.

31. Confalonieri N, Manzotti A, Pullen C. Comparison of a mobile with a fixed tibial bearing unicompartimental knee prosthesis: a prospective randomized trial using a dedicated outcome score. Knee. 2004;11:357–62. https://doi.org/10.1016/j.knee.2004.01.003.

32. Hutt JRB, Farhadnia P, Massé V, LaVigne M, Vendittoli P-A. A randomised trial of all-polyethylene and metal-backed tibial components in unicompartmental arthroplasty of the knee. Bone Joint J. 2015;97-B:786–92. https://doi.org/10.1302/0301-620X.97B6.35433.

33. Price AJ, Svard U. A second decade lifetable survival analysis of the Oxford unicompartmental knee arthroplasty. Clin Orthop Relat Res. 2011;469:174–9. https://doi.org/10.1007/s11999-010-1506-2.

34. Steele RG, Hutabarat S, Evans RL, Ackroyd CE, Newman JH. Survivorship of the St Georg sled medial unicompartmental knee replacement beyond ten years. J Bone Joint Surg (Br). 2006;88:1164–8. https://doi.org/10.1302/0301-620X.88B9.18044.

35. O'Rourke MR, Gardner JJ, Callaghan JJ, Liu SS, Goetz DD, Vittetoe DA, et al. The John Insall Award: unicompartmental knee replacement: a minimum twenty-one-year followup, end-result study. Clin Orthop Relat Res. 2005;440:27–37. https://doi.org/10.1097/01.blo.0000185451.96987.aa.

36. Naudie D, Guerin J, Parker DA, Bourne RB, Rorabeck CH. Medial unicompartmental knee arthroplasty with the miller-Galante prosthesis. J Bone Joint Surg Am. 2004;86–A:1931–5.

37. Saenz CL, McGrath MS, Marker DR, Seyler TM, Mont MA, Bonutti PM. Early failure of a unicompartmental knee arthroplasty design with an all-polyethylene tibial component. Knee. 2010;17:53–6. https://doi.org/10.1016/j.knee.2009.05.007.

38. Pandit H, Hamilton TW, Jenkins C, Mellon SJ, Dodd CAF, Murray DW. The clinical outcome of minimally invasive phase 3 Oxford unicompartmental knee arthroplasty: a 15-year follow-up of 1000 UKAs. Bone Joint J. 2015;97-B:1493–500. https://doi.org/10.1302/0301-620X.97B11.35634.

39. Whittaker J-P, Naudie DDR, McAuley JP, McCalden RW, MacDonald SJ, Bourne RB. Does bearing design influence midterm survivorship of unicompartmental arthroplasty? Clin Orthop Relat Res. 2010;468:73–81. https://doi.org/10.1007/s11999-009-0975-7.

40. Rouanet T, Combes A, Migaud H, Pasquier G. Do bone loss and reconstruction procedures differ at revision of cemented unicompartmental knee prostheses according to the use of metal-back or all-polyethylene tibial component? Orthop Traumatol Surg Res. 2013;99:687–92. https://doi.org/10.1016/j.otsr.2013.03.018.

41. Pandit H, Jenkins C, Gill HS, Barker K, Dodd CAF, Murray DW. Minimally invasive Oxford phase 3 unicompartmental knee replacement: results of 1000 cases. J Bone Joint Surg (Br). 2011;93:198–204. https://doi.org/10.1302/0301-620X.93B2.25767.

42. Zambianchi F, Digennaro V, Giorgini A, Grandi G, Fiacchi F, Mugnai R, et al. Surgeon's experience influences UKA survivorship: a comparative study between all-poly and metal back designs. Knee Surg Sports Traumatol Arthrosc. 2015;23:2074–80. https://doi.org/10.1007/s00167-014-2958-9.

43. Jeschke E, Gehrke T, Günster C, Hassenpflug J, Malzahn J, Niethard FU, et al. Five-year survival of 20,946 Unicondylar knee replacements and patient risk factors for failure: an analysis of German insurance data. J Bone Joint Surg. 2016;98:1691–8. https://doi.org/10.2106/JBJS.15.01060.

44. Argenson J-NA, Chevrol-Benkeddache Y, Aubaniac J-M. Modern unicompartmental knee arthroplasty with cement: a three to ten-year follow-up study. J Bone Joint Surg Am. 2002;84:2235–9.

Recovery After Partial Knee Arthroplasty and Daycare Surgery

12

A. Sharma, H. A. Wilson, C. O'Neill, A. Alvand,
N. Bottomley, A. J. Price, and W. F. M. Jackson

Historically, knee arthroplasty was considered a surgical procedure that required prolonged postoperative hospitalisation. In more recent years, the development of ambulatory surgery and enhanced recovery pathways across a broad range of surgical specialties has gained considerable interest. Reported benefits include improved patient satisfaction, reduced perioperative complication rates and greater cost-effectiveness.

Unlike total knee arthroplasty (TKA) which involves quite an extensive surgical dissection and a typical 2–3 day inpatient stay, unicompartmental knee arthroplasty (UKA) can be performed via a more minimally invasive approach with considerably less soft tissue trauma. For this reason, it is a procedure ideally suited to early discharge home after surgery and for many patients this procedure can be done in an outpatient setting. In addition, the literature demonstrates that it allows for safe, efficient care with fewer perioperative complications, which in turn leads to higher patient satisfaction [1, 2]. Importantly, when compared to inpatient stay there is no increased risk of complications or changes in patient outcomes with similar levels of anxiety and pain being experienced as the enhanced recovery group requiring inpatient stay [3].

Beard et al. [4] published a pilot study in which all patients were discharged within 24 hours from the time of surgery with no significant complications being noted. They commented that convalescence at home removes the patient from the threat of hospital acquired infections, permits a more functional rehabilitation and the cost for the institution is reduced, other published series have followed suit reporting similar findings.

The average reported length of stay in enhanced recovery programmes for UKA has already decreased to 1 day with good results, and in the United States health care system UKA has been performed safely with rates of discharge of up to 100% on the same day as surgery. [5, 6]

All published studies surrounding outpatient total joint arthroplasty from Europe have a well-established enhanced recovery protocol in place. As a result of their investment in time and resources, they have seen their length of stay gradually decrease to a point where day case arthroplasty has become feasible. The philosophy of marginal gains has been shown to provide success in the field of elite sport. Similarly, over the last decade, our philosophy has been to enhance patient recovery and patient satisfaction by carefully examining all the processes and individual components of the patient pathway with the aim of introducing incremental improvements to each facet. We are now in a position where we have created well defined pathways and standard

A. Sharma · H. A. Wilson · C. O'Neill · A. Alvand
N. Bottomley · A. J. Price · W. F. M. Jackson (✉)
Nuffield Orthopaedic Centre, Oxford, UK

145

A. Clavé, F. Dubrana (eds.), *Unicompartmental Knee Arthroplasty*,
https://doi.org/10.1007/978-3-031-48332-5_12

operating procedures that guide correct patient selection, reproducible anaesthetic and surgical techniques. We can select the correct patients that meet the criteria for safe same day discharge and importantly manage the medical consequences that we have created from surgery.

All patients with symptoms and radiographic features of end-stage single compartment tibiofemoral osteoarthritis (as described by the Oxford group) considered suitable candidates for UKA are assessed for suitability for daycase surgery. The inclusion criteria for discharge on the day of surgery were patients with co-morbidities that were considered stable and their home situation allowed safe discharge with appropriate care. There were no arbitrary limitations such as American Association of Anaesthesiologist (ASA) grade, age or body mass index.

Within our institute, all patients listed for surgery attend a pre-operative optimisation clinic. They are assessed by members of the orthopaedic, medical, anaesthetic, nursing, physiotherapy and occupational therapy teams allowing optimisation of co-existing medical conditions. Following medical optimisation, any patients still deemed to be at risk of unstable medical conditions who may require more intensive post-operative monitoring are excluded from the day of surgery discharge pathway. Furthermore, if a screening questionnaire reveals that a patient lives alone or has any concerns about discharge arrangements, they can be assessed by an occupational therapist.

All patients from their initial outpatient clinic and subsequent pre-operative clinic are informed about the perioperative plan in order to manage expectations and reinforce the idea of day of surgery discharge. Every patient is given consistent advice by all members of the multidisciplinary team. Written information in the form of a patient information leaflet on daycase surgery is provided to all patients, with instructions on how to make preparations for same day discharge. This principle is similarly applied on the day of surgery when the patient is reviewed by the operating surgeon, anaesthetist, nursing staff and physiotherapist.

In the pre-operative phase, sedatives are avoided as they may impair post-operative mobilisation and contribute to delays in discharge. Any premedication is intravenous as the absorption of oral analgesia may be unpredictable.

The patient should be placed early on the theatre list, aiming to complete surgery before midday in order to maximise the likelihood of same day discharge.

Our anaesthetic of choice is a general anaesthetic (GA). If there is a strong patient preference for spinal anaesthesia or contraindications to GA, then spinal anaesthesia can be performed with or without sedation. Spinal opioids are avoided. Patients undergoing GA are often supplemented with an adductor canal block under ultrasound guidance in the anaesthetic room with 20mL of 0.25% levobupivacaine. Femoral and sciatic nerve blocks are discouraged in order to avoid delays in post-operative mobilisation. Our standard pre-operative antibiotic regime of co-amoxiclav is administered before induction. Further doses of antibiotics are not given as there is good evidence to suggest that one dose of prophylactic antibiotics is sufficient [7]. Other routine intraoperative medications include intravenous tranexamic acid at induction unless contraindicated. We avoid topical tranexamic acid during UKA due to concerns regarding potential chondrotoxicity affecting the remaining compartments [8], intravenous dexamethasone, intravenous ondansetron, intravenous paracetamol and intravenous diclofenac (omitted if any contraindications to NSAIDs).

Surgery is performed in the supine position with a thigh support and a high thigh tourniquet using a standard minimally invasive approach. We use the Oxford (Biomet, Warsaw, Indiana) microplasty instrumentation for all patients. Following introduction of the final trial implants, local anaesthetic (40mL of Ropivacaine 7.5 mg/mL + 0.5 mL 1:1000 adrenaline, made up to a total volume of 100 mL with 0.9% NaCl) is infiltrated methodically into the posterior capsule, periosteum, synovium, skin margins and quadriceps using a 19-gauge spinal needle. The skin is infiltrated up to 3 cm from the margins of the wound. The tourniquet is deflated, haemostasis achieved, and subsequently the wound is closed in layers with application of a wool and crepe compression bandage. Drains are not used in our routine practice.

Post-operatively, all patients are initially recovered in main theatre recovery and promptly moved to the dedicated day case surgical unit. All patients are allowed to eat and drink freely. In the recovery ward, rescue analgesia is provided in the form of paracetamol, oxycodone, or an intravenous infusion of fentanyl if required. Morphine is avoided in order to reduce sedation, nausea and vomiting. Additional doses of tranexamic acid are given either as an inpatient or outpatient depending on the time of discharge.

Shortly following return to the day surgery unit, an assessment of sensory and motor function is performed by the physiotherapy team. If these are adequate, static quadriceps and active foot and ankle exercises are commenced. Active or passive knee flexion exercises are initially discouraged. We encourage our patients to keep their compression bandaging intact and maintain knee extension until they have returned to a designated UKA clinic on the fifth post-operative day for further review. All patients are mobilised fully weight bearing with crutches under the supervision of the physiotherapy team. Patients must also demonstrate the ability to safely negotiate steps or stairs prior to discharge. Post-operative X-rays are obtained prior to discharge. The X-ray department prioritise daycase patients in order to avoid delays to discharge. Patients are actively educated and encouraged to rest the leg in elevation to reduce post-operative swelling and when at home to walk with the assistance of crutches.

All patients are provided with detailed information on the importance of taking the prescribed post-operative analgesics, laxatives and anti-emetics. In addition, patients have direct access to a 24-hour telephone helpline service for both medical and orthopaedic advice if they experience any concerns during the time period between discharge and first planned review on the fifth

post-operative day. If for social, medical or geographic reasons patients are unable to go home on day 0, they are admitted overnight. If the patient is subsequently suitable for discharge on day 1, they receive the same post-operative instructions as those patients discharged on day 0. If the patient remains an invariant on day 2, the compression bandage is removed, knee flexion is commenced and they can be discharged when medically fit and mobilising safely. Outpatient physiotherapy can be arranged to improve range of motion or mobility in selected cases but is not our routine practice.

All patients discharged on day 0 or day 1 return to the UKA clinic on the closest weekday on the fifth post-operative day. Nurses redress the wound, and patients have a single physiotherapy session comprising additional gentle knee flexion and extension exercises along with a comprehensive booklet of exercises and advice. Surgical team review or referral to outpatient physiotherapy is available on the same day if any concerns are noted. All patients have access to physiotherapy led drop-in sessions if required.

All patients are routinely reviewed either by a surgeon or specialist physiotherapist at 6 weeks.

Following the formal introduction of the daycase pathway, we have continued to monitor our practice. In our unit we found that of all patients presenting to clinic 73% were suitable for same day discharge, and that we achieved same day discharge in 72% of these patients (118/164).

Within the first 30 post-operative days, a total of 12 (9%) of patients who went home on the same day required additional assessment, with only five (4%) required readmission. Of the five readmitted to hospital one was admitted with a significant pulmonary embolus (PE) despite receiving venous emboli prevention. Two patients were readmitted with leg swelling which were investigated with ultrasound scans, which excluded deep vein thromboses, the fourth patient had pain management issues following discharge, and went on to require a manipulation under anaesthetic (MUA) 9 weeks post-operatively, and lastly one patient required revision of the surgical wound with additional debridement with implant retention (DAIR) with bearing exchange at 3 weeks post-operatively. Of those that were reassessed as an outpatient one required additional physiotherapy for stiffness, one required oral antibiotics for a superficial wound infection, the remaining five all had minor issues that required dressing changes or reassurance.

There was no significant difference between the number of additional general practitioner (GP) appointments and Accident and Emergency (A + E) hospital admissions, between those patients that went home on the same day and those that did not.

12.1 Conclusions

Introducing an effective outpatient arthroplasty protocol requires a multidisciplinary approach. It is essential for all members of the team to be engaged with the process. The whole care pathway needs to be examined and optimised, with the principle of multiple small improvements to processes leading to substantial gains in quality for the whole care episode.

This is a constantly evolving pathway with continuous audit and improvements where necessary. From our experience to date, we feel the most important factors to achieve successful same day discharge are a well-described pathway with precise "standard operating procedures", a consistent team message and good patient education.

As an example, our delayed knee flexion program [9], allows early safe mobilisation, reduces pain and swelling at 24-48rs, and has been shown to have no detrimental consequences at 6 weeks regarding range of motion.

Within our institute, introduction of a daycase UKA pathway has provided a marked decrease in the average length of stay. The financial savings from a safe and effective day of surgery discharge pathway are considerable. It has been safe, effective, and the patient satisfaction has been high.

References

1. Cleary PD, Greenfield S, Mulley AG, et al. Variations in length of stay and outcomes for six medical and surgical conditions in Massachusetts and California. JAMA. 1991;266:73–9.
2. Kim S, Losina E, Solomon DH, Wright J, Katz JN. Effectiveness of clinical pathways for total knee and total hip arthroplasty: literature review. J Arthroplast. 2003;18:69–74.
3. Hoorntje A, Koenraadt KLM, Boeve MG, Van Geenen RCI. Outpatient unicompartmental knee arthroplasty: who is afraid of outpatient surgery? KSSTA. 2017;25:759–66.
4. Beard DJ, Murray DW, Rees JL, Price AJ, Dodd CA. Accelerated recovery for unicompartmental knee replacement—a feasibility study. Knee. 2002;9:221–4.
5. Gondusky JS, Choi L, Khalaf N, et al. Day of surgery discharge after unicompartmental knee arthroplasty: an effective perioperative pathway. J Arthroplast. 2014;29:516–9.
6. Cross MB, Berger R. Feasibility and safety of performing outpatient unicompartmental knee arthroplasty. Int Orthop. 2014;38:443–7.
7. Tan TL, Shohat N, Rondon AJ, et al. Perioperative antibiotic prophylaxsis in Total joint arthroplasty: a single dose is as effective as multiple doses. JBJS (AM). 2019;101(5):429–37.
8. Tuttle JR, Feltman PR, Ritterman SA, Ehrlich MG. Effects of tranexamic acid cytotoxicity on in vitro chondrocytes. Am J Orthop (Belle Mead NJ). 2015;44(12):E497–502.
9. Jenkins C, Jackson W, Bottomely N, Price A, Murray D, Barker K. Introduction of an innovative day surgery pathway for unicompartmental knee replacement: no need for early knee flexion. Physiotherapy. 2019;105(1):46–52.

Utility of Bilateral Single-Stage Unicompartmental Knee Arthroplasty

13

Quentin Nicolas, Arnaud Clavé, Fabien Ros, and Frédéric Dubrana

13.1 Introduction

Knee osteoarthritis is commonly a bilateral disease [1]. Sayeed et al. [2] reported that in 26% of cases with minimal disease, patients who underwent knee replacement surgery were reoperated on the opposite side within 5 years.

The expected increase in its incidence [3] combined with the legitimate desire for rapid patient recovery (particularly since the development of ERAS, enhanced recovery after surgery) and growing socioeconomic pressure have encouraged some authors to investigate bilateral single-stage knee arthroplasty.

Interest in bilateral single-stage total knee arthroplasty (SS-TKA) began in the late 1970s, primarily for patients with inflammatory arthritis [4, 5]. Abundant literature on total knee arthro-

plasty has since emerged, although its appropriateness remains widely debated [6–12]. Advocates of simultaneous procedures [9, 13–17] mention the following benefits: shorter total hospital stay, single anaesthesia, patient convenience and satisfaction, and decreased cost for the healthcare system with no increase in morbidity or mortality alongside comparable functional results. Opponents of this approach [10, 18–20] criticise its increase in perioperative complications including cardio-circulatory events and pulmonary embolism, as well as the higher rates of blood transfusion, confusion and death.

Chan et al. in 2009 [21] were the first to investigate bilateral single-stage unicompartmental (SS-UKA) knee arthroplasty. Several studies have reported that a unicompartmental procedure enables faster functional recovery with a shorter hospital stay, similar failure rate, lesser surgical trauma and lower blood loss than TKA [22–25]. Therefore, the unicompartmental procedure is considered as having a lower risk than TKA [26] and theoretically is more suitable for bilateral management. However, the literature on this subject is scarcer [18, 21, 27–35].

In this chapter, we will attempt to review the utility of bilateral single-stage unicompartmental knee arthroplasty (SS-UKA) by studying:

- The procedure's safety.
- Pain and the patient perioperative experience.
- Recovery of function.
- Cost.

Q. Nicolas · F. Ros · F. Dubrana
Service de Chirurgie Orthopédique et Traumatologique (Department of Orthopaedic Surgery and Traumatology), University Regional Hospital Centre, Brest, France

A. Clavé (✉)
Service de Chirurgie Orthopédique et Traumatologique (Department of Orthopaedic Surgery and Traumatology), Clinique Saint-George, Nice, France

Laboratoire d'Analyse et de Traitement de l'Information Médicale (LaTIM) (Laboratory of Medical Information Processing), UMR1101 INSERM-UBO (INSERM: French National Institute of Health and Medical Research), Brest, France

13.2 The Procedure's Safety

Most studies on bilateral single-stage knee arthroplasty have involved TKR (total knee replacement), with contradictory data in the literature on the procedure's safety [36, 37].

In their retrospective case–control study on 52 patients who underwent SS-UKA (104 knees) vs. 52 (unilateral) u-TKR patients, Ahn et al. [38] reported fewer perioperative complications, less blood loss, lower transfusion rates and faster clinical recovery in the SS-UKA group.

Therefore, given its less invasive characteristics, shorter surgery, anaesthesia and hospital stay, faster functional recovery and lower mortality rate [26, 39, 40], unicompartmental arthroplasty seems more appropriate for single-stage bilateral procedures than TKR.

Since the adage "first do no harm" must prevail, the evaluation of excess risk related to the procedure's bilateral nature is the subject that most interested the authors. We reviewed the various terms associated with its evaluation in the literature (see Table 13.1).

13.2.1 Estimation of Blood Losses and Transfusion Rates

In their case-control study on SS-UKA (70 knees) vs. (two stage) TS-UKA (282 knees), Berend et al. [28] did not report any blood transfusions in either group.

In a case-control study on SS-UKA (102 knees) vs. TS-UKA (102 knees), Biazzo et al. [18] found a significant difference in postopera-

Table 13.1 Summary table of various systemic and local intrahospital complications or at 6 months

		Systemic	Local
In-hospital			
	Major	• Death • AF • Myocardial infarction • Diabetes • Pulmonary embolism • Pancreatitis	• Mobilisation under general anaesthesia (GA) • Slow healing • Proximal phlebitis • Fracture
	Minor	• Minor cardiac dysrhythmia • Hypertension • Dyspnoea • Asthma • Intestinal ileus • Alteration of liver enzymes • Hypotension • Dysuria	• Distal phlebitis • Sciatica • Oedema • Wound bleeding • Disunion • Haematoma requiring its evacuation • Algodystrophy
At 6 months			
	Major	• Death • Pulmonary embolism • Atrial fibrillation • Jaundice • Heart disease	• Infection of the prosthesis • Revision of the implant • Mobilisation under GA • Proximal phlebitis
	Minor		• Oedema and haematoma • Sciatica • Unequal lower limb length • Superficial infection of the wound scar • Distal phlebitis • Algodystrophy

tive decrease in haemoglobin at D3 (3.1 g/dL vs. 2.4 g/dL) and transfusion rate (4 vs. 0, a transfusion was performed if the haemoglobin was <8 g/dL and in one patient with clinical signs of anaemia). Statistical analysis of the decrease in haemoglobin correlated with duration of surgery supports a greater decrease if surgery surpasses 90 min.

In their case-control prospective study on SS-UKA (248 knees) vs. TS-UKA (94 knees), Chen et al. [29] did not find a significant difference in fall in haemoglobin postoperatively or transfusion rate (−1.45 g/dL vs. -1.30 g/dL, 1 vs. 0 transfusions in the control group).

In their case-control study on SS-UKA (100 knees) vs. u-UKA (100 knees), Clavé et al. [30] did not find any significant difference in real blood losses (465 mL vs. 396 mL), lower haemoglobin at D3 (10.8 g/dL vs. 11.2 g/dL) or transfusion rate (3 vs. 7) between the 2 groups.

In a retrospective case-control study on SS-UKA (78 knees) vs. TS-UKA (108 knees), Feng et al. [31] concluded in a significant difference for decrease in haemoglobin at D3 postoperatively (2.9 g/dL vs. 0.6 g/dL) but no significant difference for transfusion rate (1 vs. 0).

For Romagnoli et al. [33], who conducted a retrospective case-control study on SS-UKA (382 knees) vs. 299 u-UKA, their protocol included preoperative donation of packed red blood cells (RBC). The authors found a significant difference in decrease in haemoglobin (−4 g/dL vs. -2.8 g/dL, measured at hospital discharge), but also in transfusions (24 vs. 13). There was no significant difference in autologous blood transfusion in patients in the "perioperative blood donation" group. It should be noted that the anaesthesia protocol did not include tranexamic acid in a systemic or local injection and that the lower limit for transfusion was haemoglobin <8 g/dL or clinical signs of anaemia.

In their case-control study on SS-UKA (88 knees) vs. TS-UKA (52 knees), Siedlecki et al. [34] concluded that there is no significant difference in the postoperative decrease in haemoglo-

bin (2 g/dL vs. 1.3 g/dL, no indication on the day of postoperative control) or the transfusion rate (1 vs. 3, transfusion if anaemia <7 g/dL or < 10 g/dL in patients with heart disease).

In a retrospective case-control study on SS-UKA (72 knees) vs. TS-UKA (90 knees), Tong Ma et al. [32] did not find any significant difference in postoperative haemoglobin (10.5 g/dL vs. 11.1 g/dL, no indication on the day of postoperative control) or the transfusion rate (nil in both groups).

In their retrospective cohort study on 38 SS-UKA procedures (76 knees), Akhtar et al. [27] found an average postoperative fall in haemoglobin of 1.8 g/dL (no indication on the day of postoperative control) and absence of postoperative transfusion.

The current literature seems to support a greater decrease in haemoglobin in the simultaneous procedure, without however being associated with an increased transfusion rate. Duration of surgery <90 min and use of tranexamic acid more or less in combination with a preoperative blood donation or perioperative cell-salvage protocol for patients at risk of bleeding appear to be protective factors and therefore can be advised.

13.2.2 Duration of Anaesthesia and Tourniquet Placement

For Feng et al. [31], the duration of anaesthesia in the SS-UKA group was 120.2 mins vs. 141.6 mins for the TS-UKA group (significant difference). Chen and Tong Ma(ref) found similar results in their studies.

Akhtar et al. [27] found a mean duration of tourniquet placement of 83 min for a simultaneous procedure, which is similar to that in the study by Siedlecki et al. [34].

For Chan et al. [21], the duration of tourniquet placement was 109.1 min for a simultaneous procedure versus 114.86 min for a 2-stage procedure. The authors concluded in a nonsignificant difference.

13.2.3 Perioperative Complications

Berend et al. [28] retrospectively compared the placement of unicompartmental knee replacement in 141 patients (282 knees) in sequential management and 35 patients (70 knees) in simultaneous management. They did not find a significant difference in complications and concluded in the absence of a major complication.

Chen et al. [29] compared 124 patients (248 knees) managed simultaneously and 47 (94 knees) managed sequentially. They found five minor complications and zero major complications in each group.

Romagnoli et al. [33] compared 191 SS-UKA (382 knees) and 299 u-UKA. The mortality rate at 2 years was similar (four deaths) with one case probably related to surgery in the u-UKA group. No significant difference was found in complications or revisions of the implants with at least 2 years' follow-up.

For Tong Ma et al. [32], who compared 36 SS-UKA (72 knees) and 45 TS-UKA (90 knees) with mean follow-up of 50 months, found no complication such as death, pulmonary embolism or infection of the prosthesis. Furthermore, they reported three complications in the SS-UKA group and five in the TS-UKA group with no significant difference.

In a retrospective case-control study on 51 patients with SS-UKA (102 knees) and 51 patients with TS-UKA (102 knees) by Biazzo et al. [18], no deaths, episode of confusion, VTED (venous thromboembolic disease) or hospitalisation in the ICU during the first 30 days were reported. One internal tibial plateau fracture, one TIA and one slight renal impairment were found in the SS-UKA group and two patients with algodystrophy in the TS-UKA group. The authors concluded the absence of a significant difference in complications between the two groups.

Clavé et al. [30] retrospectively compared 50 SS-UKA (100 knees) and 100 u-UKA patients;

no significant difference in terms of complications was evidenced with complication rates of 10% and 7%, respectively.

Siedlecki et al. [34] found major complication rates of 9.1% and 15.4%, respectively, and minor complication rates of 4.5% and 3.8%, respectively (no difference between the 2 cases).

Feng et al. [31], who compared the procedure's safety in a retrospective case-control study on 39 SS-UKA (78 knees) vs. 54 TS-UKA (108 knees) with 42 months' follow-up, evidenced a complication rate in the SS-UKA group of 10.3% versus 9.3% in the TS-UKA group; however, there was no significant difference.

Only the study by Chan et al. [21] found contradictory results versus the rest of the literature. In their retrospective case-control study with 159 SS-UKA (318 knees) and 80 TS-UKA (160 knees), there is a significant difference between the major complication rate in the SS-UKA group (8.2%, 13 patients) and the TS-UKA group (0%, 0 patients). Nine patients with VTED and one death subsequent to a massive pulmonary embolism were reported. It should be specified that the surgical follow-up was marked by the absence of preventive anticoagulant treatment. Furthermore, they did not find any significant difference in the rate of minor complications (2.5% for the SS-UKA group versus 3.15% for the TS-UKA group) (Table 13.2).

Take-Home Message

The current literature, although narrow and divergent, suggests that simultaneous bilateral procedures are safe and do not seem to increase the postoperative rate of complications. However, it should be specified that all the studies mentioned report non-randomisation limitations and a possible selection bias with younger patients, fewer comorbidities and volunteers/motivated participants in the simultaneous procedure groups. Therefore, it appears prudent to reiterate the utility of patient selection for a simultaneous procedure, at least early in experience.

Table 13.2 Summary table

Authors	Number of cases (solely medial UKA)	Type of arthroplasty	Study design	Complications	Follow-up
Berend et al. [28]	70 SS-UKA vs. 282 TS-UKA	Oxford	Retrospective comparative	Rate of cardiac, pulmonary problems and of similar superficial infections in the two groups	3 months
Romagnoli et al. [33]	382 SS-UKA vs. 299 u-UKA	Not specified	Retrospective comparative	No significant difference in major or minor complications	6 months
Tong Ma et al. [32]	72 SS-UKA vs. 90 TS-UKA	Oxford	Retrospective comparative	No significant difference	50 months
Chen et al. [29]	248 SS-UKA vs. 94 TS-UKA	Not specified	Prospective case-control	No significant difference	2 years
Clavé et al. [30]	100 SS-UKA vs. 100 u-UKA	Oxford	Retrospective case-control	No significant difference	Min. 2 years
Siedlecki et al. [34]	84 SS-UKA vs. 52 TS-UKA	ZUK	Retrospective comparative	No significant difference in major or minor complications	17.6 months
Chan et al. [21]	318 SS-UKA vs. 160 TS-UKA	Oxford	Retrospective comparative	8.2% major complication in the SS-UKA group. No major complication in the TS-UKA group. No anticoagulant treatment.	30 days

13.3 Perioperative Pain and Personal Experience (Tables 13.3, 13.4, 13.5 and 13.6)

Knee arthroplasty is associated with pain that is considered moderate to severe, which can delay ambulation and the patient's return home. Several studies published in the last 2 years have involved improvement of postoperative pain management and ambulation after total knee arthroplasty [23, 25, 37, 41, 42].

In this chapter, we will answer a practical question, often raised by our patients: is bilateral single-stage unicompartmental knee arthroplasty (SS-UKA) more painful than TS-UKA?

There is a paucity of data in the literature on early postoperative pain as the majority of authors who have investigated bilateral single-stage arthroplasty have focused on risk analysis.

In a retrospective cohort study, Powell et al. [15] investigated early pain in bilateral single-stage total knee arthroplasty and did not find any significant difference in the use of opioids. However, the VAS (visual analogue scale) scores were statistically different in the first 24 h after surgery. The procedure took place under general anaesthesia, with a pneumatic tourniquet and no periarticular or deep nerve block local injection.

A thesis researched at Brest University Regional Hospital Centre involved conducting a prospective case-control study including 74 patients in each group (SS-UKA vs. u-UKA) (Clavé and Ros, 48).

Their primary assessment endpoint was cumulative analgesic use in opioid equivalents during

Table 13.3 Narcotic use mean dose equivalents (1DE = 10 mg IM morphine)

		Intraoperative	0–24 postoperative	24–48h postoperative	48–72h postoperative	Cumulative for first 72h
Unilateral TKR	DE (mean ±SD)	2,1±1,67	6,08±3,26	3,40±2,60	1,67±1,29	13,43±6,92
Bilateral TKR	DE (mean ±SD)	2,01±1,47	7,14±3,66	4,44±2,85	1,69±1,61	15,09±5,84
P			0.91	0.16	0.17	0.67	0.86

Table 13.4 Analog pain scor (0 = No pain, 10 = Maximun Pain)

		Intraoperative	0–24 postoperative	24–48h postoperative	48–72h postoperative	Cumulative for first 72h
Unilateral TKR	Pain score (maen ±SD)	4,53±1,92	4,26±1,29	4,53±1,12	3,78±1,85	4,04±1,87
Bilateral TKR	Pain score (maen ±SD)	5,83±2,21	5,49±1,69	4,12±1,45	3,93±1,79	4,11±1,40
P			0.03	0.001	0.19	0.62	0.91

Table 13.5 Mean VAS score based on postoperative time and groups

Mean VAS	Control group (n=74)	Case group (n=74)	P
0–6 h	1,68(±0,35)	2,00(±0,37)	0.2
6–12 h	2,14(±0,37)	2,18(±0,34)	0.87
12–24 h	2,27(±0,35)	3,04(±0,41)	0.31
24–48 h	2,18(0,35)	2,57(±0,38)	0.13
48–72	1,15(±0,26)	1,42(±0,29)	0.17
Cumulative: 0–72 h	9,90(±0,99)	11,24(±1,11)	0.07

Table 13.6 Distribution of VAS score based on postoperative time and groups

VAS Periods	Control group (n=74)		Case group (n=74)	
H0–H6	n	%	n	%
0–3	67	90.5	65	87.8
4–6	7	9.5	9	12.2
sup 7	0	0	0	0
H6–H12	n	%	n	%
0–3	63	85.1	65	87.8
4–6	11	14.9	8	10.8
sup7	0	0	0	0
H12–H24	n	%	n	%
0–3	54	73	46	62.2
4–6	19	25.7	26	35.1
sup7	1	1.3	2	2.7
H24–H48	n	%	n	%
0–3	60	81.1	54	73
4–6	13	17.6	18	24.3
sup7	1	1.3	2	2.7
H48–H72	n	%	n	%
0–3	72	97.3	69	93.3
4–6	2	2.7	5	6.7
sup7	0	0	0	0

the first three postoperative days (Table 13.3). Surgery was performed under general anaesthesia supplemented by peripheral nerve block anaesthesia of the adductors with 50 cc of ROPIVACAINE 2% and a periarticular local injection (ROPIVACAINE 2% 100 mg, KETOPROFEN 50 mg, ADRENALINE 0.5 mg) administered in each operated knee.

The sum total of analgesic use (H0–H72) calculated in opioid equivalents found in the SS-UKA group was 21.61 mg (±3.70) versus 19.11 mg (±3.12) in the control group. The difference was not significant. Moreover, outside the H12–H24 period, use of analgesics did not differ between the two groups (Table 13.3). These results on analgesic use, moreover, are consistent with the literature. Essving et al. [43] in a similar setting (unilateral medial infiltration analgesia UKA) found analgesic use of 20 mg (±30 mg) in opioid equivalents.

The authors explained the difference in analgesic use for the H12–H24 period by the progressive regression of the combined local anaesthetics and deep nerve block, potentially more painful in

patients who underwent a bilateral surgical procedure.

No significant differences existed between the two groups concerning VAS scores in the five periods of interest or cumulative VAS scores (H0–H72) (Table 13.5); categorical analysis of postoperative VAS confirmed the more painful trend of the H12–H24 period but without significance (VAS <3: 73% of u-UKA patients vs. 62.2% of SS-UKA patients) (Table 13.6).

Take-Home Message

The single-stage bilateral procedure does not appear to be more painful or less well experienced by patients than a traditional unilateral procedure.

13.4 Functional Recovery

Most studies presenting the functional results of single-stage bilateral knee arthroplasty also involve TKA and find good clinical results [7, 9, 44], even in patients over 70 years of age [45, 46].

The literature contains less information on functional recovery for the single-stage bilateral strategy (see Table 13.7):

In their retrospective case-control study on SS-UKA (70 knees) vs. TS-UKA (282 knees) with mean final follow-up of 19.4 months and 13.9 months, respectively (significant difference), Berend et al. [28] found a significant difference for the Knee Society Function Score and Lower Extremity Activity Score in favour of the SS-UKA group (87.9 and 72.9, 11.3 and 10.2, respectively); the Knee Society Pain Scores and Knee Society Clinical Scores are similar in the two groups. However, the groups were not homogeneous with younger patients, a lower BMI (body mass index) and more favourable Knee Society Clinical Score for the SS-UKA group, which could result in a selection bias.

In their prospective case-control study on SS-UKA (248 knees) vs. TS-UKA (94 knees) with final follow-up of 2 years, Chen et al. [29] did not find any significant difference for OKS

Table 13.7 Functional recovery/score for single-stage bilateral UKA

Study name	Functional score	Case group: one-stage simultaneous strategy		Control group: two-stage strategy (TS-UKA) or unilateral surgery (u-UKA)		*p* value
		Preop score		Preop score		
			Postop score (mean duration of follow-up in months)		Postop score (mean duration of follow-up in months)	
Berend et al. [28]	Knee society clinical score	46		38		<0.0001
			91.4 (19.4)		90.1 (13.9)	NS (0.0013)
	Knee society pain score	11.6		9.5		NS
			44.6 (19.4)		46.8 (13.9)	NS (0.0013)
	Knee society function scores	58.9		55.6		NS
			87.9 (19.4)		72.9 (13.9)	<0.0001 (0.0013)
	Lower extremity activity score		11.3 (19.4)		10.2 (13.9)	<0.0001 (0.0013)
Chen et al. [29]	Oxford knee score	34		29		0.001
			18 (6)		18 (6)	NS (NS)
			17 (24)		16 (24)	NS (NS)
	Knee society knee score	44.5		47		NS
			88 (6)		88 (6)	NS (NS)
			90 (24)		90 (24)	NS (NS)
Clavé et al. [30]	OKS	27.5		25.2		NS
			41.8 (6)		40.5 (6)	NS (NS)
			44.5 (44.4)		42.2 (61.2)	NS (?)
	KOOS	56.7		52.9		
			85.28 (6)		84.1 (6)	NS (NS)
			91.8 (44.4)		87.9 (61.2)	NS (NS)
Feng et al. [31]	KSS scores	115		115		NS
			170 (12)		167.5 (12)	NS (NS)
Tong Ma et al. [32]	OKS	40.8		40.5		NS
			25.1 (1)		23.2 (1)	NS (NS)
			20 (3)		19.7 (3)	NS (NS)
			19.2 (6)		18.8 (6)	NS (NS)
			18.3 (50)		18 (50)	NS (NS)
Ros and Clavé et al. [35]	OKS	36.59		38.33		0.04

Table 13.7 (continued)

Study name	Functional score	Case group: one-stage simultaneous strategy		Control group: two-stage strategy (TS-UKA) or unilateral surgery (u-UKA)		p value
		Preop score		Preop score		
			Postop score (mean duration of follow-up in months)		Postop score (mean duration of follow-up in months)	
			46.91 (6)		47.31 (6)	NS (NS)
			49.47 (12)		48.89 (12)	NS (NS)
	Delta OKS preop-M12		10.5		12.9	0.03

functional scores, Knee Society Function Scores or Knee Society Knee Scores. Several biases existed in this study. The first is a selection bias since patients in the SS-UKA group have higher preoperative functional scores than those in the TS-UKA group. The second is a type-1 error bias since there was no randomisation, this being potentially reinforced by the inclusion of "more" motivated patients in the SS-UKA group.

In their case-control study with a control group based on a prospective matched series of SS-UKA (100 knees) vs. u-UKA (100 knees) with mean follow-up of 3.7 years and 5.1 years, respectively, Clavé et al. [30] did not find any significant difference for the OKS, KOOS and IKS functional scores. The two groups, however, do not have the same inclusion periods (maximum difference of 10 years); therefore, a bias in experience remains possible. The absence of randomisation, moreover, can also introduce a selection bias.

In their retrospective case-control study on 36 SS-UKA (72 knees) and 45 TS-UKA (90 knees) with mean follow-up of 50 months, Tong Ma et al. [32] did not find any significant difference in OKS score. A selection bias was noted with, in both groups, patients who were younger (mean age 65 years) and in "better" health (80% of the population < ASA II, mean BMI 25) than can be found in comparable series.

In a 2019 retrospective case-control study on SS-UKA (78 knees) vs. TS-UKA (108 knees) with final follow-up of 1 year, Feng et al. [31] did not find any significant difference for the KSS score. It is possible that a selection bias exists since patients in the SS-UKA group were younger and in better health than in most of these studies.

In a prospective case-control study on SS-UKA (74 patients, 148 knees) vs. u-UKA (74 patients) with final follow-up at 1 year, Ros et al. [35] (article in press) found a significant difference in favour of the case group in the analysis of OKS gain between preoperative status and M12. Given the absence of randomisation, a type-1 error remains possible, however.

13.4.1 Patient Satisfaction

For Clavé et al. [30], 96% (48/50) of patients in the SS-UKA group recommended this procedure with an excellent satisfaction rate of 74% at last follow-up (3.7 years on average) versus 94% and 79% for the control group (unilateral procedure with 5.1 years of follow-up on average). They did not find any significant difference between the groups. Results were similar in the Clavé and Ros et al. study.

13.4.2 Early Functional Recovery

In their case group (SS-UKA), Clavé and Ros et al. [35] found 62.2% of patients who made their first round trip at 24 h post-surgery and 100% at 3 days versus 68.9% and 100% for the control group (nonsignificant difference).

Concerning ascent and descent of 8 steps, Clavé and Ros et al. [35] did not find any significant difference between the 2 groups, with 33.8% of patients able to ascend a stairway at 24 h postop in the control group versus 24.3% in the case group and 100% in both groups at D3.

These data on early postoperative resumption of function could not be compared to those in the literature because, as far as we know, no other study has been conducted on this subject.

Take-Home Message

Here too, the literature on single-stage bilateral UKA provides less information compared to TKA. However, studies all converge in the same direction, with clinical scores and patient satisfaction as good as or even better than for unilateral UKA or two-stage strategies (TS-UKA). Immediate postoperative physical rehabilitation does not seem to be impacted by the bilateral nature of the procedure. These results nevertheless remain subject to criticism since the studies published have several biases, particularly younger, more motivated and healthier cohorts.

13.5 Cost

13.5.1 Duration of Stay

For Siedlecki et al. [34], total mean hospital stay was 6.7 days for the SS-UKA group vs. 13.9 days for the TS-UKA group (significant difference).

For Chen et al. [29], total hospital stay was significantly shorter by 3 days in the SS-UKA group (5 vs. 8 days).

Akhtar et al. [27] found a duration of hospital stay of 3.5 days for the simultaneous procedure versus 2 days for a unilateral procedure. They concluded in a reduced hospital stay with two-stage bilateral procedures.

For Romagnoli et al. [33], no significant difference was found for duration of hospital stay between the SS-UKA group and u-UKA group;

however, duration of rehabilitation was longer for the SS-UKA group (9.2 vs. 7.8 days).

Feng et al. [31] in 2019 also found a longer total duration of hospital stay in the TS-UKA group (7.5 vs. 4.2 days); these figures are consistent with those of Siedlecki.

For Clavé and Ros et al. [35], the medical duration of stay was evaluated based on criteria for hospital discharge so as not to be biased by delay in discharge for administrative or nonmedical reasons. Therefore, based on their study, 36.5% of patients were discharged at 24 h postoperatively, 92% at 48 h and 100% at 72 h in the control group compared to 27% at 24 h, 89.2% at 48 h and 100% at 72 h in the case group. The authors concluded in the absence of a significant difference.

13.5.2 Cost of Hospitalisation

For Siedlecki et al. [34], cost of hospitalisation was significantly higher in the TS-UKA group (€11,766.7 vs. €5626.4).

For Chen et al. [29], the hospital stay savings were 8892 USD for the SS-UKA group.

For Feng et al. [31] in 2019, the cost of hospital stay in the SS-UKA group was 11,294.2 USD versus 12,846 USD for the TS-UKA group; the difference was lower but nevertheless significant.

It should be noted that none of these studies assessed the financial impact on outpatient care (nursing, rehabilitation, cost of medical treatments at home) or societal costs, particularly regarding early return to work. There is also no study on the cost of possible increased morbidity even though studies on the risks of these procedures are reassuring in nature.

Take-Home Message

In the current literature, bilateral procedures appear economically preferable. Therefore, it is very important that health authorities take that into account and remove the current financial regulatory restraints in order to facilitate use of simultaneous bilateral procedures.

13.6   Conclusion—Take-Home Message

Bilateral single-stage unicompartmental knee arthroplasty (SS-UKA), in light of the current literature, seems to be a safe procedure for which perioperative patient experience is good, particularly thanks to good management of analgesia and pain that is ultimately well tolerated. Furthermore, immediate postoperative rehabilitation does not seem to be impacted by the bilateral aspect of the procedure. Functional scores, moreover, are identical in the medium and long terms. For all studies that examined the subject, costs for the healthcare system are decreased. However, current fee schedules imposed by France's health authorities are such that the procedures incur a loss for healthcare facilities and surgeons, preventing the study and promotion of these procedures on a larger scale.

Nevertheless, it is appropriate while awaiting larger randomised studies to remain reasonable in terms of the indications and to perform rigorous patient screening and selection.

References

1. Andersson G, Academy A, of Orthopaedic Surgeons. The burden of musculoskeletal diseases in the United States: prevalence, societal and economic cost. Rosemont, IL: American Academy of Orthopaedic Surgeons; 2008.
2. Sayeed SA, Sayeed YA, Barnes SA, Pagnano MW, Trousdale RT. The risk of subsequent joint arthroplasty after primary unilateral Total knee arthroplasty, a 10-year study. The Journal of Arthroplasty Sept. 2011;26(6):842–6.
3. Kurtz S, Ong K, Lau E, Mowat F, Halpern M. Projections of primary and revision hip and knee arthroplasty in the United States from 2005 to 2030. J Bone Joint Surg. 2007;89(4):780–5.
4. Gradillas EL, Volz RG. Bilateral Total knee replacement under one anesthetic. Clin Orthop Relat Res. 1979;(140):153–8.
5. Head WC, Paradies LH. Ipsilateral hip and knee replacements as a single surgical procedure. J Bone Joint Surg Am. 1977;59(3):352–4.
6. Bullock DP, Sporer SM, Shirreffs TG. Comparison of simultaneous bilateral with unilateral total knee arthroplasty in terms of perioperative complications. J Bone Joint Surg Am. 2003;85(10):1981–6.
7. Forster MC, Bauze AJ, Bailie AG, Falworth MS, Oakeshott RD. A retrospective comparative study of bilateral total knee replacement staged at a one-week interval. J Bone Joint Surg Br. 2006;88-B(8):1006–10.
8. Husted H, Troelsen A, Otte KS, Kristensen BB, Holm G, Kehlet H. Fast-track surgery for bilateral total knee replacement. J Bone Joint Surg. 2011;93(3):6.
9. Kim Y-H, Choi Y-W, Kim J-S. Simultaneous bilateral sequential total knee replacement is as safe as unilateral total knee replacement. J Bone Joint Surg Br. 2009;91-B(1):64–8.
10. Oakes DA, Hanssen AD. Bilateral total knee replacement using the same anesthetic is not justified by assessment of the risks. Clin Orthopa Relat Res. 2004;428(87):91.
11. Parvizi J, Sullivan TA, Trousdale RT, Lewallen DG. Thirty-day mortality after total knee arthroplasty. J Bone Joint Surg Am. 2001;83(8):1157–61.
12. Ritter MA, Meding JB. Bilateral simultaneous total knee arthroplasty. J Arthroplast. 1987;2(3):185–9.
13. Hutchinson JRM, Parish EN, Cross MJ. A comparison of bilateral uncemented total knee arthroplasty: simultaneous or staged? J Bone Joint Surg Br. 2006;88-B(1):40–3.
14. Leonard L, Williamson DM, Ivory JP, Jennison C. An evaluation of the safety and efficacy of simultaneous bilateral total knee arthroplasty. J Arthroplast. 2003;18(8):972–8.
15. Powell RS, Pulido P, Tuason MS, Colwell CW, Ezzet KA. Bilateral vs unilateral Total knee arthroplasty: a patient-based comparison of pain levels and recovery of ambulatory skills. J Arthroplast. 2006;21(5):642–9.
16. Shetty GM, Mullaji A, Bhayde S, Chandra Vadapalli R, Desai D. Simultaneous bilateral versus unilateral computer-assisted total knee arthroplasty: a prospective comparison of early postoperative pain and functional recovery. Knee. 2010;17(3):191–5.
17. Yoon H-S, Han C-D, Yang I-H. Comparison of simultaneous bilateral and staged bilateral Total knee arthroplasty in terms of perioperative complications. J Arthroplast. 2010;25(2):179–85.
18. Biazzo A, Masia F, Verde F. Bilateral unicompartmental knee arthroplasty: one stage or two stages? Musculoskelet Surg. 2019;103(3):231–6.
19. Lombardi AV, Mallory TH, Fada RA, Hartman JF, Capps SG, Kefauver CA, et al. Simultaneous bilateral Total knee arthroplasties: who decides? Clin Orthop Relat Res. 2001;392(319):29.
20. Memtsoudis SG, González Della Valle A, Besculides MC, Gaber L, Sculco TP. In-hospital complications and mortality of unilateral, bilateral, and revision TKA: based on an estimate of 4,159,661 discharges. Clin Orthop Relat Res. 2008;466(11):2617–27.
21. Chan WCW, Musonda P, Cooper AS, Glasgow MMS, Donell ST, Walton NP. One-stage *versus* two-stage bilateral unicompartmental knee replacement: a comparison of immediate post-operative complications. J Bone Joint Surg Br. 2009;(10):91-B, 1305–9.

22. Beard DJ, Davies LJ, Cook JA, MacLennan G, Price A, Kent S, et al. The clinical and cost-effectiveness of total versus partial knee replacement in patients with medial compartment osteoarthritis (TOPKAT): 5-year outcomes of a randomised controlled trial. Lancet. 2019;394(10200):746–56.
23. Lombardi AV, Berend KR, Walter CA, Aziz-Jacobo J, Cheney NA. Is recovery faster for mobile-bearing unicompartmental than total knee arthroplasty? Clin Orthop Relat Res. 2009;467(6):1450–7.
24. Newman J, Pydisetty RV, Ackroyd C. Unicompartmental or total knee replacement. J Bone Joint Surg. 2009;91(1):6.
25. Price AJ, Waite JC, Svard U. Long-term clinical results of the medial Oxford Unicompartmental knee arthroplasty. Clin Orthop. 2005;435:10.
26. Liddle AD, Judge A, Pandit H, Murray DW. Adverse outcomes after total and unicompartmental knee replacement in 101 330 matched patients: a study of data from the National Joint Registry for England and Wales. Lancet. 2014;384(9952):1437–45.
27. Akhtar KSN, Somashekar N, Willis-Owen CA, Houlihan-Burne DG. Clinical outcomes of bilateral single-stage unicompartmental knee arthroplasty. Knee Jan. 2014;21(1):310–314.
28. Berend KR, Morris MJ, Skeels MD, Lombardi AV, Adams JB. Perioperative complications of simultaneous versus staged Unicompartmental knee arthroplasty. Clin Orthop Relat Res. 2011;469(1):168–73.
29. Chen JY, Lo NN, Jiang L, Chong HC, Tay DKJ, Chin PL, et al. Simultaneous *versus* staged bilateral unicompartmental knee replacement. Bone Joint J. 2013;95-B(6):788–92.
30. Clavé A, Gauthier E, Nagra NS, Fazilleau F, Le Sant A, Dubrana F. Single-stage bilateral medial Oxford Unicompartmental knee arthroplasty: a case-control study of perioperative blood loss, complications and functional results. Orthop Traumatol Surg Res. 2018;104(7):943–7.
31. Feng S, Yang Z, Sun J-N, Zhu L, Wang S, Guo K-J, et al. Comparison of the therapeutic effect between the simultaneous and staged unicompartmental knee arthroplasty (UKA) for bilateral knee medial compartment arthritis. BMC Musculoskelet Disord. 2019;20(1):340.
32. Ma T, Tu Y-H, Xue H-M, Wen T, Cai M-W. Clinical outcomes and risks of single-stage bilateral Unicompartmental knee arthroplasty via Oxford phase III. Chin Med J. 2015;128(21):2861–5.
33. Romagnoli S, Zacchetti S, Perazzo P, Verde F, Banfi G, Viganò M. Onsets of complications and revisions are not increased after simultaneous bilateral unicompartmental knee arthroplasty in comparison with unilateral procedures. Int Orthop (SICOT). 2015;39(5):871–7.
34. Siedlecki C, Beaufils P, Lemaire B, Pujol N. Complications and cost of single-stage vs. two-stage bilateral unicompartmental knee arthroplasty: a case-control study. Orthop Traumatol Surg Res. 2018;104(7):949–53.
35. Ros Fabien, These pour le diplôme d'etat de docteur en medecine, des de chirurgie generale, universite de medecine de brest-bretagne occidentale, Prothèse unicompartimente de genou unilatérale vs bilatérale en un temps opératoire: étude cas-témoin du vécu post-opératoire et des résultats fonctionnels à court terme, 2018.
36. Liu L, Liu H, Zhang H, Song J, Zhang L. Bilateral total knee arthroplasty: simultaneous or staged? A systematic review and meta-analysis. Medicine. 2019;98(22):e15931.
37. Morrey BF. Safety of simultaneous bilateral Total knee arthroplasty: a meta-analysis. Yearbook of Orthopedics. 2008;2008(105):6.
38. Ahn JH, Kang DM, Choi KJ. Bilateral simultaneous unicompartmental knee arthroplasty versus unilateral total knee arthroplasty: a comparison of the amount of blood loss and transfusion, perioperative complications, hospital stay, and functional recovery. Orthop Traumatol Surg Res. 2017;103(7):1041–5.
39. Arirachakaran A, Choowit P, Putananon C, Muangsiri S, Kongtharvonskul J. Is unicompartmental knee arthroplasty (UKA) superior to total knee arthroplasty (TKA)? A systematic review and meta-analysis of randomized controlled trial. Eur J Orthop Surg Traumatol. 2015;25(5):799–806. https://doi.org/10.1007/s00590-015-1610-9.
40. Dalury DF, Fisher DA, Adams MJ, Gonzales RA. Unicompartmental knee arthroplasty compares favorably to total knee arthroplasty in the same patient. Orthopedics. 2009;32(4):1213–26. orthosupersite.com/view.asp?rID=38057
41. Carlsson LV, Albrektsson BEJ, Regnér LR. Minimally invasive surgery vs conventional exposure using the miller-Galante Unicompartmental knee arthroplasty. J Arthroplast. 2006;21(2):151–6.
42. Reilly KA, Beard DJ, Barker KL, Dodd CAF, Price AJ, Murray DW. Efficacy of an accelerated recovery protocol for Oxford unicompartmental knee arthroplasty—a randomised controlled trial. Knee. 2005;12(5):351–7.
43. Essving P, Axelsson K, Otterborg L, Spännar H, Gupta A, Magnuson A, et al. Minimally invasive surgery did not improve outcome compared to conventional surgery following unicompartmental knee arthroplasty using local infiltration analgesia: a randomized controlled trial with 40 patients. Acta Orthop. 2012;83(6):634–41.
44. Hooper GJ, Hooper NM, Rothwell AG, Hobbs T. Bilateral total joint arthroplasty. J Arthroplast. 2009;24(8):1174–7.

45. Adili A, Bhandari M, Petruccelli D, de Beer J. Sequential bilateral total knee arthroplasty under 1 anesthetic in patients ≥75 years old. J Arthroplast. 2001;16(3):271–8.

46. Severson EP, Mariani EM, Bourne MH. Bilateral total knee arthroplasty in patients 70 years and older. Orthopedics. 2009;32(5):316. https://doi.org/10.3928/01477447-20090501-13.

Sports and Functional Activities Following Unicondylar Knee Arthroplasty

14

David A. Crawford and Keith R. Berend

14.1 Introduction

The goal of most knee arthroplasty procedures is to decrease pain and increase function. Those patients with knee osteoarthritis (OA) have a progressive decline in their daily functioning, work and sports related activities [1]. This decline in function is important to the patients' overall health as regular exercise has been shown to reduce mortality, stimulate weight loss, reduce anxiety/depression, and improve bone density [2–4]. Studies have shown that undergoing a joint arthroplasty can reduce a patient's risk of major cardiovascular events compared to those with arthritis that do not have surgery [5]. The demands on knee arthroplasty implants continue to increase as life expectancy is higher than decades before [6], and patients want to stay active and engaged in their working activities up to and after retiring [7]. More younger patients are also seeking knee arthroplasty as a treatment for arthritis, and these younger patients are expecting to return to a high level of activity [8].

In patients with end-stage knee arthritis, the two main surgical treatment options are total knee arthroplasty (TKA) or unicondylar knee arthroplasty (UKA). While TKA is a more commonly performed procedure for knee OA, many patients with end-stage knee arthritis are candidates for unicondylar knee arthroplasty (UKA) [9].

The indications and benefits of UKA are addressed in other chapters of this book; however, some benefits of UKA related to sports and activity should be noted. Compared to TKA, UKA has been shown to have improved knee kinematics, knee range of motion, and functional outcome scores [10–12]. The preservation of the cruciate ligaments and better knee kinematics likely contribute to why a UKA tends to "feel more normal" than a TKA [13]. This more normal feeling may ultimately contribute why patients are able to return to a higher level of sport after UKA compared to TKA [8].

This chapter will review the published literature on patient activity and participation in sports following UKA.

D. A. Crawford (✉)
Joint Implant Surgeons, Inc., New Albany, OH, USA
e-mail: crawfordda@joint-surgeons.com

K. R. Berend
Joint Implant Surgeons, Inc., New Albany, OH, USA

Mount Carmel Health System,
New Albany, OH, USA

14.2 Assessing Patient's Functional Activity

There are many functional and clinical outcome scores used to assess patients following lower extremity surgery. Each of these scoring systems has varying levels of so-called ceiling effects [14]. For example, the Knee Society Functional score that is commonly used to assess functional outcome after knee arthroplasty is composed of only 3 questions: 1) walking distance, 2) stair climbing, and 3) walking aids used [15]. While this is a validated outcome score, this score would not be able to differentiate between patients that can walk an unlimited distance from those that can also golf, run, or ski.

More sports specific scoring systems that are commonly reported in arthroplasty literature include the Tegner activity level [16] (Table 14.1) and UCLA activity score [17] (Table 14.2). These scoring metrics greater separate activity levels and give examples of specific sporting activities. When interpreting functional outcomes following arthroplasty, it is also important to know whether the comparative time frame is the patient's pre-arthritic functional level or their functional level just prior to arthroplasty. This information helps answer the question of whether patients can return to their pre-symptomatic level of activity or just improve from their symptomatic arthritic level.

Table 14.1 Tegner activity level [16]

Level	Description
0	Sick leave or disability pension because of knee problems
1	Work—sedentary (secretarial, etc.)
2	Work—light labor; walking on uneven ground possible, but impossible to backpack or hike
3	Work—light labor (nursing, etc.)
4	Work—moderately heavy labor (e.g., truck driving, etc.)
5	Work—heavy labor (construction, etc.); competitive sports—cycling, cross-country skiing; recreational sports—jogging on uneven ground at least twice weekly
6	Recreational sports—tennis and badminton, handball, racquetball, down-hill skiing, jogging at least five times per week
7	Competitive sports—tennis, running, motorcars speedway, handball; recreational sports- soccer, football, rugby, bandy, ice hockey, basketball, squash, racquetball, running
8	Competitive sports—racquetball or bandy, squash or badminton, track and field athletics (jumping, etc.), down-hill skiing
9	Competitive sports—soccer, football, rugby (lower divisions), ice hockey, wrestling, gymnastics, basketball
10	Competitive sports—soccer, football, rugby (national elite)

Table 14.2 UCLA activity scale [17]

Level	Description
1	Wholly inactive, dependent on others, and cannot leave residence
2	Mostly inactive or restricted to minimum activities of daily living
3	Sometimes participates in mild activities, such as walking, limited housework, and limited shopping
4	Regularly participates in mild activities
5	Sometimes participates in moderate activities such as swimming or could do unlimited housework or shopping
6	Regularly participates in moderate activities
7	Regularly participates in active events such as bicycling
8	Regularly participates in active events, such as golf or bowling
9	Sometimes participates in impact sports such as jogging, tennis, skiing, acrobatics, ballet, heavy labor, or backpacking
10	Regularly participates in impact sports

14.3 Defining the Level of Activity

Terms such as "low impact," "high impact," "low activity," and "high activity" are often used in the literature, but the definition and consensus on these terms are vague. Patients often hear that they may return to "low-impact" activities after knee arthroplasty, but what exactly does that mean? Running is often considered a "high impact" activity, while biking and swimming are more "low impact" activities. Some surgeons have defined low activity as a Tegner level 4 or less [18]. Robertson et al. defined high activity patients as those who completed >three million gate cycles/year or 1 h of activity/day [19]. Work out of the Scripps Clinic has helped quantify the impact of certain common activities on knee arthroplasty. D'Lima et al. implanted sensors in tibial components in vivo and measured forces from inside the prosthetic knee during various activities and reported contact stresses for the following activities (Table 14.3). Interesting golf, which is often touted as a "low impact" sporting activity, produced some of the highest joint forces. Rowing was the only activity to have less than bodyweight force on the knee [20].

Table 14.3 Tibial forces after TKA during specific activities [20]

Activity	Multiple of body weight
Cycling	1.3
Treadmill	2.05
Walking on ground	2.6
Rowing	0.85
Tennis—Forehand	3.6
Tennis—Backhand	3.1
Jogging	4.3
Golf driving swing—Leading leg	4.5
Golf driving swing—Opposite leg	3.2

14.4 Activity Level After UKA

Once patients become symptomatic with knee arthritis, their activity level decreases. Fisher et al. who found that only 25% of patients who underwent UKA were still participating in activities that they did before symptom onset [1]. Correspondingly, pre-surgery UCLA activity levels in patients undergoing UKA is low, ranging from 3.3 to 5.3. [1, 21–23]. The goal of UKA is to improve patient's pain and increase their activity from prior to surgery. However, we should also aim to return patients to as close to pre-symptom level as possible.

A few studies have compared post-operative UKA activity to pre-symptom activity. Walker et al. compared patients sporting activity after UKA to their activity level prior to any restricting symptoms of osteoarthritis. They found that 93% of patients were involved in at least one physical activity prior to the onset of symptoms and 92% of patients participated in at least one sporting activity after surgery. This 1% decline represented 6 patients who had quit their pre-symptoms sports, but 5 patients who began new sports after surgery [22]. Fisher et al. found that 93% of patients after UKA were able to return to their same level of activity as before knee arthritis symptoms [1], while others have found slightly less patients returning to their pre-symptom level of activity at 80.1% [24]. Ho et al. compared UCLA activity score prior to knee pain and after UKA. They found that there was a significant decline in UCLA from 8.1 pre-knee pain to 7.4 after surgery [25]. However, a score 7.4 is still quite high correlating to an activity level between "regularly participating in active events such as bicycling" and "regularly participating in active events such as golf or bowling" [17].

Most studies have compared post-operative activity level to the patients' immediate pre-

Table 14.4 Published results reporting rate of return to activity following UKA

Study	Number of subjects	Return to activity rate (%)
Fisher et al. [1]	66	93
Naal et al. [21]	83	95
Walker et al. [22]	45	98
Walker et al. [23]	93	93
Ho et al. [25]	36	87

operative activity level (Table 14.4). Overall activity level does tend to increase after UKA with significant improvements in UCLA to mean scores of 6.3 to 7.1. [1, 22, 23, 26] and Tegner activity levels of 2.6 to 4.0 [26–29].

Patients may want to know what specific sports they can expect to be able to return to after UKA. Common sports activities that increase after UKA are swimming, hiking, aerobics, golf, and dancing. However, patients may also expect a decreased participation in certain sports such as skiing, jogging, tennis, and soccer [1, 22, 26]. Time to return to sporting activities varies between patients. Walker et al. found that in those patient that returned to activity, 27% did so by the first month, 56% within 3 months, and 77% by 6 months after surgery [22].

14.5 Effect of Activity Level on UKA Implant Survivorship

Historically, the recommended activity level following knee arthroplasty has been guided by physician gestalt and consensus statements rather than objective publications of deleterious effects from specific activities [30]. In a consensus statement by the Knee Society in 2001, the recommended activities following knee arthroplasty were bowling, golfing, walking, swimming, and dancing [31].

The concern from surgeons about high patient activity level is that certain activities may shorten the survivorship of the arthroplasty due to accel-

erated polyethylene wear and aseptic loosening [32, 33]. A person with an average activity level produces approximately 1.0 million knee cycles/year where highly active individuals about 3.2 million knee cycles/year [34]. The concern over polyethylene wear in arthroplasty has slowed since polyethylene manufacturing has improved with decreased wear and oxidation [35]. Furthermore, polyethylene wear in UKA is not as much of an issue as in TKA. In the mobile bearing Oxford knee (Zimmer Biomet, Warsaw, IN), for example, the 20-year wear was shown to be only 0.4 mm [36]. Polyethylene wear is also a relatively infrequent failure mode in UKA, representing only 4% of UKA revisions [37].

In TKA literature, there are conflicting studies on activity level and the relationship to implant failure. Some studies have shown a positive correlation between activity level and arthroplasty failure [38–40], while others have not demonstrated any correlation [41, 42]. There has been limited research on the specific question of activity level and failure in UKA. One of the few studies was published by Al et al., who evaluated the effect of activity level on survivorship of the Oxford knee. They separated patients by postoperative Tenger score, with 4 or less being low activity and 5 or greater being high activity. They found that the high activity group had 40% less revisions than the low activity group. Each 1 point increase in Tenger score was associated with around 30% fewer revisions. They further found, which may be intuitive, that the more active patients were younger [18]. Greco et al. reported on 340 patients under the age of 50 years old that underwent a medial UKA with the Oxford mobile bearing implant. At a mean of 6.1 years, only 2% of patients had a revision for aseptic loosening and there were no revision for polyethylene wear [43].

14.6 Summary

Patients who undergo UKA can expect to return to most activities they participated prior to knee symptoms. Certain activities such as skiing and jogging may decline, while others such as swimming may increase. There does not appear to be a negative effect of increased activity on the survivorship of UKA.

References

1. Fisher N, Agarwal M, Reuben SF, Johnson DS, Turner PG. Sporting and physical activity following Oxford medial unicompartmental knee arthroplasty. Knee. 2006;13(4):296–300.
2. American College of Sports Medicine Physicians Statement. The recommended quantity and quality of exercise for developing and maintaining cardiovascular and muscular fitness in healthy adults. Med Sci Sports Exerc. 1990;22:265.
3. Macnicol MF, McHardy R, Chalmers J. Exercise testing before and after hip arthroplasty. J Bone Joint Surg. 1980;62:326.
4. Ries MD, Philbin EF, Groff GD, et al. Improvement in cardiovascular fitness after total knee arthroplasty. J Bone Joint Surg Am. 1996;78:1696.
5. Ravi B, Croxford R, Austin P, Lipscombe L, Bierman A, Harvey P, Hawker G. The relation between total joint arthroplasty and risk for serious cardiovascular events in patients with moderate-severe osteoarthritis: propensity score. BMJ. 2013;347:f6187.
6. Arias E, Heron M, Xu J. United States Life Tables, 2013. Natl Vital Stat Rep. 2017;66(3):1–64.
7. Maxwell JL, Keysor JJ, Niu J, et al. Participation following knee replacement: the MOST cohort study. Phys Ther. 2013;93(11):1467–74.
8. Witjes S, van Geenen RC, Koenraadt KL, van der Hart CP, Blankevoort L, Kerkhoffs GM, Kuijer PP. Expectations of younger patients concerning activities after knee arthroplasty: are we asking the right questions? Qual Life Res. 2017;26(2):403–17.
9. Berend KR, Berend ME, Dalury DF, Argenson JN, Dodd CA, Scott RD. Consensus statement on indications and contraindications for medial unicompartmental knee arthroplasty. J Surg Orthop Adv. 2015;24(4):252–6.
10. Banks SA, Fregly BJ, Boniforti F, Reinschmidt C, Romagnoli S. Comparing in vivo kinematics of unicondylar and bi-unicondylar knee replacements. Knee Surg Sports Traumatol Arthrosc. 2005;13:551–6.
11. Hollinghurst D, Stoney J, Ward T. No deterioration of kinematics and cruciate function 10 years after medial unicompartmental arthroplasty. Knee. 2006;13:440–4.
12. Li MG, Yao F, Joss B, et al. Mobile vs. fixed bearing unicondylar knee arthroplasty: a randomized study on short term clinical outcomes and knee kinematics. Knee. 2006;13:365–70.
13. Laurencin CT, Zelicof SB, Scott RD, Ewald FC. Unicompartmental versus total knee arthroplasty in the same patient: a comparative study. Clin Orthop Relat Res. 1991;273:151–6.
14. Steinhoff AK, Bugbee WD. Knee Injury and Osteoarthritis Outcome Score has higher responsiveness and lower ceiling effect than Knee Society Function Score after total knee arthroplasty. Knee Surg Sports Traumatol Arthrosc. 2016;24(8):2627–33.
15. Insall JN, Dorr LD, Scott RD, Scott WN. Rationale of the knee society clinical rating system. Clin Orthop Relat Res. 1989;248:13–4.
16. Tegner Y, Lysholm J. Rating systems in the evaluation of knee ligament injuries. Clin Orthop Relat Res. 1985;198:43–9.
17. Amstutz HC, Thomas BJ, Jinnah R, et al. Treatment of primary osteoarthritis of the hip: a comparison of total joint and surface replacement arthroplasty. J Bone Joint Surg Am. 1984;66:228.
18. Ali AM, Pandit H, Liddle AD, Jenkins C, Mellon S, Dodd CA, Murray DW. Does activity affect the outcome of the Oxford unicompartmental knee replacement? Knee. 2016;23(2):327–30.
19. Robertson NB, Battenberg AK, Kertzner M, Schmalzried TP. Defining high activity in arthroplasty patients. Bone Joint J. 2016;98-B(1 Suppl A):95–7.
20. D'Lima DD, Steklov N, Patil S, Colwell CW Jr. The Mark Coventry Award: in vivo knee forces during recreation and exercise after knee arthroplasty. Clin Orthop Relat Res. 2008;466(11):2605–11.
21. Naal FD, Fischer M, Preuss A, et al. Return to sports and recreational activity after unicompartmental knee arthroplasty. Am J Sports Med. 2007;35:1688–95.
22. Walker T, Gotterbarm T, Bruckner T, Merle C, Streit MR. Return to sports, recreational activity and patient-reported outcomes after lateral unicompartmental knee arthroplasty. Knee Surg Sports Traumatol Arthrosc. 2015;23(11):3281–7.
23. Walker T, Streit J, Gotterbarm T, Bruckner T, Merle C, Streit MR. Sports, physical activity and patient-reported outcomes after medial unicompartmental knee arthroplasty in young patients. J Arthroplast. 2015;30(11):1911–6.
24. Pietschmann MF, Wohlleb L, Weber P, Schmidutz F, Ficklscherer A, Gülecyüz MF, et al. Sports activities after medial unicompartmental knee arthroplasty Oxford III—what can we expect? Int Orthop. 2013;37(1):31–7.
25. Ho JC, Stitzlein RN, Green CJ, Stoner T, Froimson MI. Return to sports activity following UKA and TKA. J Knee Surg. 2016;29(3):254–9.
26. Jahnke A, Mende JK, Maier GS, Ahmed GA, Ishaque BA, Schmitt H, Rickert M, Clarius M, Seeger JB. Sports activities before and after medial unicompartmental knee arthroplasty using the new Heidelberg sports activity score. Int Orthop. 2015;39(3):449–54.
27. Pandit H, Jenkins C, Gill HS, Barker K, Dodd CA, Murray DW. Minimally invasive Oxford phase 3 unicompartmental knee replacement: results of 1000 cases. J Bone Joint Surg Br. 2011;93(2):198–204.

28. Weston-Simons JS, Pandit H, Kendrick BJ, Jenkins C, Barker K, Dodd CA, Murray DW. The mid-term outcomes of the Oxford domed lateral unicompartmental knee replacement. Bone Joint J. 2014;96-B(1):59–64.
29. Yim JH, Song EK, Seo HY, Kim MS, Seon JK. Comparison of high tibial osteotomy and unicompartmental knee arthroplasty at a minimum follow-up of 3 years. J Arthroplast. 2013;28(2):243–7.
30. Swanson EA, Schmalzried TP, Dorey FJ. Activity recommendations after total hip and knee arthroplasty: a survey of the American Association for hip and Knee Surgeons. J Arthroplast. 2009;24(6):120–6.
31. Healy WL, Iorio R, Lemos MJ. Athletic activity after joint replacement. Am J Sports Med. 2001;29(3):377–88.
32. Harris WH. Wear and periprosthetic osteolysis: the problem. Clin Orthop Relat Res. 2001;393:66–70.
33. Horikoshi M, Macaulay W, Booth RE, Crossett LS, Rubash HE. Comparison of interface membranes obtained from failed cemented and cementless hip and knee prostheses. Clin Orthop Relat Res. 1994;309:69–87.
34. Seedhom B, Dowson D, Wright V. Wear of solid phase formed high density polyethylene in relation to the life of artificial hips and knees. Wear. 1973;24:35–51.
35. Grupp TM, Fritz B, Kutzner I, Schilling C, Bergmann G, Schwiesau J. Vitamin E stabilised polyethylene for total knee arthroplasty evaluated under highly demanding activities wear simulation. Acta Biomater. 2017;48:415–22.
36. Kendrick BJ, Simpson DJ, Kaptein BL, Valstar ER, Gill HS, Murray DW, et al. Polyethylene wear of mobile-bearing unicompartmental knee replacement at 20 years. J Bone Joint Surg Br. 2011;93(4):470–5.
37. Van der List JP, McDonald LS, Pearle AD. Systematic review of medial versus lateral survivorship in unicompartmental knee arthroplasty. Knee. 2015;22(6):454–60.
38. Lavernia CJ, Sierra RJ, Hungerford DS, et al. Activity level and wear in total knee arthroplasty: a study of autopsy retrieved specimens. J Arthroplast. 2001;16(4):446–53.
39. Odland AN, Callaghan JJ, Liu SS, Wells CW. Wear and lysis is the problem in modular TKA in the young OA patient at 10 years. Clin Orthop Relat Res. 2011 Jan;469(1):41–7.
40. Rohrbach M, Lüem M, Ochsner PE. Patient and surgery related factors associated with fatigue type polyethylene wear on 49 PCA and DURACON retrievals at autopsy and revision. J Orthop Surg Res. 2008;22(3):8.
41. Bisschop R, Brouwer RW, Van Raay JJ. Total knee arthroplasty in younger patients: a 13-year follow-up study. Orthopedics. 2010;33(12):876.
42. Diduch DR, Insall JN, Scott WN, et al. Total knee replacement in young, active patients: long-term follow-up and functional outcome. J Bone Joint Surg Am. 1997;79(4):575–82.
43. Greco NJ, Lombardi AV Jr, Price AJ, Berend ME, Berend KR. Medial Mobile-Bearing Unicompartmental Knee Arthroplasty in Young Patients Aged Less Than or Equal to 50 Years. J Arthroplast. 2018;33(8):2435–9.

Complications of Unicompartmental Knee Replacement

15

Stefano Campi

15.1 Introduction

Complications after unicompartmental knee replacement occur with a similar incidence than after TKA. However, their management can be difficult in the hands of low volume surgeons, who unfortunately tend to experience more than expert surgeons. The higher susceptibility to revision and the scepticism towards UKR of many orthopaedics surgeons are a threat for patients undergoing UKR, especially if they encounter a complication. It is therefore really important to recognise and manage the most common complications of UKR and protect patients from unnecessary revisions and/or overtreatment. A second opinion from an experienced UKR surgeon can be really helpful in dealing with complex situations.

The most common causes of failure and complications of UKR will be discussed in this chapter.

S. Campi (✉)
Department of Medicine and Surgery, Università Campus Bio-Medico di Roma, Fondazione Policlinico Universitario Campus Bio-Medico, Rome, Italy

15.2 Progression of Osteoarthritis in the Retained Compartments

Progression of osteoarthritis in the retained compartments represents the most common cause of failure of UKA in the majority of clinical series, with an incidence between 0.9 and 7% [1–3] [4–6]. It represent the third cause of failure in the National Joint Registry of England and Wales, with a revision rate of 2.27 for 100 component years [7].

The causes of OA progression in the lateral compartment are still controversial.

Overcorrection of the mechanical axis of the lower limb is considered as a relevant cause by many authors, causing overload of the lateral compartment of the knee. This complication is due to an error in the surgical technique implying the release or damage of the medial collateral ligament, inadequate bone resections, or the use of thick inserts with LCM stretching. However, OA progression is frequently observed in knees that are not overcorrected [1]. Overcorrection is probably one of the possible causes of OA progression, but not the only one [8].

It has been suggested that OA progression is time dependent. However, long-term studies did not show an increase of this complication over time [9].

Other factors, such as BMI or chondrocalcinosis, have been suggested as possible causes of OA

A. Clavé, F. Dubrana (eds.), *Unicompartmental Knee Arthroplasty*,
https://doi.org/10.1007/978-3-031-48332-5_15

progression, but this hypothesis has not been supported by clinical studies [10, 11].

Finally, it has been suggested that lateral OA is mainly related to the conditions of the lateral compartment at the moment of the operation, and that the missed diagnosis of chondral damage can cause the subsequent failure of the implant [8]. Consequently, in the author's opinion, it is mandatory to obtain stress-views or Rosenberg views besides standard, weight-bearing radiographs. The use of MRI is controversial and still debated.

The progression of osteoarthritis is usually diagnosed on standard weight-bearing X-rays. In some cases, stress X-rays or Rosenberg views are needed to highlight this complication (Fig. 15.1). Joint space narrowing or its disappearance are the most relevant radiographic finding. In contrast, the presence of marginal osteophytes is not specific and it is common also in the presence of preserved cartilage [12].

Clinically, the main symptom is pain, which can correspond to the affected compartment or be referred elsewhere. It is important to notice that the radiographic evidence of lateral OA is not always associated with pain.

There are two treatments for symptomatic progression of OA. The first is revision to TKA. This can be performed extending the old incision through a medial parapatellar approach. The second option is the addition of a lateral UKR. Thus technically more demanding, the latter is an effective procedure which should be preferred in patients that have been happy with their medial UKR for years [13]. This operation can be performed through a lateral approach or extending the medial skin incision and performing a lateral parapatellar approach, or using a TKA approach.

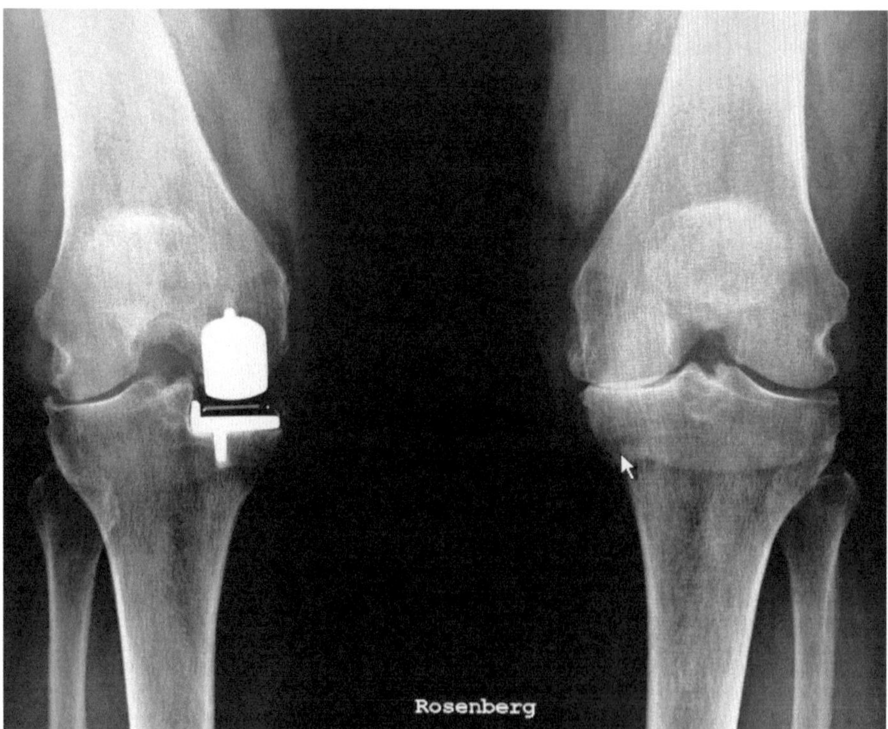

Fig. 15.1 Osteoarthritis progression in the lateral compartment shown on Rosenberg views, with lateral joint space narrowing, sclerosis, and marginal osteophytes

15.3 Infection

Periprosthetic joint infections are relatively uncommon in partial knee replacement, with an incidence around 1% [14]. The diagnostic algorithm is the same as in total knee replacement and should be based on the most recent guidelines.

Acute infections can be treated with a DAIR procedure, while late infections usually require a revision to total knee replacement. This can be performed either as a single-stage or a two-stage procedure. The author's preference is to perform a two-stage procedure. In the first-stage, beside implant removal, it is important to perform also the total knee resections to remove the retained cartilage, as it can be contaminated with bacteria [15]. A standard spacer, either fixed or articulating, is implanted and followed by i.v. and/or oral antibiotics. Once the infection is cleared, the second stage can be performed.

15.4 Aseptic Loosening

Aseptic loosening is a frequent cause of failure in the joint registries. However, it is really uncommon in case series from high volume centres. This discrepancy has different possible explanations. First, revisions for unexplained pain are frequently categorised as loosening even in the absence of clear evidence of such complication. Second, the wrong interpretation of periprosthetic radiolucent lines (RL) is frequent among surgeons that are not familiar with UKR. Radiolucent lines are frequently encountered in the X-rays of well-functioning UKRs (Fig. 15.2). It is paramount to distinguish physiological and pathological radiolucencies. A physiological RL is usually less than 2 mm in thickness, non-progressive, with a sclerotic margin. Physiological RL are not correlated with loosening and do not affect the survival of the implant. In contrast, a progressive, poorly defined radiolucent line that is thicker than 2 mm is considered "pathological" and correlated with failure

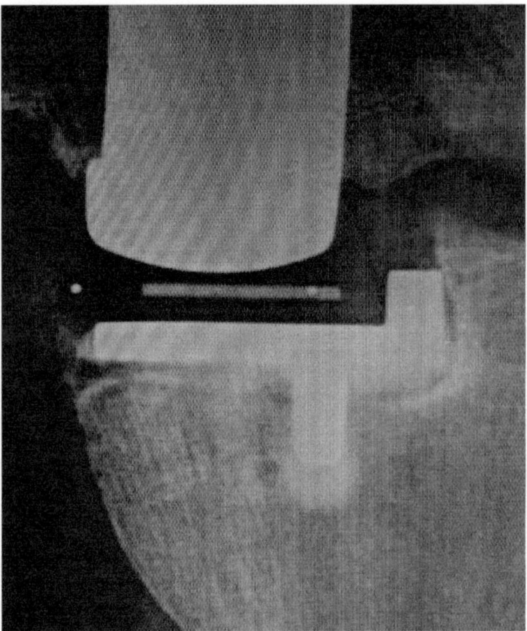

Fig. 15.2 Physiological radiolucent lines around the tibial component of a well-functioning mobile-bearing UKR. Physiological RL are usually less than 2 mm in thickness, non-progressive and with a sclerotic margin

of fixation or infection [16]. It has to be noticed that the presence of RL is common in all cemented implants; however, it is more evident in UKR than TKR because of the absence of a central keel. Furthermore, the presence of RLs is influenced by the X-ray alignment, so that even few degrees of inclination of the beam can hide or show them.

While failure, the diagnosis of tibial loosening is usually evident on standard X-ray, the loosening of the femoral component is less frequent but also less easy to diagnose. If there is the suspect of femoral loosening, a lateral X-ray with the knee in flexion and then in extension can highlight this problem showing position changes of the component.

In case of aseptic loosening is generally revision to TKR. The revision of UKR to UKR is option in early loosening. However, this indication is controversial and should be performed is selected cases by experienced surgeons.

15.5 Fracture

Perioperative medial condyle fracture is a rare but known complication of UKRs [17]. The aetiology of fracture is likely to be multifactorial.

Technical errors such as a deep tibial resection, a medialised positioning of the tibial component, the damage of the posterior cortical bone, and the use of a heavy hammer are known risk factors [18]. In addition, patient characteristic such as small sizes and poor bone quality can increase the risk of fracture. The risk seems higher in specific subset of patients such as the Asian population, in which the size and morphology of the proximal tibia can predispose to fracturing of the medial condyle.

A careful surgical technique can significantly reduce the risk of this complication.

Most of the fractures are diagnosed intraoperatively or in the first 4–8 weeks after surgery, when patients increase mobilisation and weight-bearing.

A standard X-ray is usually enough for the diagnosis (Fig. 15.3).

Some surgeons have experienced and increased number of fracture using cementless, mobile-bearing UKRs. This is probably related to the interference generated around the keel of the tibial component during implantation. Even though this complication is rare, the suspect should be higher when cementless UKRs are used, especially at the beginning of the learning curve.

The conservative treatment with restricted weight-bearing is usually effective for undisplaced or minimally displaced fractures diagnosed within 3 months after surgery. In case of displaced fractures (with stable tibial component over the fragment), open reduction and internal fixation with screws and/or buttress plate are the preferred treatment. In case of late diagnosis or loose components, revision to TKR with stemmed components is usually required [18].

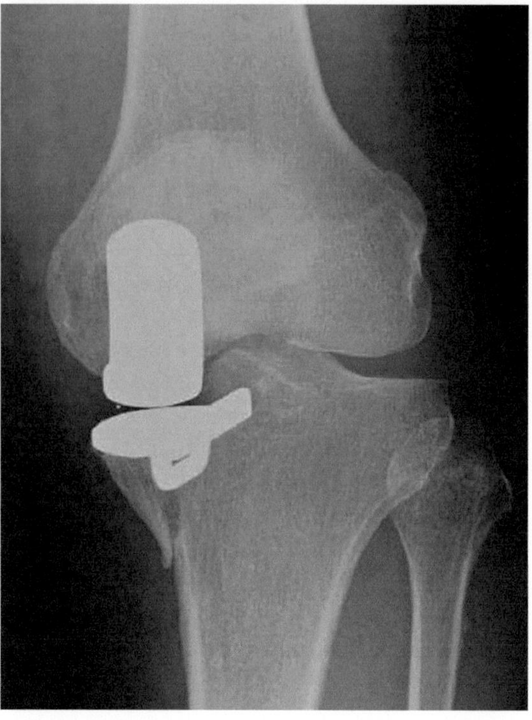

Fig. 15.3 X-ray of a periprosthetic fracture of the tibial condyle after medial unicompartmental knee replacement, diagnosed 4 weeks after the operation

15.6 Bearing Dislocation in Mobile Bearing Designs

Bearing dislocation is a relatively uncommon complication of mobile-bearing designs. With the recent design and surgical technique improvements, the dislocation rate is around one on 200 cases (0.5%) [2]. Bearing dislocations tend to occur early. Primary dislocations are usually caused by a surgical error: inadequate osteophyte removal, poor gap balancing, MCL damage, retained cement, or a femoral component sited too far from the sagittal wall allowing the bearing to spin. A "loose" bearing is often a reason of concern for surgeons that are not familiar with the procedure. However, this is rarely a cause of

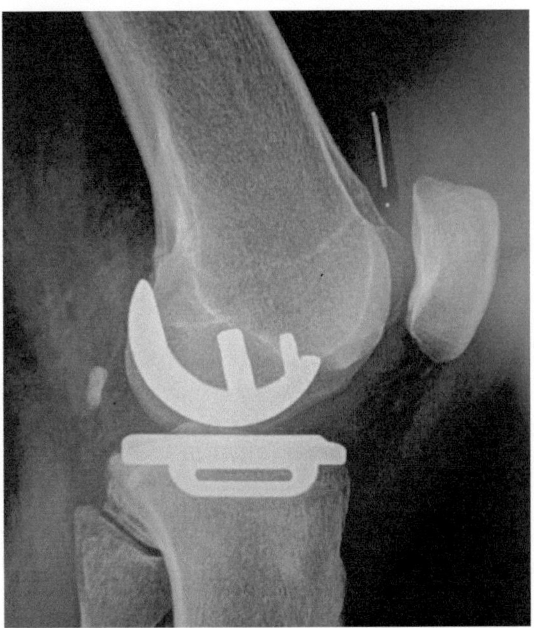

Fig. 15.4 Lateral view showing a dislocated bearing in the supra-patellar pouch

dislocation. In contrast, a bearing that is too tight increases the risk of dislocation [18]. A bearing dislocation can also result from a trauma or twisting injury of the knee.

A bearing dislocation is usually characterised by acute pain and functional impairment. However, it can be relatively silent in some cases. Bearing dislocations are usually noticeable on a standard X-ray (Fig. 15.4).

In most cases, the treatment consists in the arthrotomy, joint examination to assess and address possible causes of dislocation, and bearing exchange. In case of recurrent dislocation or severe imbalancing of the gaps, revision to TKA can be necessary.

15.7 Unexplained Pain

Unexplained pain is the second most common cause of revision of UKR according to the NJR, while it is relatively uncommon in case series from high volume centres (0.6% of revisions) [19].

Anteromedial pain is not uncommon in the first 6–12 months after the operation, and it resolves spontaneously in the vast majority of cases. One possible cause is related to bone overload and remodelling in the proximal tibia after the operation [20]. These cases must be treated conservatively with active monitoring and reassurance of the patient. A second opinion from an expert surgeon can be helpful for managing complex patients. Some studies report benefits from the off-label use of high dosages of clodronate [21].

A relevant pain in the anteromedial region in the first 2–3 months after the surgery can also be caused by a tibial condyle fracture. This should be always suspected and ruled out with appropriate imaging.

Possible causes of persistent pain are component malpositioning with significant overhang (causing soft tissue irritation), retained cement fragments or loose bodies, impingement, tendinopathies, meniscal tears, progression of OA in the retained compartment. However, the most frequent cause of unexplained pain is a wrong indication to surgery. The results of UKR in partial thickness cartilage loss are not predictable and correlated with a higher incidence of persistent pain [22]. The surgical treatment should always be reserved to patients with end-stage OA, with no exceptions. The bone-on-bone contact is not always revealed by standard, weight-bearing X-rays and has to be confirmed with further imaging (stress X-rays, Rosenberg views). If a patient with unexplained pain has been operated elsewhere, it is fundamental to review the preoperative imaging. In case the operation was performed on a partial thickness disease, a revision is likely to be ineffective. In these cases of "overtreatment", further operations usually lead to disappointing results and should be avoided. Better results are achieved with pain therapy.

Adequate imaging is important to assess component positioning. An overhang greater than 2 mm can hypothetically cause soft tissue irritation and pain. However, this is not always the case. The nature and features of pain should be

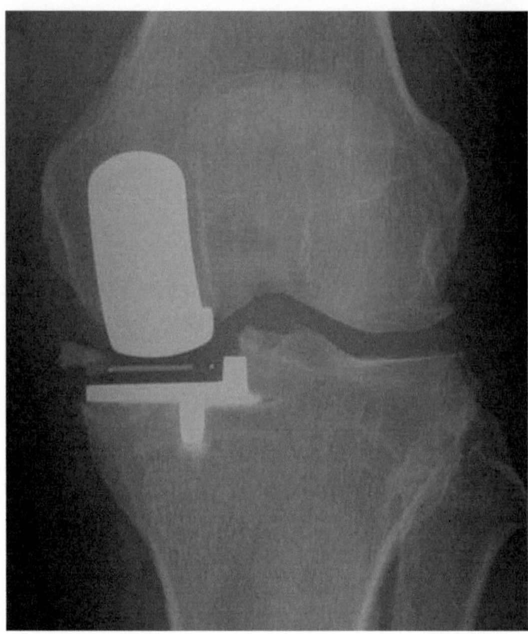

Fig. 15.5 X-ray showing a retained cement fragment medial to the bearing. This patient initially experienced mechanical symptoms, which settled in few weeks' time after the fragment moved in the posterior recess

evaluated meticulously to confirm this hypothesis. An injection with local anaesthetics over the tender spot can be useful to confirm the diagnosis.

Malalignment of the components is frequently observed in X-rays of well working implants. Therefore, it is really important to rule out other possible causes of failure (including the indication to surgery) before considering revision surgery.

In contrast, overcorrection of limb alignment, overstuffing of the medial compartment, and MCL stretching are less tolerated and often cause problems on the short- or long-term follow-up.

Retained cement fragments or loose bodies are not uncommon, especially when using a minimally invasive approach (Fig. 15.5). The patients usually refer mechanical symptoms while walking, with sharp, occasional pain. In some cases, the symptoms resolve spontaneously over time. However, if there is evidence of a loose fragment and the patients is symptomatic, arthroscopic removal is a viable and effective option.

Arthroscopy can be useful also when a meniscal tear is suspected, or in case of proper "unexplained pain" when other possible causes of failure have been investigated.

When a revision is needed, conversion to TKR is usually the most reliable option. However, selected cases in the hands of expert surgeons can be treated with partial revision.

As a general rule, in case of unexplained pain, a UKR should be treated with the same approach and threshold to revision of a TKR: early revisions (less than 2 years post-op) should be avoided, unless there is an obvious cause of failure.

References

1. Emerson RH Jr, Higgins LL. Unicompartmental knee arthroplasty with the oxford prosthesis in patients with medial compartment arthritis. J Bone Joint Surg Am. 2008;90(1):118–22.
2. Pandit H, Jenkins C, Gill HS, Barker K, Dodd CA, Murray DW. Minimally invasive Oxford phase 3 unicompartmental knee replacement: results of 1000 cases. J Bone Joint Surg Br. 2011;93(2):198–204.
3. Khan OH, Davies H, Newman JH, Weale AE. Radiological changes ten years after St. Georg sled unicompartmental knee replacement. Knee. 2004;11(5):403–7.
4. Kim KT, Lee S, Kim JH, Hong SW, Jung WS, Shin WS. The survivorship and clinical results of minimally invasive Unicompartmental knee arthroplasty at 10-year follow-up. Clin Orthop Surg. 2015;7(2):199–206.
5. Pandit H, Hamilton TW, Jenkins C, Mellon SJ, Dodd CA, Murray DW. The clinical outcome of minimally invasive phase 3 Oxford unicompartmental knee arthroplasty: a 15-year follow-up of 1000 UKAs. Bone Joint J. 2015;97-B(11):1493–500.
6. Campi S, Pandit HG, Dodd CAF, Murray DW. Cementless fixation in medial unicompartmental knee arthroplasty: a systematic review. Knee Surg Sports Traumatol Arthrosc. 2017;25(3):736–45.
7. National Joint Registry for England, Wales and Northern Ireland. 13th annual report., 2016.
8. Pandit H, Spiegelberg B, Clave A, McGrath C, Liddle AD, Murray DW. Aetiology of lateral progression of arthritis following Oxford medial unicompartmental knee replacement: a case-control study. Musculoskelet Surg. 2016;100(2):97–102.
9. Price AJ, Waite JC, Svard U. Long-term clinical results of the medial Oxford unicompartmental knee arthroplasty. Clin Orthop Relat Res. 2005;435:171–80.

10. Murray DW, Pandit H, Weston-Simons JS, Jenkins C, Gill HS, Lombardi AV, Dodd CA, Berend KR. Does body mass index affect the outcome of unicompartmental knee replacement? Knee. 2013;20(6):461–5.

11. Hernigou P, Pascale W, Pascale V, Homma Y, Poignard A. Does primary or secondary chondrocalcinosis influence long-term survivorship of unicompartmental arthroplasty? Clin Orthop Relat Res. 2012;470(7):1973–9.

12. Waldstein W, Kasparek MF, Faschingbauer M, Windhager R, Boettner F. Lateral-compartment osteophytes are not associated with lateral-compartment cartilage degeneration in arthritic Varus knees. Clin Orthop Relat Res. 2017;475(5):1386–92.

13. Pandit H, Mancuso F, Jenkins C, Jackson WFM, Price AJ, Dodd CAF, Murray DW. Lateral unicompartmental knee replacement for the treatment of arthritis progression after medial unicompartmental replacement. Knee Surg Sports Traumatol Arthrosc. 2017;25(3):669–74.

14. Liddle AD, Judge A, Pandit H, Murray DW. Determinants of revision and functional outcome following unicompartmental knee replacement. Osteoarthr Cartil. 2014;22(9):1241–50.

15. Goodfellow JOCJ, Dodd CAF, Murray DW. Unicompartmental arthroplasty with the Oxford knee. New York: Oxford University Press; 2006.

16. Gulati A, Chau R, Pandit HG, Gray H, Price AJ, Dodd CA, Murray DW. The incidence of physiological radiolucency following Oxford unicompartmental knee replacement and its relationship to outcome. J Bone Joint Surg Br. 2009;91(7):896–902.

17. Ji JH, Park SE, Song IS, Kang H, Ha JY, Jeong JJ. Complications of medial unicompartmental knee arthroplasty. Clin Orthop Surg. 2014;6(4):365–72.

18. Goodfellow J, O'Connor J, Pandit H, Dodd C, Murray D. Unicompartmental arthroplasty with the Oxford knee, vol. 1. 2nd ed. Goodfellow Publishers Limited; 2015.

19. Mohammad HR, Strickland L, Hamilton TW, Murray DW. Long-term outcomes of over 8,000 medial Oxford phase 3 Unicompartmental knees-a systematic review. Acta Orthop. 2018;89(1):101–7.

20. Pegg EC, Walter J, Mellon SJ, Pandit HG, Murray DW, D'Lima DD, Fregly BJ, Gill HS. Evaluation of factors affecting tibial bone strain after unicompartmental knee replacement. J Orthop Res. 2013;31(5):821–8.

21. Frediani B, Giusti A, Bianchi G, Dalle Carbonare L, Malavolta N, Cantarini L, Saviola G, Molfetta L. Clodronate in the management of different musculoskeletal conditions. Minerva Med. 2018;109(4):300–25.

22. Pandit H, Gulati A, Jenkins C, Barker K, Price AJ, Dodd CA, Murray DW. Unicompartmental knee replacement for patients with partial thickness cartilage loss in the affected compartment. Knee. 2011;18(3):168–71.

What to Do If a Medial Unicompartmental Knee Arthroplasty Fails

16

F. -X. Gunepin, L. Tristan, G. Le Henaff, O. Cantin, and T. Gicquel

16.1 Introduction

The rate of revision surgery for unicompartmental knee arthroplasty (UKA) can be very different in the literature and vary by a factor of 1 to 2 depending on the publication: from 91% survival at 20 years in a series on the Oxford implant to 21% failure at 15 years for the Australian register [1]. The UK register lies between the two with 88% survival at 10 years. However, all authors agree that survival increases with the expertise of the centres and practitioners [2].

Early failures tend to result from improper indication or incorrect surgical technique with a few complex regional pain syndromes. In the long term, causes of failure are progression of osteoarthritis (OA) in the other knee compartments or wear of the polyethylene insert. Complications such as fracture or infection occur more randomly.

Analysing the causes of medial UKA failure is relatively difficult because retrospective studies involve implants of different design and insertion. North European and Australian registers have evidenced this [3–6].

When a medial unicompartmental knee arthroplasty fails, it is sometimes difficult to diagnose loosening of the implant. Certainly, unexplained pain can be an early manifestation of loosening of the implant, excess stress or micro-mobility processes. The combination of unexplained pain and loosening, all series combined, represents 2/3 to 3/4 of the causes of revision surgery. The Oxford teams make a distinction between technical error and improper indication [4, 7].

Dislocation of the polyethylene (PE) insert is specific to implants with a mobile insert (Table 16.1).

In all cases, it is necessary to seek to identify this failure in order to offer the patient the most appropriate therapeutic solution for his/her situation.

The reason for consultation is the onset of pain more or less associated with deterioration of a functional result that was previously satisfactory. The context can be sudden (trauma, dislocation of the PE) or slowly progressive (wear). The combination with inflammatory signs should suggest sepsis, which will require prompt aggressive management to save the implant.

Unexplained pain should suggest the hypothesis of an unstable implant.

F. -X. Gunepin (✉) · L. Tristan
G. L. Henaff · O. Cantin
Clinique Mutualiste de la porte de L'Orient,
Lorient, France

T. Gicquel
Clinique Mutualiste de la porte de L'Orient,
Lorient, France

Department of Orthopaedic Surgery and
Traumatology, Rennes University Teaching Hospital,
Rennes, France

A. Clavé, F. Dubrana (eds.), *Unicompartmental Knee Arthroplasty*,
https://doi.org/10.1007/978-3-031-48332-5_16

Table 16.1 Aetiology of UKA failures

	Oxford (%)	NJR UK (%)	Epinette/SFHG[a] (%)	Australian register (%)
Unexplained pain	65	25	5.5	12
OA progression	10	20	15	14
Loosening of the implant (T/F/ T + F)	10 (7 and 3)	32	44 (25/6/13)	54
Dislocation/wear of the PE insert	7	6	12	4.8 (2, 8/2)
Infection	6	5	2	4
Technical error	2	6	11.5	3
Fracture	2	2	4	2

[a] SFHG: French Society of Hip and Knee Surgery

16.2 Specific Case of Allergy

To date, there has been no published report on UKA failure due to allergy, but many situations of pain and inflammation remain unexplained. The processes of an allergic complication in knee arthroplasties are regularly described. The diagnosis should be considered in a consultation by questioning the patient on their history of atopic dermatitis, asthma or metal intolerance (belt buckle, expansion band of a wristwatch, costume jewellery, earrings).

The operator may want to use the questionnaire developed by the SFHG [8] (https://www.sfhg.fr/accueil/fiches-d-information/allergies-et-prothèses/) to aid management. In case of doubt, an assessment should be performed. It is based on conducting skin patch tests [8–9]. The sensitivity of these tests is an imperfect reflection of the biological reality, and a skin allergy is not necessarily correlated with joint allergy. Whatever the reason, the preoperative hypothesis of possible allergy should lead the surgeon to consider the choice of implant; the unavailability of a titanium or surface-treated UKA should lead him/her to consider using a total arthroplasty or to continue with further investigations by conducting a MEmory Lymphocyte Immuno Stimulation Assay (MELISA), the only specific test for metal allergy but of limited access (no laboratory in France) [10].

> Before a joint implant is inserted, completion of an allergy screening questionnaire is advisable. In cases of unexplained loosening of the implant or pain, the hypothesis of an allergic origin should be considered.

16.3 Measures to Be Taken on Wear Progression

Wear progression can occur in patellofemoral or lateral tibiofemoral OA. The therapeutic solutions range from total knee arthroplasty or replacement of the deteriorated compartment. In the case of lateral or patellofemoral unicompartmental implants, the surgeon should refer to conventional indications for these procedures. The only factor that should be considered is the degree of wear on a medial UKA. Any alteration in the internal implant should suggest use of total knee arthroplasty.

For a lateral UKA, the preoperative axis of the limb should be in valgus position, and it is logical to maintain slight postoperative valgus in order not to overload the medial UKA, which is by definition an older implant and therefore potentially already involved. Other criteria, of course, should be followed: reducibility of the valgus deformity, conserved joint amplitude and efficient ligament system [11].

For patellofemoral arthroplasty, indications are rare. They can be considered in light of UKA deterioration with the onset of patellofemoral pain in combination with Iwano radiological stage 3 or 4. The central pivotal point should be intact, and joint amplitude should be conserved or with limited and reducible stiffness (<10°). The axis of the lower limb should be close to normal [12].

Once the indication has been established, the approach will be chosen based on the one performed for medial UKA.

> Wear progression in the lateral compartment can benefit from revision by external UKA subject to a reducible genu valgum.

16.4 TKR After UKA

In cases of UKA failure, revision surgery with TKR is the most common approach. In the SFHG series combining 425 failures of UKA alone, 36 underwent revision by UKA, i.e. 8.5% [13], and in a series by Lewis, this figure rose to 11.2% (follow-up of 45,615 UKA in the Australian register). The implant should be chosen following an attentive clinical and paraclinical assessment.

Clinically, it is necessary to assess the morphotype, joint amplitudes, muscle capital and competence of the different ligament structures. The surgeon should note the position and size of scars and the existence and extent of any joint effusion (which can be punctured and drained). Every effort should be made to obtain the previous surgery report.

The paraclinical assessment consists of standard X-ray views (anteroposterior and profile with weightbearing, patellofemoral series). Long-leg radiographs are advisable to provide details of the limb axis, but also the presentation of the tibial and femoral diaphysis in order to use a stem approach. In case of doubt on the intactness of the collateral ligament planes, X-rays with stress on the joint should be performed.

Other investigations (needle puncture, scintigraphy, CT scan, etc.) will be used as needed and oriented by the possible diagnoses: loosening of the implant, sepsis, allergy.

Choice of the TKR should also consider present or potential loss of bone substance (fixation method). The choice can involve:

- First-line implant more or less under stress.
- First-line implant with a stem or augment.
- Specific case of a first-line implant with an autologous bone graft augment.
- An implant for revision surgery more or less under weightbearing.

Medial UKA implants should be kept as long as possible during revision surgery to give the surgeon the most precise view of the lower limb axis and joint space height [14].

Lewis et al. studied the impact of different solutions on TKR survival for UKA revision through data from the Australian register [15]. They did not find any difference in survival between posterior-stabilised or non-weightbearing implants. On the contrary, they showed with a statistically significant difference that use of a stem (with or without augments/blocks) increased survival at 10 years (87% versus 81% without a stem). They also noted, irrespective of the TKR used (posterior-stabilised or non-weightbearing, with or without a stem, with or without augments/blocks), that the survival of cemented implants is systematically better than cementless implants.

Scott et al. showed that the use of augments and stems is more common in UKA revision surgery with metal backs than for full polyethylene tibial implants, which are more economical in terms of bone tissue resection [16].

During placement of a TKR for medial UKA failure, the lateral compartment is often the healthy one. The reference for the mechanical sectioning guide is therefore the lateral tibial glenoid surface with a conventional section of 10 mm in height below the reference level. At this stage, the operator can assess the difference between the section and the healthy area of bone under the medial tibial implant. It is this difference that should guide the operator in the choice of revision technique. This assessment is made preoperatively based on anteroposterior X-ray views with one magnification or a CT scan. Perioperatively, mechanical guides, but also navigation, can be used. Crawford et al. recommend the systematic use of sealed implants. They use the fixation of stems and augments when the medial tibial section is more than 5 mm above the lateral section [17]. A study by Marinier et al., SOFCOT 2017 congress, confirmed that, beyond cutting of 14 mm, a first-line implant risks being insufficient [18].

Deficiency of the medial collateral ligament should be analysed. If it involves incompetency related to UKA failure, revision of the UKA should enable restoration of the MCL tension, and Table 16.2 can be used. If not, it will be necessary to plan the use of stress implants, which

must be available in the operating room at the slightest doubt.

Perioperatively, it is conventional to start with tibial resection with the medial implant in position. The probe marker is placed in the healthy compartment, which is most often in the lateral compartment. It is then possible to evidence the level of resection under the lateral compartment (at 10 mm for most implants), and to verify at what level resection will be performed in the medial level. At that stage, it is necessary to refer to the table. Below a 5-mm defect, the cut can descend and be compensated by thicker polyethylene. This is all the more relevant when the tibia is large in size (Diagram 16.1). This can sometimes be problematic in small sizes because lowering of the section can result in a decrease in the weightbearing area of the tibial implant. It is in this situation that an autologous bone graft augment may be useful.

If the difference between resection height laterally and in the medial healthy area is greater than 5 mm, it would be necessary to choose a stem more or less in combination with an augment (which can sometimes also be performed at the expense of the lateral resection).

Table 16.2 Choice of TKR type for UKA revision

Bone defect compared to the lateral section	Bone quality	
	Good	Mediocre or poor[a]
≤5 mm	Cemented primary implant (Fig. 16.1a)	Cemented primary implant with a short (or long) stem (Fig. 16.1b)
>5 mm	Cemented primary implant with a short (or long) stem and augment[b] (Fig. 16.1c)	Cemented primary implant with a long stem and augment (Fig. 16.1d)

[a] Bone quality and BMI (body mass index)
[b] Possibility of using an autologous bone graft

The unpredictable nature of UKA revision, related to perioperative discovery, makes it necessary to have a TKR with stem and augment. At the slightest doubt over the quality of the MCL, it would also be necessary to have a weightbearing revision TKR.

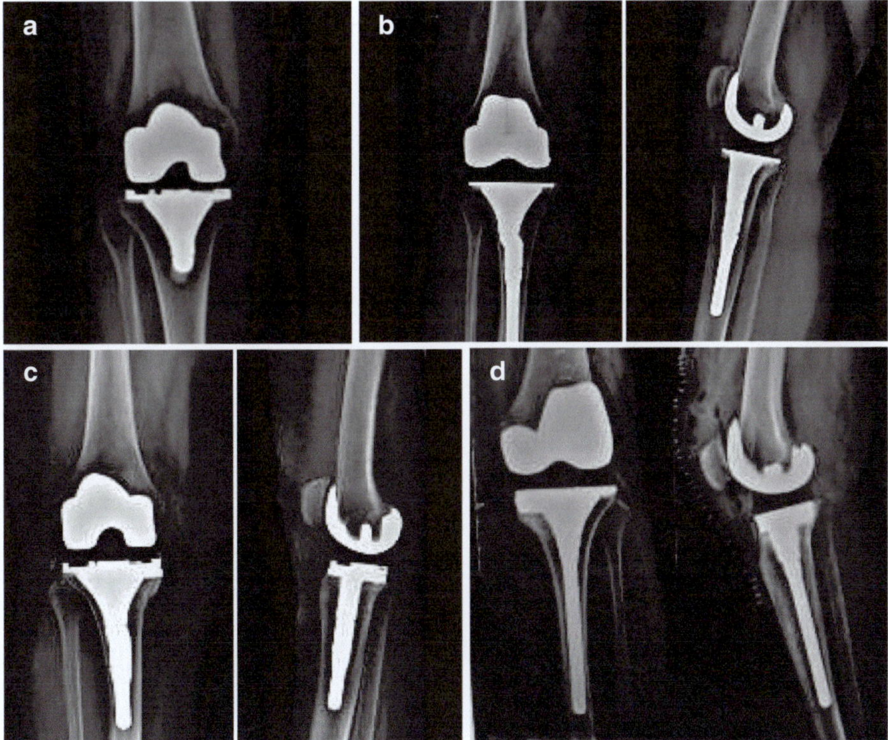

Fig. 16.1 Choice of TKR type for UKA revision: (**a**) primary, (**b**) primary with short (or long) stem, (**c**) primary with short (or long stem) and augment, (**d**) primary with long stem and augment

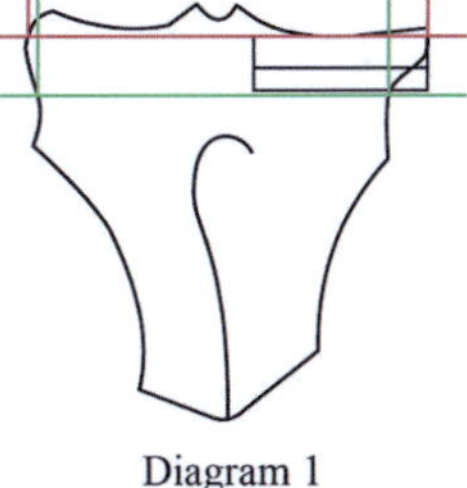

In red: initial tibial width

In green: tibial width after resection in the healthy area (under the UKA)

⟶ Loss of width can result in a harmful decrease in the tibial size and inadequacy with the femoral implant

Diagram 1

Diagram 16.1 If the tibial cut is to big the loss of width can result in a harmful decrease in the tibial implant size and inadequacy with the femoral implant

16.5 Principle of the Autologous Bone Graft Augment/Block

Whenever use of an augment is necessary, and if bone quality is satisfactory, the lateral tibial resection can be used as an autologous bone graft augment. This makes it possible for the surgeon to work in the conditions of a first-line total arthroplasty. The difference between the sched-uled height of the lateral cut and the medial cut in the healthy area must be assessed. This difference provides the thickness of the defect to be filled. It is necessary to start with subchondral resection laterally and then to perform sectioning at the height of the defect to be filled medially and then a final resection to reach the height of the final lateral resection (Diagrams 16.2a, 16.2b and 16.2c).

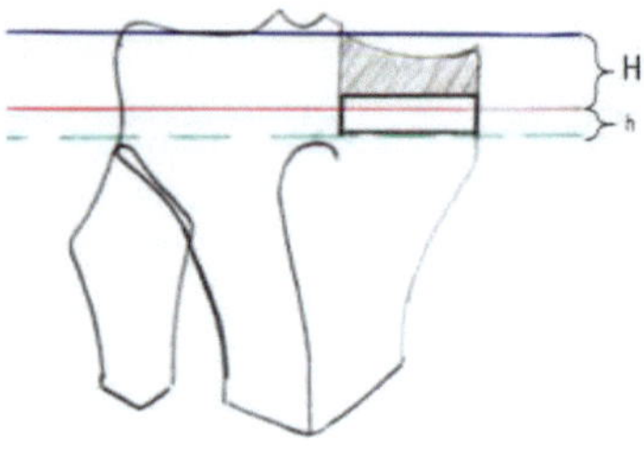

In blue: Tibial section guide reference level. B

In red: Level of tibial section on a first-line implant. R

In green: Level of resection to find healthy bone under the medial UKA. V

B-R= H; R-V = h

Diagram 16.2a How to calculte the thickness of the bone graft augment

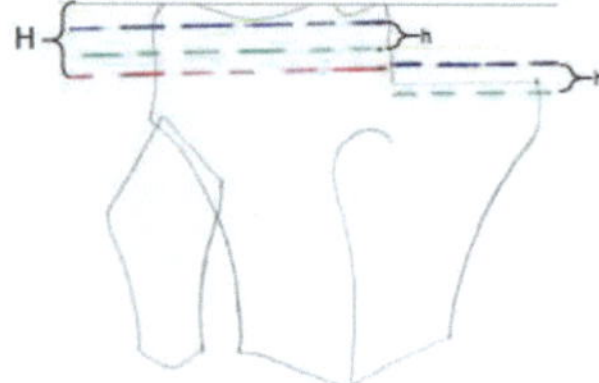

In blue: First cut removing subchondral bone

In green: Second cut of height h to make an autologous bone graft augment

In red: Third cut at height H at the level of the future tibial baseplate

Diagram 16.2b Preparation of the bone graft augment

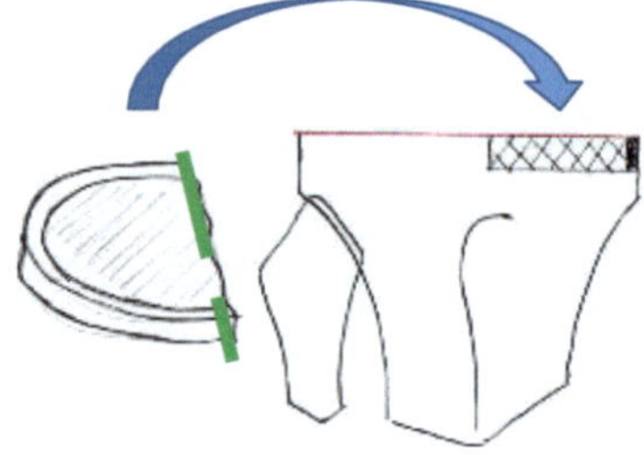

The bone graft augment is prepared (sagittal section) and then positioned in the medial compartment

An autologous bone graft augment is an alternative to metal block/augment, which enables bone saving provided that the bone is of good quality. The delicate phase is preparation of the tibial baseplate.

Diagram 16.2c Positionning of the bone graft augment

The bone graft must be sized and positioned in the medial compartment. Temporary stabilisation with a pin is performed. The guide for preparation of the tibial baseplate is positioned. It is recommended to prepare tibial stamping for baseplates with a different wing by making a saw cut so as not to risk splitting the graft. After this preparation, temporary pins can be replaced with compression screws, taking care not to enter into contact with the imprint of the tibial baseplate (Fig. 16.2). Even for satisfactory bone quality, it is recommended to use a sealed tibial baseplate [15–19].

> An autologous bone graft augment is an alternative to metal block/augment, which enables bone saving provided that the bone is of good quality. The delicate phase is preparation of the tibial baseplate.

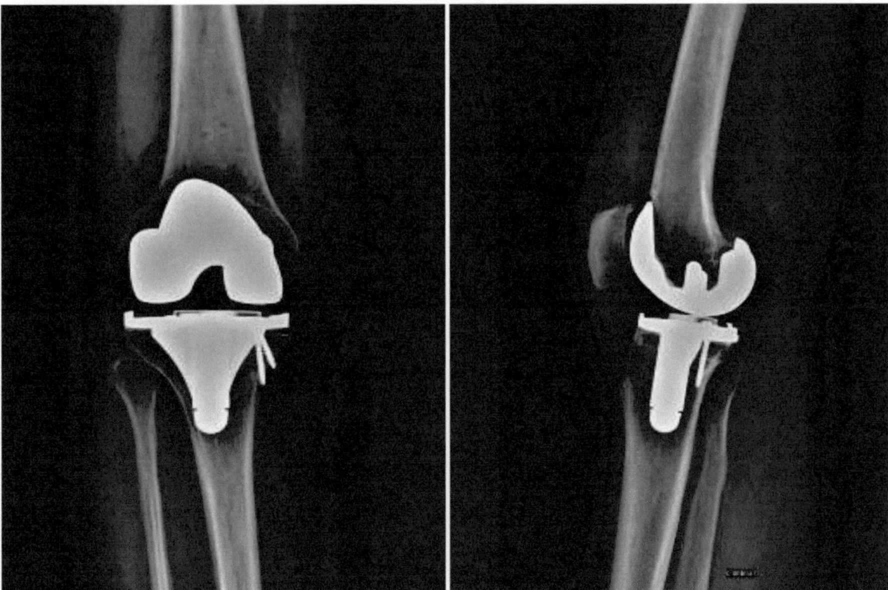

Fig. 16.2 First-line TKR revision with a medial autologous bone graft augment affixed by screws and use of navigation

16.6 UKA and Sepsis

The occurrence of sepsis in UKA is governed by the principles of infection management in a knee implant. The strategy will be based on the conditions in which the infection occurred. The diagnosis of infection is suggested based on clinical findings and a warm swollen knee that is painful on mobilisation, weightbearing and may progress until total functional disability. General signs are not always present, and the clinical presentation may be asymptomatic, particularly for chronic forms. Conversely, the existence of a discharge or fistula is almost always a point of certainty.

Needle puncture of the knee and a laboratory assessment should be performed systematically. The speed of erythrocyte sedimentation and C-reactive protein elevation can remain low, but various information should be crosschecked (Table 16.3, [20]).

The infection can be:

- Acute: early postoperative (up to one month postoperatively) or haematogenic of early diagnosis (less than one month between the start of symptoms and diagnosis).

- Chronic in all cases when symptoms progress for more than four months.

In cases of *acute infection*, imaging has little utility [21]. Surgical management should be as early as possible with lavage synovectomy and change of the polyethylene implant if possible (difficulty in cases of a solid or fully sealed polyethylene implant). Antibiotic therapy should be the subject of a multidisciplinary discussion with the infectious disease specialist and bacteriologist. Either the microorganism is known upstream of surgery (needle puncture, blood cultures) and antibiotic therapy will be immediately targeted, or the microorganism is unknown and antibiotic therapy will be probabilistic, broad spectrum and by intravenous route, until the results of perioperative samples. It should be remembered that survival at 1 year after conservative treatment is 76% in a series by Chalmers [22].

In cases of *chronic infection*, imaging has a more important place but its specificity is tricky to assess (simple scintigraphy or radiolabelled WBC, CT scan) and surgery consists of removing the implants. The strategy for surgery in one or two stages remains debated. TKR results

Table 16.3 From The Journal of Arthroplasty Vol. 27 No. 8 Suppl. 12,012

	n	Cutoff	% Sensitivity	% Specificity
ESR	172	21 mm/h	79,2 [73–85]	73,0 [66–80]
CRP	158	14 mg/L	82,6 [77–89]	80,7 [75–87]
Synovial WBC	96	6200/µL	90,0 [84–96]	96,5 [93–100]
PMN	91	60%	90,9 [85–97]	93,8 [89–99]

ESR: erythrocyte sedimentation rate = VS.
Synovial WBC: number of leucocytes per microliter of needle puncture fluid
PMN: polymorphonuclear neutrophils = altered white blood cells found in histological bone samples

after sepsis in UKA or TKR are identical irrespective of the strategy (77% survival at 2 years for Bauer [23]).

The existence of risk factors increases the probability of infection during initial surgery, but also for revision surgery [21–23].

The occurrence of acute or chronic infection is always a serious event. Even with optimal management, the risk of failure in revision surgery is 25% at 2 years.

16.7 Specific Case of Dislocation of the Polyethylene Implant

This complication is the result of mobile implants and therefore requires a dedicated chapter. Its incidence is low, assessed at 1.2 per 1,000 patients/year in the UK national register of implants.

It should be considered based on sudden deterioration of the clinical result; this requires prompt consultation with the patient. Diagnosis is confirmed by a clinical examination and X-ray assessment: anteroposterior view of the knee (Fig. 16.3) profile and long-leg radiography. It is essential to have the surgical report with details of the implants inserted.

Once these details have been collected, it is necessary to determine which of the possible

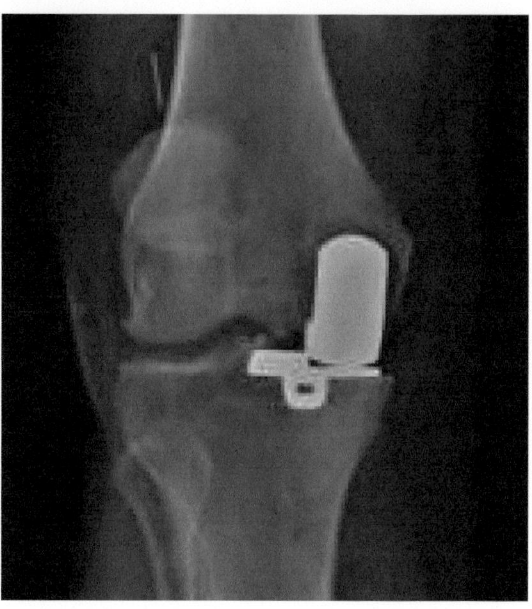

Fig. 16.3 Anteroposterior view of the knee with weightbearing and PE dislocation

causes is responsible in the case analysed. Fig. 16.4 can guide this analysis.

Apart from defects in the implant's design, the dislocation depends on two major categories: defects in mechanical stress of the implant compartment and obstacles to proper movement of the insert.

In these two major groups, we find causes related to the indication for UKA, a perioperative technical issue and secondary causes, occurring most often sometime after implant surgery.

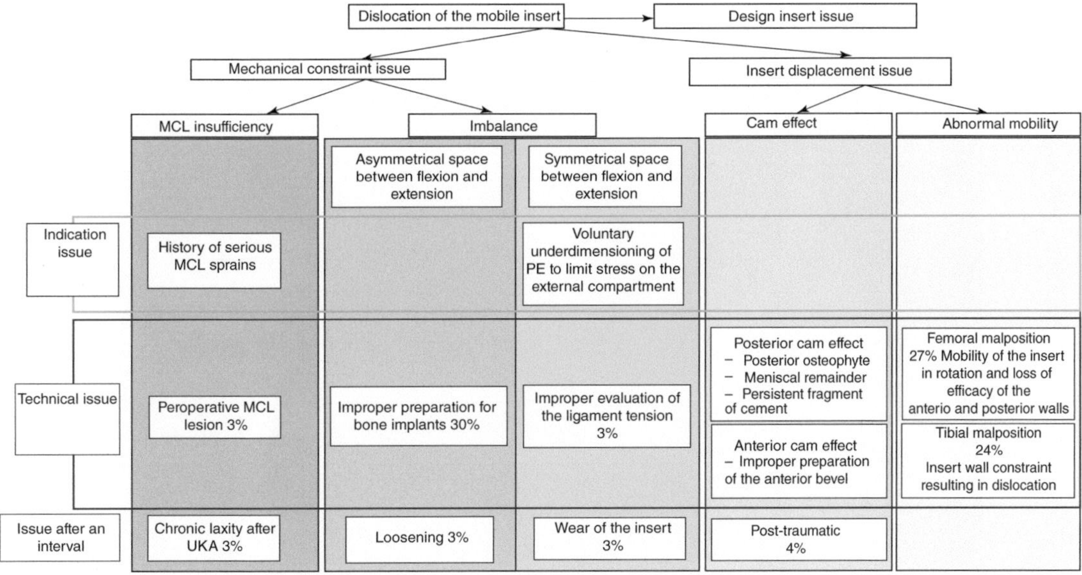

Fig. 16.4 Decision Tree in case of PE dislocation

Analysis of the causes of dislocation in an Asian series found 87% dislocation attributable to a perioperative technical issue. Once the cause was determined, the latter guides the technique to use to restore optimal knee function.

Technical Conduct

The Oxford team first proposes, depending on the cases, reduction by external procedure, which makes it possible to resolve the issue under anaesthesia. In most cases, however, arthrotomy is the rule [24].

Different situations are to be differentiated for revision on dislocation of an UKA insert:

– In cases with a CAM effect, which may be observed perioperatively in some cases, the procedure consists of removing the bone fragments or cement responsible for a conflict. Another insert can then be reintroduced and control of good stability should be performed on complete mobility of the knee to ensure the absence of any other cause.

– In cases of MCL insufficiency, the anatomical conditions are no longer met to enable good mechanical motion of the implant, therefore revision should be planned with TKR (Fig. 16.5), adjusting the stress on the implant depending on the cases.

In cases of asymmetry of the joint spaces in flexion and extension, revision by TKR makes it possible to correct these differences during bone resection. Cases of malposition of an implant also require a change of implant.

Lastly, in cases where no other anomaly is found, and the space in flexion and extension is identical, it is necessary to determine if the insert is too thin or too thick.

In most cases, the surgeon will try with an insert increased by 1 mm. Here too, testing of complete mobility with the trial insert makes it possible to verify the absence of dislocation by a "nutcracker" effect in flexion or extension.

In all cases where the UKA is kept, the crucial stage lies in tests of the insert size in flexion and extension. It is necessary to make certain that the sensation of retention of the ancillary material size in flexion and extension is the same. It is important to be wary of an insert that has to be greatly increased in size, which can suggest rupture of the MCL. In our experience, another obstacle consists of first testing with the trial mobile inserts. It can be very difficult to remove

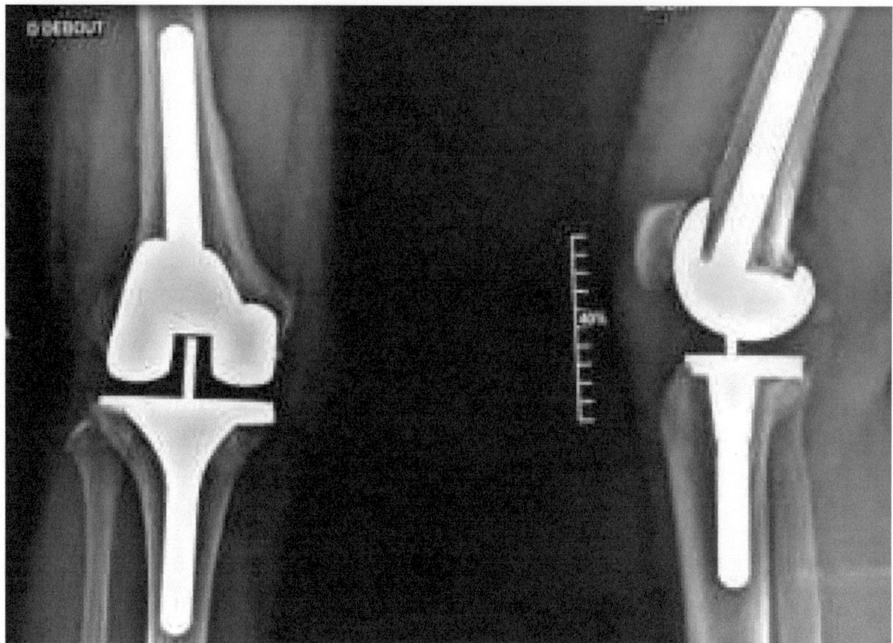

Fig. 16.5 Constraint TKA with a metal augment in the medial compartment

them in some cases. They are used after testing in flexion and extension with the size of the trial insert of the ancillary material.

16.8 Fracture and Sinking (Fig. 16.6)

Fractures and sinking of the implant are rare complications (0% to 10%) depending on the series and almost exclusively affect the tibia [17]. The causes are multifactorial and often combine:

– Defect in indication (osteoporosis or major osteopenia, BMI, axis).
– Technical defect (sagittal cut is too large or too high, impaction of the tibial implant).
– Postoperative trauma.

In cases of osteosynthesis, use of a plate produces better results according to Seeger et al. [25] (Fig. 16.7).

A perioperative sagittal fracture during impaction of a tibial baseplate is not a systematic indication for a switch to TKR. If satisfactory osteosynthesis is possible, UKA can be maintained. Mobilisation and postoperative relief of weight-bearing will be assessed on a case-by-case basis.

If the indication for TKR is chosen, the selection criteria will be those mentioned in Table 16.2.

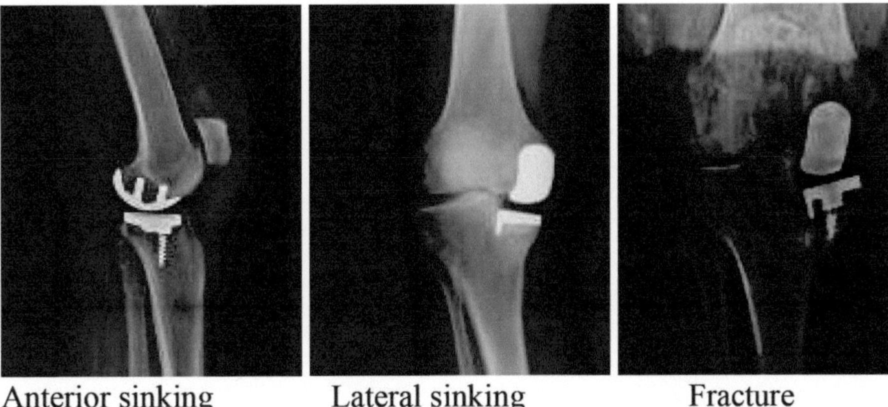

Fig. 16.6 Fracture and sinking. It is necessary to analyse the stability of the tibial implant. If stability of bone/implant is maintained and the fracture is not displaced, treatment can be conservative with relief of weightbearing with/without mobilisation. In cases of fracture with displacement, osteosynthesis can be considered if the implant has remained solid with the bone. If not, it will be necessary to plan revision of the UKA

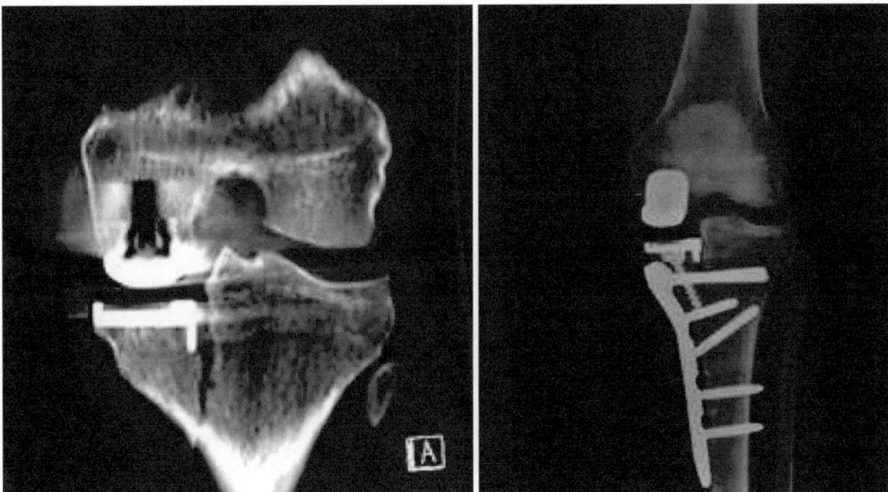

Fig. 16.7 Postoperative CT scan for unexplained pain and post-osteosynthesis control

16.9 Conclusion

The number of UKA is constantly increasing due to this surgical procedure's excellent functional results. Failures are also increasing too, although the curve is not parallel because of relevant indications and reliable techniques.

Failure occurs most often due to loosening of the tibial implant, but attentive screening to detect the cause is vital because revision surgeries for unexplained pain are those which produce less optimal results [26].

Recourse to total arthroplasty is the most widely used solution. In the tibia, it is necessary to use implants sealed with a stem and augment whenever necessary.

References

1. Johal S, Nakano N, Baxter M, Hujazi I, Pandit H. Unicompartmental knee arthroplasty: the past, current controversies, and future perspectives. J Knee Surg. 2018;31(10):992–8. https://doi.org/10.1055/s-0038-16255961.

2. Hansen EN, Ong KL, Lau E, Kurtz S, Lonner JH. Unicondylar knee arthroplasty has fewer complications but higher revision rates than total knee arthroplasty in a study of large united states databases. J Arthroplast. 2019;34(8):1617–25. https://doi.org/10.1016/j.arth.2019.04.004.

3. Australian Joint Registry: AOANJRR. https://aoanjrr.sahmri.com/documents/10180/677574/Table+KP8.png.

4. Kennedy JA, Palan J, Mellon SJ, Esler C, Dodd CA, Pandit HG, Murray DW. Most unicompartmental knee replacement revisions could be avoided: a radiographic evaluation of revised Oxford knees in the National Joint Registry. Knee Surg Sports Traumatol Arthrosc. 2020;28:3926–34. https://doi.org/10.1007/s00167-020-05861-5.

5. Epinette JA, Brunschweiler B, Mertl P, Mole D, Cazenave A. French Society for Hip and Knee: unicompartmental knee arthroplasty modes of failure: wear is not the main reason for failure: a multicentre study of 418 failed knees. Orthop Traumatol Surg Res. 2012;98(6 Suppl):S124–30. https://doi.org/10.1016/j.otsr.2012.07.002. Epub 2012 Aug 24

6. Dahl W, Robertsson O, Lidgren L, Miller L, Davidson D, Graves S. Unicompartmental knee arthroplasty in patients aged less than 65. Acta Orthop. 2010;81(1):90–4. https://doi.org/10.3109/17453671003587150.

7. Goodfellow J, Goodfellow J, O'Connor J, Pandit HG, Dodd C, Murray DW. Unicompartmental arthroplasty with the oxford knee. Oxford: Goodfellow Publishers Lim; 2015.

8. Mertl P, Cazenave A. https://www.sfhg.fr/accueil/fiches-d-information/allergies-et-prothèses/.

9. Dietrich KA, Mazoochian F, Summer B, Reinert M, Ruzicka T, Thomas P. Intolerance reactions to knee arthroplasty in patients with nickel/cobalt allergy and disappearance of symptoms after revision surgery with titanium-based endoprostheses. J Dtsch Dermatol Ges. 2009;7(5):410–3. https://doi.org/10.1111/j.1610-0387.2008.06987.x. Epub 2009 Jan 15

10. Stejskal V, Hudecek R, Stejskal J, Sterzl I. Diagnosis and treatment of metal induced side effects. Neuro Endocrinol Lett. 2006;27(Suppl 1):7–16.

11. Servien E, Merini A, Lustig S, Neyret P. Lateral uni-compartmental knee replacement: current concepts and future directions. Knee Surg Sports Traumatol Arthrosc. 2013;21(11):2501–8. https://doi.org/10.1007/s00167-013-2585-x.

12. Romagnoli S, Marullo M, Massaro M, Rusteni E, D'Amario F. Corbella M : Bi-unicompartmental and combined uni plus patellofemoral replacement: indications and surgical technique. Joints. 2015;3(1):42–8.

13. Epinette JA, Leyder M, Saragaglia D, Pasquier G, Deschamps G, Société Française de la Hanche et du Genou. Is unicompartmental-to-unicompartmental revision knee arthroplasty a reliable option ? Case-control study. Orthop Traumatol Surg Res. 2014;100(1):141–5. https://doi.org/10.1016/j.otsr.2013.10.013.

14. Weißenberger M, Petersen N, Bölch S, et al. Revision of unicompartmental knee arthroplasty using the in situ referencing technique. Oper Orthop Traumatol. 2020;32(4):273–83. https://doi.org/10.1007/s00064-020-00656-w.

15. Lewis PL, Davidson DC, Graves SE, De Steiger RN, Donnelly W, Cuthbert A. Unicompartmental knee arthroplasty revision to TKA: are tibial stems and augments associated with improved survivorship? J Arthroplast. 2019;34(8):1617–25. https://doi.org/10.1016/j.arth.2019.04.004.

16. Scott CE, Powell-Bowns MF, MacDonald DJ, Simpson P, Wade F. Revision of unicompartmental to total knee arthroplasty: does the unicompartmental implant (metal-backed vs. all-polyethylene) impact the total knee arthroplasty? J Arthroplast. 2018;33(7):2203–9. https://doi.org/10.1016/j.arth.2018.02.003.

17. Crawford DA, Berend KR, Lombardi AV. Management of the failed medial unicompartmental knee arthroplasty. J Am Acad Orthop Surg. 2018;26(20):e426–33. https://doi.org/10.5435/jaaos-d-17-00107.

18. Marinier ES, Peltier A, Gaillard R, Cheze L, Servien E, Neyret P, Lustig S. Conséquence de la hauteur de la coupe osseuse tibiale sur la laxité du genou dans le plan frontal : étude biomécanique cadavérique. Revue de Chirurgie Orthopédique et Traumatologique. 2017;103(7):S27. https://doi.org/10.1016/j.rcot.2017.09.015.

19. Leta TH, Lygre SH, Skredderstuen A, Hallan G, Gjertsen J-E, Rokne B, Furnes O. Outcomes of unicompartmental knee arthroplasty after aseptic revision to total knee arthroplasty. J Bone Joint Surg. 2016;98(6):431–40. https://doi.org/10.2106/jbjs.o.00499.

20. Society of Unicondylar Research and Continuing Education. Diagnosis of periprosthetic joint infection after unicompartmental knee arthroplasty. J Arthroplast. 2012;27(8):46–50. https://doi.org/10.1016/j.arth.2012.03.033.

21. de Santé HA. Recommandations de la Haute Autorité de Santé. Prothèse de hanche ou de genou: diagnostic et prise en charge de l'infection dans le mois suivant l'implantation : Méthode Recommandation pour la pratique clinique. 2014. https://www.has-sante.fr/upload/docs/application/pdf/2014-03/rbp_argumentaire_prothese_infectees_vd_.pdf.

22. Chalmers B, Kapadia M, Chiu Y, Henry M, Miller A, Carli A. Treatment and outcome of periprosthetic joint infection in unicompartmental knee arthro-

plasty. J Arthroplast. 2020;35(7):1917–23. https://doi.org/10.1016/j.arth.2020.02.036.

23. Bauer T, Piriou P, Lhotellier L, Leclerc P, Mamoudy P, Lortat-Jacob A. Résultats des changements de prothèse de genou pour infection multicentrique portant sur 107 cas d'infections sur prothèse totale de genou. Revue de Chirurgie Orthopédique et Traumatologique. 2006;92(7)

24. Bae JH, Kim JG, Lee SY, Lim HC, Yong I, MUKA Study Group. Epidemiology of bearing dislocations after mobile-bearing unicompartmental knee arthroplasty: multicenter analysis of 67 bearing dislocations. J Arthroplast. 2020;35(1):265–71. https://doi.org/10.1016/j.arth.2019.08.004.

25. Seeger JB, Jaeger S, Röhner E, Dierkes H, Wassilew G, Clarius M. Treatment of periprosthetic tibial plateau fractures in unicompartmental knee arthroplasty: Plates versus cannulated screws. Arch Orthop Trauma Surg. 2013;133:253–7.

26. Kerens B, Boonen B, Schotanus MG, Lacroix H, Emans PJ, Kort NP. Revision from unicompartmental to total knee replacement: the clinical outcome depends on reason for revision. Bone Joint J. 2013;95–B:1204e8.

Results and Registry Data for Unicompartmental Knee Replacements

A. Rahman, A. D. Liddle, and D. W. Murray

The results of unicompartmental knee replacement can be gathered from three main sources: reports from national registries, observational studies, and randomised controlled studies. These all have advantages and disadvantages.

National registries have very large numbers, but tend only to track a single outcome measure rate of revision. As the numbers are very large, statistically significant associations are often found, but these do not imply causation. There are also large numbers of observational studies. Although most are short term, we will focus on those reporting 10-year outcomes or more. There are very few randomised studies available. While their results are very reliable, they tend to have highly selected populations, and hence are not necessarily generalisable to all patients and surgeons.

We will first compare the results of unicompartmental (UKR) and total (TKR) knee replacements, as this is critical in determining whether UKR should be done at all. We will then review the clinical results of UKR in general and focus on the results of the Oxford UKR (OUKR) in more detail, as there are many more publications on this implant than any other in current use.

17.1 Registry-Based Comparisons of UKR and TKR: Interpretations and Limitations

All national registries have found that the revision rate of UKR is about three times that of TKR. As a result, they tend to conclude that UKR has a poorer outcome than TKR, discouraging surgeons from using UKR. This conclusion is not justified; the main reason the revision of UKR is higher than that of TKR is that the threshold for revision is much lower. Therefore, higher revision rate of UKR does not necessarily suggest that UKR has a worse outcome than TKR.

The New Zealand Joint Registry (NZJR) collects data about revision rates and post-operative Oxford Knee Score (OKS) 6 months after the operation. The OKS assesses overall knee joint pain and function and is categorised into 'Poor', 'Fair', 'Good' and 'Excellent' [1]. Data from the NZJR demonstrates that UKR not only have more *Excellent* results, but also fewer *Poor* results than TKR (Fig. 17.1). Therefore, the higher revision of UKR cannot be because UKR has a poorer outcome [2].

A. Rahman (✉) · D. W. Murray
Oxford Orthopaedic Engineering Centre, NDORMS, University of Oxford, Oxford, UK

Nuffield Orthopaedic Centre, Oxford, UK
e-mail: azmi.rahman@ndorms.ox.ac.uk

A. D. Liddle
MSk Lab, Imperial College London, London, UK

Department of Trauma and Orthopaedics, Imperial College Healthcare NHS Trust, London, UK

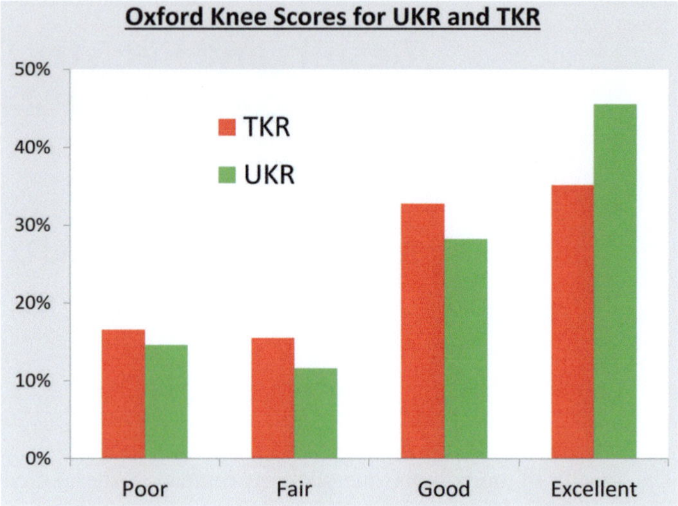

Fig. 17.1 TKR revision rate classified by Oxford knee score categories, based on data from the New Zealand Joint Registry. Graph adapted from Goodfellow et al. (2010) [2]

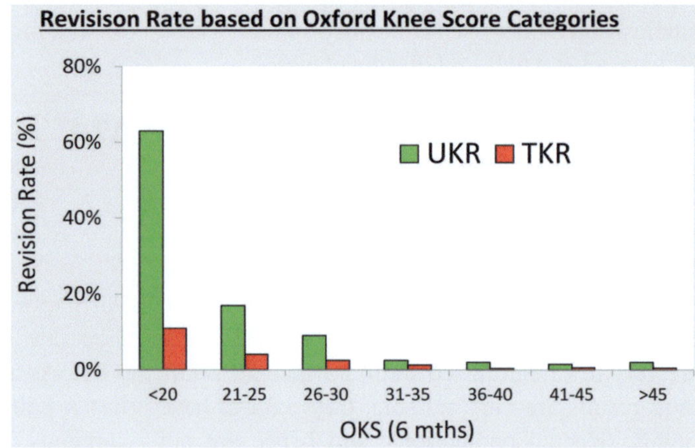

Fig. 17.2 Revision rates for UKA and TKA having different PROMS results at 6 months post-surgery [2]

The NZJR also compares patients' 6-month OKS with their subsequent revision rate (Fig. 17.2). It found that whatever the outcome score, the subsequent revision rate of UKR is about five times higher than that of TKR. This suggests that factors independent of outcome scores increase the UKR revision rate. These factors would be closely related to the threshold for revision. The most striking difference in revision rate occurs in patients who have a worse score post-operatively than pre-operatively (i.e. those who have a post-operative OKS less than about 20). These patients have a 10% chance of being revised if they have a TKR, and a 60% chance of being revised if they have a UKR.

This very large difference is not surprising because a revision of UKR is usually a simple conversion to a primary TKR and the outcome would generally be expected to be good, whereas a revision of a TKR is usually complex, requiring stems, wedges, and stabilised implants, and the outcome is unpredictable. We therefore conclude that the higher revision rate of UKR is not because they have poorer outcomes (Fig. 17.1 demonstrates UKRs have better outcomes at least in the short and medium term), but because they have a lower threshold for revision.

Most surgeons would agree that the relative ease of revision (if there was a problem) is an advantage of the UKR over the TKR. The consequence of it being easy to revise is that the threshold for revision is lower, and therefore the revision rate is higher. The higher revision rate of UKR should thus not be considered to be a serious problem, as it is a manifestation of an advantage.

Patients may have a poor result after UKR or after a TKR. If a patient has a poor result after a TKR, the knee will probably not be revised. National registries will classify this to be a success, whereas the patient will consider this to be a failure. Conversely, if a patient has a poor result following a UKR, it will probably be revised and have a successful outcome. National registries will classify this as a failure, whereas the patient will consider this to be a success. A patient-centred approach to knee replacements should place a greater emphasis on patient beliefs rather than registry conclusions.

17.2 Matched Comparisons with UKR and TKR Registry Data

When national registries compare different implants, they usually analyse unmatched data. However, UKR is generally implanted in younger and fitter patients than TKR [3, 4]. Younger and fitter patients are more likely to have higher revision rates and lower complication rates. Hence, a fair comparison between UKR and TKR requires matched patients. Liddle et al. (2014) compared adverse events in matched UKR and TKR [5]. The data was obtained from the National Joint Registry of England, Wales, Northern Ireland and the Isle of Man (NJR) and other national databases. Over 100,000 UKR and TKR were matched at a 1:3 ratio using propensity score analysis on 20 outcome measures. It was found that there were many advantages of UKR compared to TKR. For example, the length of stay was 1.38 (CI 1.33–1.43) days shorter, and the re-admission rate within the first year (incidence rate ratio 0.65, CI 0.58–0.72), the intraoperative complication rate (OR 0.73 CI 0.58–0.91),

and the transfusion rate (OR 0.25, CI 0.17–0.37) were all less. Complications also occurred less frequently with UKR: for example, the odds ratio of thromboembolism was 0.49 (CI 0.39–0.62), infection was 0.5 (CI 0.38–0.66), stroke was 0.37 (CI 0.16–0.86), and myocardial infarct was 0.53 (CI 0.30–0.90).

The mortality following UKR was also significantly lower than following TKR. In the first 30 days, the hazard ratio was 0.23 (CI 0.11–0. 50, $p < 0.001$); in the first 90 days, it was 0.46 (CI 0.31–0.69, $p < 0.001$). This difference in mortality was not just observed in the short term. The survival curves progressively separated for 4 years and thereafter remained parallel, suggesting the effect of surgery on mortality lasted for 4 years. At 8 years, the mortality following UKR was 0.87 (CI 0.80–0.94 $p < 0.001$) that of TKR (Fig. 17.3a, b).

In this matched comparison, it was found that the revision rate in UKR was 2.1× that of TKR, and the overall reoperation rate was 1.3× higher. To put the adverse outcomes in perspective, it was concluded that if 100 patients receiving TKR received a UKR instead, the results would be around one less death and three more revisions in the first 4 years after surgery.

Liddle et al. in a separate matched study compared the patient-reported outcomes of about 15,000 UKR and TKR [7]. The primary outcome measure was the post-operative Oxford knee score at 6 months after the operation. The OKS was significantly better for the UKR (UKR 38 vs. TKR 36, $p < 0.0001$). The difference in OKS is relatively small; however, many more patients achieved excellent OKS (>41) with UKR (odds ratio 1.59, CI 1.47–1.73, $p < 0.001$). EQ-5D data was also collected, and a significantly better overall score was achieved with UKR ($p < 0.001$). The four subscales relating to mobility, pain, function, and self-care were significantly better, and no statistical difference was found in the anxiety subscale. The level of patient satisfaction was also assessed, and patients were 1.3× more likely to be report excellent satisfaction with UKR than TKR.

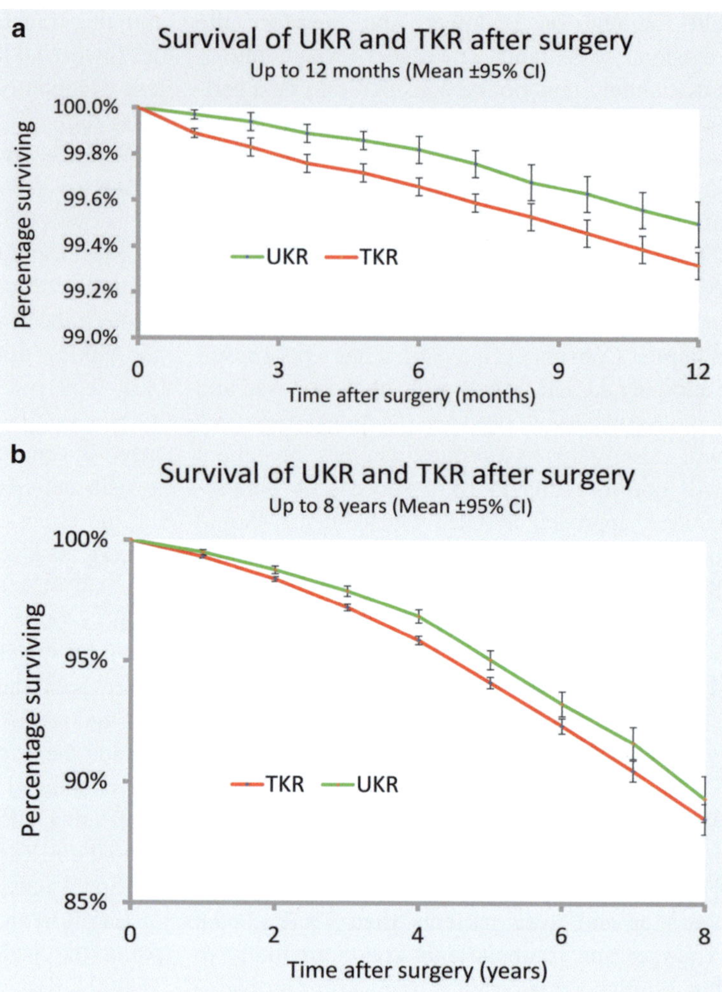

Fig. 17.3 Post-operative mortality for matched UKA and TKA (**a**) for the first year and (**b**) for 8 years, from UK registry data [6]. (Courtesy of AD Liddle)

17.3 Randomised Control Trials Comparing UKR and TKR

The 5-year results of the Total Or Partial Knee Arthroplasty Trial (TOPKAT) were recently published [8]. In this randomised study of 528 patients, the primary outcome measure was the OKS. UKR was significantly better than TKR at 1 year after surgery, and better at 5 years (though the difference was not statistically significant). UKR was also significantly better when the whole 5 year period was taken together. The most marked difference was a higher proportion of patients achieving 'Excellent' outcomes (OKS > 41) [9].

Nearly all other outcome measures favoured the UKR, and several were statistically significant: at 5 years, EQ-5D VAS was 75.4 vs. 71.1 ($p = 0.004$), self-reported knee improvement was 95.2% vs. 90.1% ($p = 0.016$), and self-reported likelihood of willing to have operation was 91.2% vs. 84.3% ($p = 0.010$).

The most remarkable finding of the study was that the revision rate of UKR was not higher than that of TKR at 5 years. When analysed based on intention to treat, it was actually lower following UKR, although not significantly (3% $n = 8$ v 5% $n = 12$), and when analysed based on the treatment it was the same (4% $n = 10$ v 4% $n = 10$). Various other endpoints were studied, including a composite failure measure, defined as reoperation or revision surgery or no appreciable improvement in OKS. At 5 years, there were 26 (9.9%) failures in the UKR group and 37 (14.0%) failures in the TKR group ($p = 0.118$). The death rate at 5 years was also lower following UKR (2.3%, $n = 6$) than following TKR (4.2%, $n = 11$), although the difference was not significant.

A detailed health economic analysis was also undertaken, and this showed that UKR was both more effective (0.24 additional quality adjusted life years, 95% CI 0.046 to 0.434), and had lower healthcare costs for surgery and aftercare (−£910, 95% CI −1503 to −317) than TKR, during the 5 years of follow-up.

A longer but small 15-year randomised controlled trial comparing 52 fixed bearing UKR and 50 TKR found similar outcomes: patients with UKR reported higher *Excellent* Bristol knee scores (71.4% UKR vs. 52.6% TKR) and higher survivorship based on revision or failure (89.8% vs. 78.7%). However, this study was underpowered to test for statistical significances [10].

17.4 Comparative Cohort Studies Between UKR and TKR

We were only able to identify a few matched cohort studies.

Burn et al. (2018) matched 590 UKR to 590 TKR from prospective cohorts and assessed OKS and EQ-5D outcomes over 10 years after surgery [11]. At 1 year, UKR patients reported significantly better OKS [40.3 (CI 39.5–41.0) vs. 35.9 (CI 35.0–37.6)] and EQ-5D [0.82 (CI 0.80–0.83) vs. 0.74 (CI 0.72–0.76)] scores. When OKS was divided into pain and function sub-scores, both remained significantly better for UKR [OKS pain: 23.8 (CI 23.3–24.2) vs. 22.0 (21.5–22.5), OKS function: 16.5 (CI 16.2–16.7) vs. 14.1 (13.8–14.5)]. These differences persisted and remained statistically significant throughout the 10 years.

A recent study compared the early postoperative outcomes of matched 150 UKR and 150 TKR, assessing the Numeric Pain Rating Scale (NPRS), American Knee Society Score (KSS), and Forgotten Joint Score (FJS) [12]. At 2 weeks, UKR had significantly better NPRS (3.7 vs. 7.8, $p < 0.001$), KSS (86.5 vs. 81.4, $p < 0.001$), and FJS (90.5 vs. 79.5, $p < 0.001$). These significant differences persisted at 6 weeks.

Considerably more literature is available comparing non-matched cohorts. However, readers should take greater caution in interpreting findings. A 2019 meta-analysis analysed 36 cohort studies covering a wide range of outcome measures [13]. It found UKR procedures were 23.8 (CI 9.8–37.8) minutes shorter than TKR, required 1.7 (CI 1.2–2.3) days shorter hospital stays, enabled 8.7 (CI 5.6–11.8) degrees greater range of movement, and had better pain and function scores.

17.5 Decreasing the Revision Rate in UKR

A striking finding is that in registry studies, UKR has substantially higher revision rates than TKR, whereas in randomised studies and matched cohort studies, there are no marked differences. There can be various reasons for this, but probably the most important are surgeon-related factors.

In national registries, most surgeons are found to be doing very small numbers of UKR, whereas in published series, surgeons tend to do large numbers of UKR. The data from the NJR would suggest that about half the surgeons doing knee replacement do some UKR [6]. For those doing UKR, the most common number implanted per year is one, the second is two, and the third is three; the average number is five (Fig. 17.4).

When the number of UKR performed per surgeon per year was compared to revision rate, it was found that surgeons doing small numbers had a high revision rate. Surgeons doing one or two UKR per year have a 4% failure rate per year, which would equate to about 60% survival at 10 years. The revision rate dramatically decreases with increasing numbers. Surgeons doing about 10 UKR per year have a revision rate of 2% per year, whereas those doing ≥30 UKR per year have a revision rate of 1% per year (Fig. 17.5).

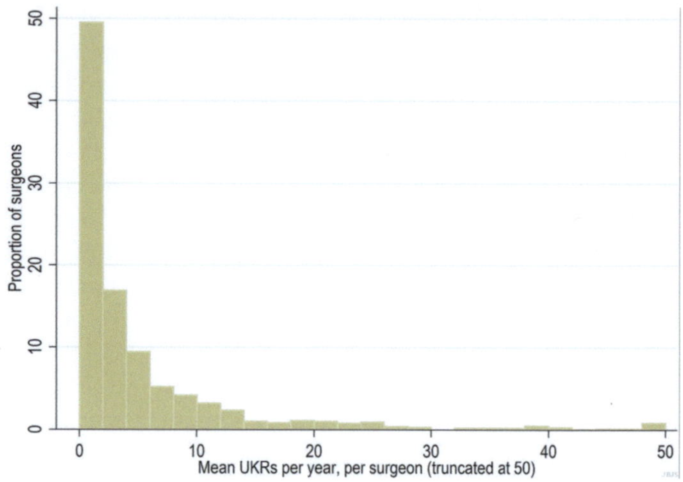

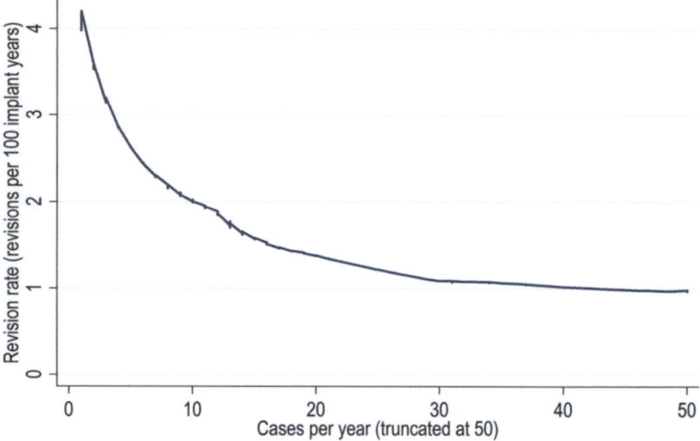

Fig. 17.4 Histogram demonstrating the distribution of UKR caseload among surgeons performing UKR in England and Wales [6]. (Courtesy of AD Liddle)

Fig. 17.5 LOWESS curve demonstrating the effect of increasing caseload on revision rates following UKR (up to 50 cases), based on NJR data [6]. (Courtesy of AD Liddle)

Surgeons cannot easily increase the size of their knee replacement practice. Hence, the only way they can increase the numbers of UKR they do is by increasing the proportion of UKR in their knee replacement practice, which we have defined as 'usage' of UKR. Figure 17.6 shows the relationship between revision rate and usage of UKR for the Oxford knee based on NJR data. Fixed bearing UKR has a relatively similar curve that drops to a minimum at 20%, and then steadily increases rather than dropping further [14].

In Fig. 17.6, the shape of the graph is not what would be expected. As Kozinn and Scott's (1989) ideal indications for UKR are satisfied in perhaps 5% of patients [15], one would expect the revision rate to increase above 5% usage, but it does not. The average usage in the NJR is about 10%

[4]. Surgeons doing less than this have a very high revision rate, and they should either consider stopping doing UKR, or doing more. A minimum acceptable usage is about 20% [16]. With the Oxford UKR (OUKR), the revision rate decreases until surgeons are doing about 50% of their knees as UKR (Fig. 17.7). At this rate, a matched study of UKR and TKR shows that the revision and reoperation rates of UKR and TKR are similar [14].

Hamilton, in a meta-analysis of the outcome of published studies of the OUKR compared the influence of caseload and usage on revision rate [16]. He found that high-usage ($\geq$20%) surgeons had low revision rates, whether their caseload was high or low, and conversely low-usage (<20%) surgeons had high revision rates whether

Fig. 17.6 Annual revision rate plotted against the proportion of a surgeon's knee replacement practice that are UKR [14]. (Courtesy of AD Liddle)

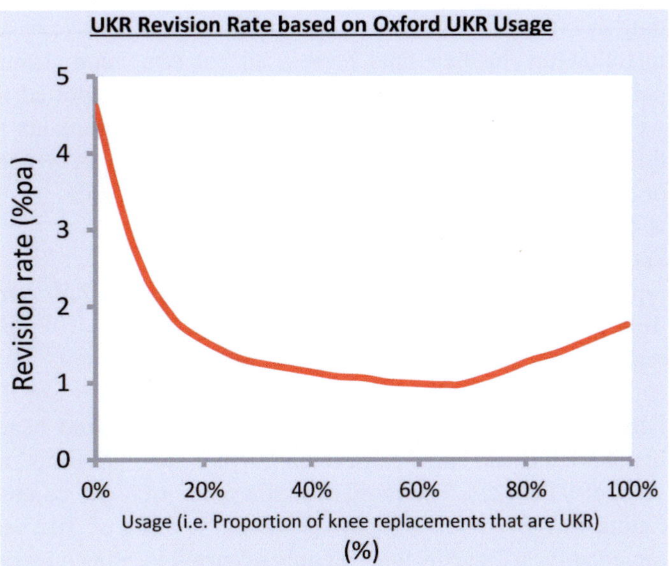

their caseload was high or low.[1] This suggests that usage is more important than caseload in decreasing revision rate.

Usage is a manifestation of indications. Surgeons following very narrow indications will have a very low usage and will probably have poor results, whereas surgeons following broad indications will have high usage and probably better results. The indications for fixed bearing UKR are relatively poorly defined. However with the mobile-bearing OUKR, the indications are well defined, evidence based, and are satisfied in about 50% of cases needing knee replacements [17, 18]. Therefore, to obtain optimal results with the OUKR, surgeons should adhere to the recommended indications and have a usage of over 20% and ideally somewhere in the region of 50%. Surgeons with low usage are likely to be using UKR in inappropriate patients. There is a common but incorrect perception that UKR should be used for early arthritis, when the surgeon feels disease in not severe enough for TKR, and where the surgeon expects a TKR may not perform well [19]. In early arthritis, without bone-on-bone

contact, UKR is also unreliable and should not be performed [20].

A 2018 health economics study compared the lifetime health and financial benefits of UKR to TKR and how they vary with surgeon usage [8]. Overall, UKR dominated TKR for both males and females in all age groups as it provided a greater lifetime health gain at a lower cost. However, surgeon usage had a marked effect on the findings. If the usage was <10%, then there was no lifetime health gain of UKR over TKR [ΔQALY: -0.04 (CI -0.32 to 0.21)] even though the costs were less [ΔCosts £ -127 (CI -429 to 127)]. If the usage was >10%, there were substantial benefits of UKR with both greater lifetime health gain [ΔQALY: 0.26 (CI 0.12 to 0.40)] and lower lifetime costs [ΔCosts (£ -758 (-939 to -579))].

17.6 Long-Term Results of UKR (≥20 Years)

The longest series of UKR we are aware of is a series of 125 medial mobile-bearing Phase 1 Oxford UKR implanted in 104 patients by Dr. U. Svard and his colleagues in Sweden begin-

---

[1]In this meta-analysis, high caseload was defined as >12 UKR per year, and low caseload was defined as ≤12 UKR per year.

ning in 1983 (Table 17.1). No patients were lost to follow-up. In their final review, all but two patients were revised or deceased. The two that were alive were followed up at over 30 years. In this study, failure was defined as either a revision or a 'poor' result (based on the HSS knee score) at last follow-up or death. Overall, the Oxford knee was a successful and definitive knee replacement in 84% of patients over their lifetime [21]. As far as we know, no other knee replacement has had such complete follow-up, and such good lifetime results. Prior to this publication, a standard follow-up had been done of his 683 UKR and these achieved a 20-year survival of 91% [22]. The most common mode of failure was progression of disease laterally, but remarkably, at 20 years this had only occurred in 2.3% of patients. This demonstrates that if the operation is done appropriately in appropriate patients, progression of arthritis is not inevitable. This comes as important evidence for surgeons who do not use UKR, as most are concerned about revision for progression of arthritis.

There are publications of 20-year results of three fixed bearing devices (Table 17.2). The 20-year survival of the Miller-Galante UKR was reported by Argenson to be 74% (CI 67–71) in an independent series of 160 implants [23]. Common causes of failure in the second decade were patella femoral problems and wear. A designer series of 68 Miller-Galante UKR by Foran had a higher 90% survival [24]. A single surgeon series of 103 Marmor UKR was followed by O'Rourke for a minimum of 21 years, with a survival of 84% (CI 76–92%) at 20 years, and 72% (CI 58–95%) at 25 years. A series of St Georg Sled UKR from Bristol has been reported at various time intervals. Ansari reported a

10-year survival of 88% in 461 implants [25], and from those reaching 10 years, Steele reported that 86% survived to 20 years in 203 implants [26]. The overall survival at 20 years can hence be calculated to be approximately 75%.

17.7 Mid-Term Results for Fixed Bearing UKR (~10 Years)

Most of the studies reporting 10-year results of fixed bearing UKR are on the Miller-Galante, Marmor, and St Georg UKRs, which are no longer commonly used (Table 17.2). A wide range of 10-year survivals, from 70% to 94%, have been reported in various cohorts. The only fixed bearing UKR implants in common use, as reported by the NJR, with published 10-year survival is the ZUK (now sometimes called Physica ZUK). There are many other devices in use for which 10-year data is not currently available.

The ZUK is an evolution of the Miller-Galante. Three publications report the 10-year survival rates which range between 94 and 98% [27–29] (Table 17.4). Unfortunately, none of the papers reports the number of cases at risk at 10 years, so it is impossible to assess the reliability of these estimates. The numbers at risk may have been relatively low as the average follow-up was relatively short. Only one paper quoted the 'loss to follow up' rate and one appeared to overestimate the survivorship by incorrectly assuming it was the same the percentage of cases not revised. The indications and contraindications used for UKR by the different groups are also different.

Table 17.1 Survival of the Phase 1 and Phase 2 Oxford UKR (10-year results)

Implant	Principal surgeon or author	Date	References	No. of knees	Age	Time (years)	Survival (%)	No. of revisions	Reasons for revision
Phase 1–2	U Svard	2006	[22]	683	70	20	92		
Phase 1–2	Svard	2001	[44]	124	70	10	95		
Phase 2	Emerson	2010		54	64	20	84	9	
Phase 1–2	Emerson	2008	[45]	54	64	10	85	5	Disease progression (7), loosening (1), impingement (1)
Phase 1–2	Murray	1998	[46]	143	71	10	98	1	Disease progression (2), infection (1), pain (1), loosening (1)
Phase 2	Rajesekhar	2004	[47]	135	70	10	94		
Phase 1–2	Kumar	1999	[48]	100	71	10	85	7	Patient selection (see text, 4), disease progression (2), fracture (1)
Phase 1–2	Price	2005	[49]	52	56	10	91		
Phase 1–2	Price	2005	[49]	512	71	10	96		
Phase 2	Vorlat	2006	[50]	149	66	10	84	24	
Phase 1–2	Koskinen	2007	[51]	1113	64	10	85		
Phase 1–2	Lidgren	2010	[52]	749		10	86		
Phase 1–3	Price	2011	[53]	683	70	15	92	29	Disease progression (10), loosening (9), infection (5), pain (3), bearing dislocation (2)

17.8 Mid-Term Results for Mobile-Bearing OUKR (~10 Years)

The Phase 3 Oxford UKR is the version of the OUKR that is currently used. It is available with both cemented fixation, introduced in 1998, and cementless fixation, introduced in 2004 (Table 17.3). A review of Oxford Phase 3 UKR in 2017 found 15 studies which had a follow-up of 10 years or longer. It assessed a total of 8658 implants and found a 10-year survival of 93% and a 15-year survival of 89% [30]. Revisions were due to progression of the arthritis to the lateral component (1.42%), aseptic loosening of the implant (1.25%), dislocation of the mobile bearing (0.58%), and pain (0.57%). Complications were rare at 0.83%. The studies reported an average weighted 10-year OKS score of 40 (out of 48) and an average weighted KSS-objective score of 86 (out of 100).

Before the cementless Oxford Phase 3 UKR was generally released, 2 small randomised trials were undertaken [31, 32]. These showed similar second year migration, as assessed by radio-stereometric analysis, with both cemented and cementless components. In addition, they found markedly decreased incidence of tibial radiolucent lines with the cementless components, sug-

Table 17.2 Survival and outcomes for fixed-bearing UKR (10-year results)

Implant	Principal surgeon or author	Date	References	Number of knees (Lateral)	Age	Follow-up (years)	Survival (%)	No. of revisions	Reason for revision	Outcome measure	Latest score
Genesis	Heyse	2012	[54]	261 (78)	54	10	94	15	Wear/loosening (6), disease progression (4), pain (4), instability (2)	KSS-Fcn	92.0–97.2
Marmor	O'Rourke	2005	[55]	136	71	21 (minimum)	84	19	Disease progression (9), loosening (8), pain (2)	KSS-Fcn	53
Marmor	Squire	1999	[56]	140 (15)	68	15	87	14	Disease progression (7), tibial subsidence (6), pain (1)	KSS-Obj	71
Marmor	Tabor	1998	[57]	67	61	10	84	11	Subsidence (6), disease progression (2), inflammatory disease (2), not stated (1)	KSS-Fcn	77 (5–100)
Marmor	Cartier	1996	[58]	207	65	10	93	7	Not given	KSS (both)	75% 'excellent'
Marmor, C1,C2	Heck	1993	[59]	294 (39)	68	10	91	16	Loosening (11), disease progression (4), infection (1)	HSS	50% 'excellent'
Marmor	Marmor	1988	[60]	60 (7)	63	10	70	21	Loosening (11), disease progression (8), other (2)	Various	-
Miller-Galante	Argenson	2013	[23]	160	66	20	74	19	Disease progression (12), loosening (2), wear (5), infection (1	KSS-Fcn	88 (45–100)
Miller-Galante	Rachha	2013	[61]	74	64	10	93	5	Disease progression (2), pain (2), infection (2)	KSS-Fcn	75.5 (45–90)
Miller Galante	Foran	2012	[24]	62 (3)	68	15	93	5	Disease progression (2), pain (1), component dissociation (1), not stated (1)	HSS	80% 'excellent'
Miller-Galante	John	2011	[62]	94 (9)	67	10	94	7	Disease progression (5), loosening (2)	BKS	43.6 (28–50)
Miller-Galante	Naudie	2004	[63]	113	68	10	90	11	Disease progression (4), wear (3), loosening (2), pain (1), traumatic ligament rupture (1)	KSS-Fcn	80 (20–100)
St Georg	Ansari	1997	[25]	461	70	10	88	19	Not given	Not given	
St Georg	Steele	2006	[26]	203	67	10–20 (second decade)	86	18	Disease progression (7), bearing wear (3), aseptic loosening (4), component fracture (2), infection (2)	Not given	
UNIX	Hall	2013	[64]	85 (20)	65	10	92		Not given	OKS	38

gesting improved fixation. A multi-centre 10-year study of the first 1000 cementless UKR found 97% survival (CI 92–100%), and no significant differences in survival or clinical outcome between designer and independent centres [33]. In 2019, a single-centre case series of 1000 cementless OUKR found a 10-year survival of 98% (CI 96–99%), with a mean 10-year OKS of 41, and KSS-objective of 89 [34] (Table 17.3).

Multiple studies have directly compared the cemented and cementless OUKR. A 10-year matched registry study of 14,814 OUKR found significantly greater survival [cemented 90% (CI 88–92%), cementless 93% (CI 90–96%)]. Of the causes of revision, the greatest improvement was in implant loosening (58% reduction, from 1.00% in cemented to 0.42% in cementless)[35]. A follow-up study of these 14,814 implants was done to assess the effect of surgeon caseload on outcomes. It found that cementless Oxford had lower risk of revision across all surgical caseload groups (Hazard Ratios: low-volume 0.74, medium-volume 0.79, high-volume 0.80)[2] [36].

A separate study comparing detailed patient outcomes for 267 cemented and 278 cementless OUKR at 5 years found superior outcome scores for the cementless with OKS (43 vs. 41, $p = 0.008$) and EQ-5D-5L index (0.87 vs. 0.81, $p = 0.0001$, higher is better). The most remarkable difference, however, was in pain. Four independent pain measures recorded significantly less pain with the cementless: ICOAP (5 vs. 11, $p < 0.0001$, lower is better), OKS pain (18.2 vs. 16, $p < 0.0001$, higher is better), AKSS pain (46.2 vs. 43.1, higher is better), and EQ-5D (0.492 vs. 0.789, $p < 0.0001$, lower is better). Across all patients, 61% of those with the cementless OUKR had no pain, compared to 43% of those with the cemented [37].

Following the success of the cementless OUKR (which had a dual peg femoral component), the cemented OUKR was modified to include the same design. The first 100 cases of Dual Peg cemented OUKR had good outcomes similar to the Phase 3 [38]. A 5-year matched registry study of 2834 Single Peg and 2834 Dual Peg cemented Oxfords found a 26% decrease in revision (Single Peg 5.2%, Dual Peg 3.8%), with significant >50% reductions in revisions for aseptic loosening (Single Peg 0.4%, Dual Peg 0.1%, $p = 0.03$) and pain (Single Peg 0.8%, Dual Peg 0.3%, $p = 0.01$) [39].

In 2012, new microplasty instrumentation was introduced, facilitating improved positioning of the femoral component and preventing impingement. Comparative cohort studies found the microplasty instrumentation reduce average surgery time by 15%, reduce the time range of procedures [40, 41], reduce malalignment [41, 42], and reduce the rate of bearing dislocation [42]. The broader clinical benefits were established by a five-year matched registry study of 7953 microplasty and 7953 non-microplasty procedures, which found a significant 31% reduction in revision rate with microplasty (97% vs. 95%, Hazard Ratio 0.77, $p = 0.008$) [43].

17.9 Registry Reports on Fixed and Mobile-Bearing UKR

In 2019, the UK National Joint Registry found that the Oxford UKR comprises more than half all UKR performed in the UK, at 68098. This is followed by the ZUK UKR at 14973, and Sigma HP UKR at 10445, both of which have a fixed bearing. Other implants had a total implant number below 10,000 [3]. The general conclusion from registry data is that both good mobile and fixed bearing devices perform very well, on a national basis, at least up to 10 years. With the mobile-bearing device, the indications are well defined and are satisfied in about 50% of knees requiring replacement. With fixed bearing devices, the indications and contraindications are not well defined.

---

[2] Low volume was defined as <10 cases/year, medium volume 10–29 cases/year, and high volume $\geq$ 30 cases/year.

Table 17.3 Survival and outcomes for Phase 3 and cementless Oxford UKR (10-year results)

Implant	Principal surgeon or author	Date	References	Number of knees	Age	Follow-up (years)	10 year Survival (%)	No. of revisions	Reason for revision	Outcome measure	Latest score
Phase 3	Kristensen	2012	[65]	794	64	10	95	49	Disease progression (16), loosening (11), pain (10), infection (4), fracture (2), other (6)		
Phase 3	Jones	2012	[66]	1000	67	10	94				
Phase 3	Lim	2012	[67]	400	69	10	94	14	Bearing dislocation (12), disease progression (1), infection (1)	OKS KSS-O KSS-F	37.8 85.1 86.9
Phase 3	Davidson	2012	[68]	124			90				
Phase 3	Keys	2013	[69]	107			97				
Phase 3	Briant-Evans	2013	[70]	827		10	91	41			
Phase 3	Faour-Martin	2013	[71]	416	59	10	95	29	Infection (15), bearing dislocation (2), persistent pain (8), Aseptic loosening (4)	KSS-O KSS-F	90.2 88.6
Phase 3	Yoshida	2013	[72]	1279	77	10	96	25	Aseptic loosening (12), bearing dislocation (10), periprosthetic fracture (2), lateral progression (1)	OKS	40.8
Phase 3	Kristensen	2013	[73]	695	64	10	85	51	Progression (16), aseptic loosening (11), pain (10), infection (4), periprosthetic fracture (2), malposition (2), instability (4), other (2)		
Phase 3	Nagy	2013		107		10	97				
Phase 3	Kim	2015	[74]	166		10	91	16	Bearing dislocation (8), bearing fracture (1), aseptic loosening (5), periprosthetic fracture (1), infection (1)	KSS-O KSS-F	85.4 80.5
Phase 3	Emerson	2016	[75]	213	67	10	88	20	Lateral progression (9), aseptic loosening (4), chronic haemarthrosis (3), bearing dislocation (1), bearing fracture (1), other (2)	KSS-O KSS-F	93 78
Phase 3	Lisowski	2016	[76]	138	72	10	92	11	Lateral progression (6), PFJ progression (2), pain (2), bearing dislocation (1)	OKS KSS	41.9 81
Phase 3	Bottomley	2016	[77]	1084	67	10	93	46	Lateral progression (13), aseptic loosening (12), bearing dislocation (7), infection (7), pain (5), periprosthetic fracture (1), other (1)		
Cementless	Campi (9 surgeons)	2018	[33]	1000	66	10	97	25	Lateral progression (9), bearing dislocation (6), periprosthetic fracture (2), pain (4), aseptic loosening (1)	OKS	41.7
Cementless	Mohammad (2 surgeons)	2020	[78]	1000	66	10	98	15	Lateral progression (4), bearing dislocation (7), periprosthetic fracture (1), pain (2), aseptic loosening (1)	OKS KSS-O KSS-F	41.2 89.1 80.4

Table 17.4 Survival and outcomes for the Physica ZUK UKR (10-year results)

Implant	Principal surgeon or author	Date	References	Number of knees (lateral)	Age	Follow-up (years)	Survival (%)	No. of revisions	Reason for revision	Outcome measure	Latest score
ZUK	Nicolai	2019	[27]	452 (14)	67	10	98	6	Disease progression (3), MCL Rupture (1), arthrofibrosis (1), subsidence (1)	KSS-Obj KSS-Fn	93.4 91.0
ZUK	Grave	2018	[28]	460	66	10	94	11	Infection (4), pain (3), disease progression (2), synovitis (1)	OKS	77% 'excellent'
ZUK	Vasso	2015	[29]	136	67	10	97.1	4	Infection (2), lateral progression (1), pain (1)	IKS	87.2 (71–100)

References

1. Kalairajah Y, et al. Health outcome measures in the evaluation of Total hip arthroplasties—a comparison between the Harris hip score and the Oxford hip score. J Arthroplast. 2005;20(8):1037–41.
2. Goodfellow JW, O'Connor JJ, Murray DW. A critique of revision rate as an outcome measure: reinterpretation of knee joint registry data. J Bone Joint Surg Br. 2010;92(12):1628–31.
3. The New Zealand Joint Registry. Twenty Year Report: January 1999 to December 2018. 2019.
4. National Joint Registry. 16th Annual report 2019—National Joint Registry for England. Northern Ireland and the Isle of Man: Wales; 2019.
5. Liddle AD, et al. Adverse outcomes after total and unicompartmental knee replacement in 101,330 matched patients: a study of data from the National Joint Registry for England and Wales. Lancet. 2014;384(9952):1437–45.
6. Liddle AD. Failure of unicompartmental knee replacement [DPhil]. Oxford: University of Oxford; 2014.
7. Liddle A, et al. Patient-reported outcomes after total and unicompartmental knee arthroplasty: a study of 14,076 matched patients from the National Joint Registry for England and Wales. Bone Joint J. 2015;97-B(6):793–801.
8. Beard DJ, et al. The clinical and cost-effectiveness of total versus partial knee replacement in patients with medial compartment osteoarthritis (TOPKAT): 5-year outcomes of a randomised controlled trial. Lancet. 2019;394(10200):746–56.
9. Beard DJ, et al. Total versus partial knee replacement in patients with medial compartment knee osteoarthritis: the TOPKAT RCT. 2020;24:20.
10. Newman J, Pydisetty RV, Ackroyd C. Unicompartmental or total knee replacement: the 15-year results of a prospective randomised controlled trial. J Bone Joint Surg Br. 2009;91(1):52–7.
11. Burn E, et al. Ten-year patient-reported outcomes following total and minimally invasive unicompartmental knee arthroplasty: a propensity score-matched cohort analysis. Knee Surg Sports Traumatol Arthrosc. 2018;26(5):1455–64.
12. Blevins JL, et al. Postoperative outcomes of total knee arthroplasty compared to unicompartmental knee arthroplasty: a matched comparison. Knee. 2020;27(2):565–71.
13. Wilson HA, et al. Patient relevant outcomes of unicompartmental versus total knee replacement: systematic review and meta-analysis. BMJ. 2019;364:l352.
14. Liddle AD, et al. Narrow indications predict poor outcomes in unicompartmental knee replacement, in International Society of Arthroplasty Registers (ISAR) annual meeting. UK: Stratford-upon-Avon; 2013.
15. Stern SH, Becker MW, Insall JN. Unicondylar knee arthroplasty: an evaluation of selection criteria. Clin Orthop Relat Res. 1993;286:143–8.
16. Hamilton TW, et al. The interaction of caseload and usage in determining outcomes of Unicompartmental knee arthroplasty: a meta-analysis. J Arthroplast. 2017;32(10):3228–3237.e2.
17. Hamilton TW, et al. Evidence-based indications for Mobile-bearing Unicompartmental knee arthroplasty in a consecutive cohort of thousand knees. J Arthroplast. 2017;32(6):1779–85.
18. Willis-Owen CA, et al. Unicondylar knee arthroplasty in the UK National Health Service: an analysis of candidacy, outcome and cost efficacy. 2009;16:473–8.
19. Kennedy JA, et al. Most unicompartmental knee replacement revisions could be avoided: a radiographic evaluation of revised Oxford knees in the National Joint Registry. Sports Traumatology, Arthroscopy: Knee Surgery; 2020.
20. Hamilton T, et al. Radiological decision aid to determine suitability for medial unicompartmental knee arthroplasty. Bone Joint J. 2016;98-B(10_Supple_B)):3–10.
21. Price AJ, Svard U. 30-year survival of the Oxford Mobile bearing Unicompartmental knee arthroplasty. Arthroscopy. 2017;33(10):e115–6.
22. Price AJ, Svard U. 20-year survival and 10-year clinical results of the Oxford medial UKA. In 73rd Annual Meeting of the AAOS. Chicago; 2006, p. Il.
23. Argenson JN, et al. Modern unicompartmental knee arthroplasty with cement: a concise follow-up, at a mean of twenty years, of a previous report. J Bone Joint Surg Am. 2013;95(10):905–9.
24. Foran JR, et al. Long-term survivorship and failure modes of unicompartmental knee arthroplasty. Clin Orthop Relat Res. 2013;471(1):102–8.
25. Ansari S, Newman JH, Ackroyd CE, St. Georg sledge for medial compartment knee replacement. 461 arthroplasties followed for 4 (1-17) years. Acta Orthop Scand. 1997;68(5):430–4.
26. Steele RG, et al. Survivorship of the St Georg sled medial unicompartmental knee replacement beyond ten years. J Bone Joint Surg Br. 2006;88(9):1164–8.
27. Gill JR, Nicolai P. Clinical results and 12-year survivorship of the Physica ZUK unicompartmental knee replacement. Knee. 2019;26(3):750–8.
28. Winnock de Grave P, et al. Outcomes of a fixed-bearing, medial, cemented Unicondylar knee arthroplasty design: survival analysis and functional score of 460 cases. J Arthroplast. 2018;33(9):2792–9.
29. Vasso M, et al. Unicompartmental knee arthroplasty is effective: ten year results. Int Orthop. 2015;39(12):2341–6.
30. Mohammad HR, et al. Long-term outcomes of over 8,000 medial Oxford phase 3 Unicompartmental knees-a systematic review. Acta Orthop. 2018;89(1):101–7.
31. Kendrick BJL, et al. Cemented versus cementless Oxford unicompartmental knee arthroplasty using radiostereometric analysis. Bone Joint J. 2015;97-B(2):185–91.
32. Pandit H, et al. Improved fixation in cementless unicompartmental knee replacement: five-year results of

a randomized controlled trial. J Bone Joint Surg Am. 2013;95(15):1365–72.

33. Campi S, et al. Ten-year survival and seven-year functional results of cementless Oxford unicompartmental knee replacement: a prospective consecutive series of our first 1000 cases. Knee. 2018;25(6):1231–7.

34. Mohammad HR, et al. Ten-year clinical and radiographic results of 1000 cementless Oxford unicompartmental knee replacements. Knee Surg Sports Traumatolo Arthrosc. 2020;28(5):1479–87.

35. Mohammad HR, et al. Comparison of the 10-year outcomes of cemented and cementless unicompartmental knee replacements: data from the National Joint Registry for England, Wales, Northern Ireland and the Isle of Man. Acta Orthop. 2019:1–6.

36. Mohammad HR, et al. The effect of surgeon caseload on the relative revision rate of cemented and Cementless Unicompartmental knee replacements: an analysis from the National Joint Registry for England, Wales, Northern Ireland and the Isle of Man. J Bone Joint Surg Am. 2020;102(8):644–53.

37. Rahman A, et al. Pain and function following Cementless and cemented Unicompartmental knee replacement: a 5 year comparison. In: Virtual EFORT congress. Vienna, Austria; 2020.

38. White SH, Roberts S, Jones PW. The twin peg Oxford partial knee replacement: the first 100 cases. Knee. 2012;19(1):36–40.

39. Mohammad HR, et al. A matched comparison of revision rates of cemented Oxford unicompartmental knee replacements with single and dual peg femoral components, based on data from the National Joint Registry for England, Wales, Northern Ireland and the Isle of Man. Acta Orthop. 2020;91

40. Berend K, et al. New instrumentation reduces operative time in medial unicompartmental knee arthroplasty using the Oxford Mobile bearing design. Reconstruct Rev. 2015;5(4)

41. Tu Y, et al. Superior femoral component alignment can be achieved with Oxford microplasty instrumentation after minimally invasive unicompartmental knee arthroplasty. Knee Surg Sports Traumatol Arthrosc. 2017;25(3):729–35.

42. Gaba S, et al. Early results of Oxford Mobile bearing medial Unicompartmental knee replacement (UKR) with the Microplasty instrumentation: an Indian experience. Arch Bone Joint Surg. 2018;6(4):301–11.

43. Mohammad HR, et al. New surgical instrumentation reduces the revision rate of unicompartmental knee replacement: a propensity score matched comparison of 15,906 knees from the National Joint Registry. Knee. 2020;27(3):993–1002. In Press

44. Svard UC, Price AJ. Oxford medial unicompartmental knee arthroplasty. A survival analysis of an independent series. J Bone Joint Surg Br. 2001;83(2):191–4.

45. Emerson RH Jr, Higgins LL. Unicompartmental knee arthroplasty with the oxford prosthesis in patients with medial compartment arthritis. J Bone Joint Surg Am. 2008;90(1):118–22.

46. Dawson J, et al. Questionnaire on the perceptions of patients about total knee replacement. J Bone Joint Surg Br. 1998;80:63–9.

47. Rajasekhar C, Das S, Smith A. Unicompartmental knee arthroplasty. 2- to 12-year results in a community hospital. J Bone Joint Surg Br. 2004;86(7):983–5.

48. Kumar A, Fiddian NJ. Medial unicompartmental arthroplasty of the knee. Knee. 1999;6:21–3.

49. Price AJ, et al. Oxford medial unicompartmental knee arthroplasty in patients younger and older than 60 years of age. J Bone Joint Surg Br. 2005;87(11):1488–92.

50. Vorlat P, Verdonk R, Schauvlieghe H. The Oxford unicompartmental knee prosthesis: a 5-year follow-up. Knee Surg Sports Traumatol Arthrosc. 2000;8(3):154–8.

51. Koskinen E, et al. Unicondylar knee replacement for primary osteoarthritis: a prospective follow-up study of 1,819 patients from the Finnish arthroplasty register. Acta Orthop. 2007;78(1):128–35.

52. Robertsson O, et al. Knee arthroplasty in Denmark, Norway and Sweden. A pilot study from the Nordic arthroplasty register association. Acta Orthop. 2010;81(1):82–9.

53. Price AJ, Svard U. A second decade lifetable survival analysis of the Oxford unicompartmental knee arthroplasty. Clin Orthop Relat Res. 2011;469(1):174–9.

54. Heyse TJ, et al. Survivorship of UKA in the middle-aged. Knee. 2012;19(5):585–91.

55. O'Rourke MR, et al. The John Insall award: unicompartmental knee replacement: a minimum twenty-one-year followup, end-result study. Clin Orthop Relat Res. 2005;440:27–37.

56. Squire MW, et al. Unicompartmental knee replacement. A minimum 15 year followup study. Clin Orthop Relat Res. 1999;367:61–72.

57. Tabor OB Jr, Tabor OB. Unicompartmental arthroplasty: a long-term follow-up study. J Arthroplast. 1998;13(4):373–9.

58. Cartier P, Sanouiller JL, Grelsamer RP. Unicompartmental knee arthroplasty surgery. 10-year minimum follow-up period. J Arthroplast. 1996;11(7):782–8.

59. Heck DA, et al. Unicompartmental knee arthroplasty. A multicenter investigation with long-term follow-up evaluation. Clin Orthop Relat Res. 1993;286:154–9.

60. Marmor L. Unicompartmental knee arthroplasty. Ten- to 13-year follow-up study. Clin Orthop Relat Res. 1988;226:14–20.

61. Rachha R, Veravalli K, Sood M. Medium term results of the miller-Galante knee arthroplasty with 10 year survivorship. Acta Orthop Belg. 2013;79(2):197–204.

62. John J, Mauffrey C, May P. Unicompartmental knee replacements with miller-Galante prosthesis: two to 16-year follow-up of a single surgeon series. Int Orthop. 2011;35(4):507–13.

63. Naudie D, et al. Medial unicompartmental knee arthroplasty with the miller-Galante prosthesis. J Bone Joint Surg Am. 2004;86-A(9):1931–5.

64. Hall MJ, Connell DA, Morris HG. Medium to long-term results of the UNIX uncemented unicompartmental knee replacement. Knee. 2013;20(5):328–31.
65. Wagner-Kristensen P. Follow up on 800 patients having a medial Oxford prosthesis at Vejle hospital, Denmark. Oxford: Oxford Global Masters Symposium; 2012.
66. Jones L, et al. 10 year survivorship of the medial Oxford unicompartmental knee arthroplasty. A 1000 patient non-designer series - the effect of surgical grade and supervision. Osteoarthr Cartil. 2012;20:S90–1.
67. Lim HC, et al. Oxford phase 3 unicompartmental knee replacement in Korean patients. J Bone Joint Surg Br. 2012;94(8):1071–6.
68. Davidson JA, et al. A district general hospital experience of Oxford partial knee replacement in the young patient. Oxford: Oxford Global Masters Symposium; 2012.
69. Nagy M, Keys GW. Long-term outcome of unicompartmental knee replacement in a district general hospital (paper 234). Chicago: AAOS; 2013.
70. Briant-Evans T, et al. The Oxford phase 3 medial unicompartmental knee replacement. 10 year results from an independent Centre: survival, function and risk factors for revision. In: British Association for Surgery of the Knee (BASK) Annual Meeting. Derby, UK; 2013.
71. Faour-Martin O, et al. Oxford phase 3 unicondylar knee arthroplasty through a minimally invasive approach: long-term results. Int Orthop. 2013;37(5):833–8.
72. Yoshida K, et al. Oxford phase 3 unicompartmental knee arthroplasty in Japan—clinical results in greater than one thousand cases over ten years. J Arthroplast. 2013;28(9 Suppl):168–71.
73. Kristensen PW, Holm HA, Varnum C. Up to 10-year follow-up of the Oxford medial partial knee arthroplasty—695 cases from a single institution. J Arthroplast. 2013;28(9 Suppl):195–8.
74. Kim KT, et al. The survivorship and clinical results of minimally invasive unicompartmental knee arthroplasty at 10-year follow-up. Clin Orthop Surg. 2015;7(2):199–206.
75. Emerson RH, et al. The results of Oxford unicompartmental knee arthroplasty in the United States: a mean ten-year survival analysis. Bone Joint J. 2016;98-B(10 Supple B):34–40.
76. Lisowski LA, et al. Ten- to 15-year results of the Oxford phase III mobile unicompartmental knee arthroplasty: a prospective study from a non-designer group. Bone Joint J. 2016;98 B(10 Supple B):41–7.
77. Bottomley N, et al. A survival analysis of 1084 knees of the Oxford unicompartmental knee arthroplasty: a comparison between consultant and trainee surgeons. Bone Joint J. 2016;98-B(10 Supple B):22–7.
78. Mohammad HR, et al. Ten-year clinical and radiographic results of 1000 cementless Oxford unicompartmental knee replacements. Knee Surg Sports Traumatol Arthrosc. 2020;28(5):1479–87.